THE PRACTICE OF CLINICAL NEUROPSYCHOLOGY

STUDIES ON NEUROPSYCHOLOGY, DEVELOPMENT, AND COGNITION

Series Editor:

Linas Bieliauskas, Ph.D.
University of Michigan, Ann Arbor, MI, USA

To those who have supported me. My wife, Janette; children, Annalise and Vincent; and my prodigious family of origin who are literally too numerous to name. — G.J.L.

To the neuropsychologist who gently reminded me of A.R. Luria's comment that our work is not about lesions (or business), but patients. — J.C.C.

To my parents, who created me; to my wife, who helped to shape me; to my children, who have completed me. I love you all. — R.L.H.

THE PRACTICE OF CLINICAL NEUROPSYCHOLOGY

A SURVEY OF PRACTICES AND SETTINGS

Edited by

GREG J. LAMBERTY
JOHN C. COURTNEY
AND
ROBERT L. HEILBRONNER

SWETS & ZEITLINGER
PUBLISHERS

LISSE ABINGDON EXTON (PA) TOKYO

Library of Congress Cataloging-in-Publication Data

Applied for

Cover design: Magenta Grafische Producties, Bert Haagsman
Typesetting: Grafische Vormgeving Kanters, Sliedrecht, The Netherlands

Published by: Swets & Zeitlinger Publishers
www.szp.swets.nl

ISBN 90-265-1940-0

Contents

From the Series Editor

The Practice of Clinical Neuropsychology represents a much-needed contribution to the 'applied' end of our growing series on *Neuropsychology, Development, and Cognition*. In emphasizing the need to translate theory and science into practice, it is not unusual to sometimes neglect the maze of obstacles and blinds which face the enterprise of applying what we have learned. Dr. Lamberty, his fellow editors, and the contributors to this volume have done a masterful job of reviewing the general parameters of clinical practice as well as issues in its development, both in terms of training and clinical extension. The treatment of current issues ranges from being as down-to-earth as dealing with a business structure in general, and managed care in particular, while also offering helpful hints on conducting research in private practice settings and engaging the internet to practice advantage. The last section of this book surveys the many and varied modes of practice and offers hints on improving efficiency and satisfaction for the patient and the practitioner, often based on hard-learned life lessons. I believe the reader who is interested in how the applied aspects of clinical neuropsychology have developed, are enacted, and have differentiated to meet the current practice environment will learn much of value. It will stimulate a re-examination of how applied Clinical Neuropsychology has arrived where it is as well as its adaptation to the changing environments which will guide where it is going. This volume will hopefully help to encourage that journey to grow smoother and more rewarding.

Linas Bieliauskas
Ann Arbor, October, 2002

Preface

This volume represents the culmination of several years of effort on the part of its contributors and editors. The time course of its completion is a testimonial to the vagaries of the lives of busy clinical practitioners. The title of this volume might lead one to believe that it is a definitive guide to *The Practice of Neuropsychology*, but such is clearly not the case. The book *is* decidedly about the *practice* of neuropsychology. That is, the daily machinations of conducting a clinical practice and/or working as a neuropsychologist. My conception of the volume was that it should provide information for those interested in practice-related issues generally, as well as specific information about how neuropsychologists in various practice settings ply their trade.

Well before my anointment as the editor for this project, a volume for private practitioners of neuropsychology was proposed to Linas Bieliauskas. Dr. Bieliauskas determined that such a volume could serve as a valuable reference for practicing neuropsychologists, and the proposal was enthusiastically approved. When the originally proposed project stalled, I was asked if I might be interested in such a project given that I was transitioning from pseudo-academia to full-time practice. Not seeing the wisdom of simplicity, I agreed to take on the project, provided that the scope of the volume could be widened to include the practice of neuropsychology in a more inclusive sense. My belief at the time was that neuropsychologists often wore numerous hats and were employed in many different settings. To focus solely on private practitioners seemed somewhat limiting. Such a volume might indeed be practical, but it seemed that the field's newer practitioners, and perhaps those interested in looking for a change in their practice life, would be better served by a survey of practice settings and topics germane to all who practice in this area. Of course, as the project trudged on, it became apparent that editing a volume while maintaining a busy practice was a heavy burden, so I enlisted the assistance of two trusted and valued colleagues, John Courtney, and Robert L. Heilbronner. Their support and effort was instrumental in getting this volume ready for publication.

To say that the contributors to this volume have been patient and dedicated would indeed be an understatement. Many of the contributors have joked with me about the fact that the final iteration of their chapter bears little resemblance to their current positions and practice life. I have assured them that the 'snapshots' provided will nonetheless be of great interest to the readership. Most of us understand that it is the rare practice that doesn't change and evolve on a nearly constant basis. The insights and personal accounts of our authors are the essence of what *The Practice of Neuropsychology* was envisioned to be — an informative and collegial conversation with enthusiastic practitioners of clinical neuropsychology. We believe there is much to be learned in such conversations and it is our hope that there are many pearls within the pages of this text for any given reader.

Fortunately, most neuropsychologists are benevolent and good-humored individuals, so we, as a group have awaited the publication of this tome and are very pleased to see it in print. We hope that the material contained within these covers is useful to its readers and that the next edition can be compiled within a less impressive span of time.

Greg J. Lamberty

Foreword

This book is about, for, and by, practicing neuropsychologists, and, as such, defines a diverse landscape and has a broad agenda. As we enter the first new century of clinical neuropsychology, our scope of practice has never been larger, and the settings in which neuropsychologists perform services extend from the gridiron to the operating room, and from the courtroom to the classroom. Despite this diversity, recent trends in education and training have moved toward better defining the core knowledge, experience, skills, and identities that characterize the contemporary clinical neuropsychologist. This is truly an interesting time to witness the development, and the growing pains, of our field.

This book provides insights and wisdom about neuropsychological practice from a series of contributors who have walked the walk. The first section provides an introductory overview of the field as it exists today, and links trends in practice to developments in education and training. The second section addresses current issues facing clinical neuropsychology, including issues related to business practices and managed care, neuropsychology in the electronic age, and the importance of integrating research or program evaluation activities into clinical practice. The third section provides personal accounts of neuropsychological practice in a variety of settings. Each of these chapters provides a sort of socialization experience for clinicians who want to learn more about neuropsychology in the schools, in rural and community-based settings, in a broad range of hospitals, and in private practice.

In recent years, some of our professional organizations have refined definitions of what it means to be a clinical neuropsychologist and have found such 'intensive' definitions to be desirable if for no other reason than to educate the public about who we are and what we are trained to do. The contributors to this book take this latter point further by adopting an 'extensive' definition of the field and of those practicing within it. Collectively, the contributors show that clinical neuropsychology cannot be defined by setting, or procedure, or referral question. Instead, the nature and breadth of the field is revealed through descriptions about how important clinical problems can be addressed through the thoughtful application of knowledge about brain-behavior relationships.

Some chapters in this book may find their way into graduate neuropsychological assessment courses, but most will hold primary value for revealing personal insights into the continuing process of professional development we all experience. The book will be particularly valuable to young professionals who are in the process of deciding what to do with themselves. It may help these readers in the process of forging their professional identity or in certain aspects of setting up a practice. But the book will also help any neuropsychologist who practices in an insular setting to more fully appreciate and understand the richness and diversity of our specialty.

Russell M. Bauer, Ph.D., ABPP/Cn
Gainesville, FL

PART I

PRACTICE, TRAINING AND EVOLUTION OF CLINICAL NEUROPSYCHOLOGY

Chapter 1

THE PRACTICE OF CLINICAL NEUROPSYCHOLOGY

Greg J. Lamberty

Introduction

Clinical neuropsychologists comprise a relatively small lot when compared to other specialists in the healthcare marketplace. If the membership of *Division 40* (Clinical Neuropsychology) of the *American Psychological Association* (APA) or the *National Academy of Neuropsychology* (NAN) were used as an estimate, there are roughly 4000 individuals purporting to practice clinical neuropsychology in the United States. In comparison, there are 7000 members of Division 12 of the APA (Clinical Psychology), 17,000 members of the American Academy of Neurology, over 40,000 members of the American Psychiatric Association, and even 14,000 podiatrists (according to the American Podiatric Medical Association). I begin with this simple acknowledgement because, regardless of how important the issues and practices discussed in this volume are to clinical neuropsychologists, most of our colleagues in various health care fields are oblivious to our concerns. This state of affairs is changing slowly as the aforementioned groups (NAN and Division 40) are lobbying vigorously and educating their ranks in ways that will hopefully improve the professional lives of members — but more on this later.

To the extent that there was a field of practice that could be called clinical neuropsychology in the decades of the 1960s and 1970s, it was undertaken largely by individuals working within academic medicine. Today's elder statesmen (who are typically not so very elderly) learned at the guiding hand of our modern field's pioneers who established their laboratories in the 1950s and 1960s. From the beginning of this relatively short history, neuropsychology has flourished as a practice field because of its utilitarian focus. Neuropsychologists did things that others simply weren't trained to do, or did not know about. In other words, they offered something unique. For example, in the early days, detection of 'brain damage' and the ability to identify lesion laterality were important services. It was through the unique combination of careful clinical observation and the application of psychometric theory that instruments and methods were developed to define the subject matter of our field. Today, the focus of clinical neuropsychology has evolved into characterizing patients' neurobehavioral strengths and limitations and working with referral sources to recommend and provide optimal treatments for their patient's concerns. The forensic arena has also emerged as a major focus, with sometimes markedly different goals. In contrast to traditional clinical settings, the neuropsychologist in the forensic setting serves as an expert whose role is to provide information to a third party, and not necessarily to the patient that is being evaluated.

Through it all, neuropsychology has remained primarily a study of the relationship between brain and behavior. While different schools of thought within the field have sought to elucidate these relationships in different ways, the end goal has been the same — a better understanding of how pathological conditions affect observable behavior. A secondary, but vitally important goal in this enterprise is how to run a viable practice. As this volume will show, there are many modes of practice in clinical neuropsychology. Some neuropsychologists make a good deal of money and others just get by. Increasingly, however, the bottom line in neuropsychology is a financial one. Salaries, commissions, and departmental appropriations exist only as long as there are receivables to support them. When it became clear in the early 1990s that the public had increasing expectations that health care was to become a business, the need for accountability increased, while professional income decreased. Thus, the 'salad days' of clinical practice in neuropsychology have long past.

In this chapter, a number of issues that affect the practitioner of clinical neuropsychology will be highlighted. There is nothing particularly systematic about this treatment. In conversations with colleagues, lurking on various neuropsychology list servers, and considering my own idiosyncratic view of the practice world, I have come to view the topics herein as important. Similarly, the editors have requested that the various chapter contributors include their own experiences in their chapters. As such, the format and voice of some contributions will appear a bit mixed. It is our hope that this style, while a bit nontraditional, will afford the reader a more accessible view of areas that might otherwise be less than stimulating when presented in stilted, academic language. Following the exposition of all that is important in the practice of neuropsychology, the structure of the volume will be briefly reviewed.

Current Issues in the Practice of Clinical Neuropsychology

Identity

Try as we might to present ourselves as independent, serious, scientifically-based brain scientists, we are, after all, psychologists in the eyes of the public and our non-neuropsychologist colleagues. In fact, the majority of NPs are trained as clinical psychologists as pointed out by Sweet & Moberg in Chapter 3. Most NPs are licensed as psychologists, and most have non-MD doctoral degrees (e.g., Ed.D., Ph.D., Psy.D.). As such, we struggle with the appropriate placement of ourselves among the firmament of healthcare specialists.

Art vs. science

In many respects, a field that can entertain vigorous 'art versus science' debates is a field that has made significant progress over its history. In today's neuropsychology, few would argue against the importance of having a sizable normative database against which a given individual's performance can be compared. The real debate concerns how tenaciously a neuropsychologist adheres to one tradition to the exclusion of another. The extremes of this debate are represented by dyed-in-the-wool empiricists on one hand, and clinicians on the other hand. The empiricists believe that the ultimate answers to vexing clinical questions lie within meticulously kept databases. They would suggest that we are only as far from the truth as our data allow and that the ultimate answers will be in the form of actuarial decision algorithms, bolstered by freshly obtained test data from large, impeccably administered batteries of empirically validated measures. They believe that few questions need be asked following such a process and that the truth is in the tests. Without the right tests and data, one cannot know the truth.

At the other end of the spectrum are the sage clinicians, who are appreciative of nuance and mindful of a career's worth of cases in which a single idiosyncratic behavior betrayed the reluctant brain's wish to keep the truth obscured. According to the sages, little need be done beyond 'the interview.' The truth is in clinical artistry and can only be found by looking in the right places, many or most of which are inaccessible to common technicians armed with hopelessly inadequate tests. Truth is in the clinician and without the appropriate experience and insight, one cannot access the truth.

The extremes of this debate are discriminatory by nature, but the data-oriented approach has the potential to be more egalitarian. That is, more people have access to data than to insight and clinical wisdom. Clearly, we are moving toward being a predominantly data-based enterprise. It appears that most neuropsychologists understand the necessity of this trend. Nevertheless, we would be seriously remiss to discount the importance of clinical acumen and the ability to identify pathognomonic signs through observation and interaction with patients.

As much as any single source in the past several years, the *Daubert versus Merrell Dow Pharmaceutical* (1993) ruling has served as a catalyst for improving the scientific rigor of opinions offered when any expert testifies in court. This case, coupled with the Federal cases that have adapted it more recently, is widely cited as the standard that requires expert opinions to be supported by scientific 'facts.' Determination of scientific validity in this context should consider issues of falsifiability, support from the peer-reviewed literature, knowledge of error rates, and general acceptance by the field's practitioners[1] (Lees-Haley & Cohen, 1999). Of course, data can be fickle and there are many circumstances that demonstrate how the reification of test scores can result in erroneous, and potentially harmful diagnostic impressions. When challenged to defend the importance of clinical judgment and skill, I often remind my data-oriented NP colleagues that they might one day find themselves in a position of needing a neuropsychologist for a family member or friend. I ask them to reflect on what they think is important in selecting such an individual. This scenario usually gives them pause to consider factors that 'go beyond the data.'

Clinical neuropsychology is not a field of practice with which the public is very familiar. To the extent that the field garners any public attention, it is often in the forensic arena. If most people hear about neuropsychology in the context of a highly publicized trial, it is troubling to think what they might take away from such exposure. The artist versus scientist dichotomy is no more evident than in the courtroom and while the *Daubert* decision has been presented as the end to 'soft science' testimony, the jury is clearly still out regarding this point. It is interesting to hear from colleagues how surprised they were to find that their science and expertise seemed to be ignored in a particular trial. In Chapter 10, David Bush nicely illustrates the fact that while neuropsychologists are well positioned to offer expert opinions in forensic cases, there is inevitably a strongly emotional aspect to legal proceedings that can be very difficult from which to dissociate oneself. In other words, the truth as we know it is not always heard by a jury or by the public. When this happens, we are challenged with making the truth more clear, while maintaining personal and scientific integrity. Once again, this requires flexibility and an understanding that there are many ways to communicate knowledge obtained from good science and practice.

Defining standards for neuropsychology

In the realm of controversies that generate heat, but little light, we have the issue of training and credentialing in neuropsychology. Fortunately, like many intra-disciplinary squabbles, this issue appears to be of concern mainly to those of us in neuropsychology practice. It is fortunate because most patients and referral sources could scarcely be less interested or informed, though many would doubtless be troubled by the rancorous exchanges that characterize this 'debate.' Still, the fact that our customers don't seem to pay much attention to this issue does not mean that it lacks relevance.

---

1 General acceptance as a standard of proof is known as the *Frye standard* (Frye v. United States, 293 F. 1013 (D.C. Cir 1923)).

In Chapter 2, Bieliauskas and Steinberg describe a set of standards (a.k.a. "The Houston Conference"; Hannay et al., 1998) that are thought by many in clinical neuropsychology to represent desirable aspirational goals that will serve the field of clinical neuropsychology as it matures and moves forward. The fact that opposition has been expressed regarding the adoption of the Houston Conference standards cannot be denied, though few published documents have emanated from this opposition to date. One recent paper critiques the Houston model in terms of what it doesn't specify in the way of curricular recommendations (Ardila, 2002).

It would appear that much of the opposition to the Houston Conference has to do with perceived exclusivity in selecting conference participants and what this means for the representativeness of the document for the field in general. Outsiders looking in would probably note that important individuals and groups from within our field fall on different sides of the training and credentialing 'debate.' The divide does not seem to represent fundamental differences of opinion regarding what neuropsychologists should offer to the public or what constitutes good neuropsychology. Rather, there is an inexorable concern about who is directing the future of the field, largely a result of the apparent deep and abiding personality conflicts among certain members of the profession. Of course, this is my opinion and those with stakes on either side of this debate would likely present a somewhat different picture of the importance of these matters. Interested readers are directed to Chapter 2 in this volume and to Ardila's (2002) recent publication for further background on this issue.

The bottom line for practitioners who presents themselves as neuropsychologists is that they need a license to practice psychology in their state of residence. Therefore, at present, the true minimum standard for practicing neuropsychology is state licensure as a psychologist (with the exception of the State of Louisiana, where there is licensure specifically for neuropsychologists). With the exception of grandfathered Master's level practitioners, all states now require that psychologists possess a doctoral degree from a regionally accredited university in order to practice independently. Individual states are less universal in requiring that the program be accredited by the APA, though degrees from APA accredited programs are generally thought to meet the education standards of all states. As standards and credentials become more important in terms of protecting the public and limiting liability, individual states' standards for postdoctoral training and supervision have generally become more demanding.

The National Academy of Neuropsychology (NAN) has deemed that a more thorough, but still basic, definition of a clinical neuropsychologist is desirable (NAN; http://nanonline.org/paio/defneuropsych.shtm). It is hard to argue against the wisdom of such a definition. While board certification in various medical specialties is often regarded as evidence that a person is what they say they are, such is not the case in clinical neuropsychology. Reasonable parties can argue whether this state of affairs is desirable, but the fact is, a relatively small proportion of practicing neuropsychologists are currently board certified, by any board. The NAN definition would thus provide a simple reference that could be used by consumers, referral sources, attorneys, or others seeking to assure that a person is at least minimally qualified as a neuropsychologist. As mentioned above, previous definitions have been viewed as unduly restrictive and somewhat prejudiced with respect to the mention of specific boards.

I will resist the temptation to examine critically the issue of board certification in clinical neuropsychology. As with many such issues, the market will likely determine whether board certification is 'necessary,' and subsequently which board(s) provide the best assurance of competence and/or excellence in practice. The requirements for board certification vary as a function of a given board. The components of the process (credentials review, written exams, work samples, oral exams) are seen by some as an indication of the 'validity' of the product, though this assertion has not been put to an empirical test. Such a study would, of course, be fraught with difficulty and the results would likely be disputed.

Realistically, in the practice of psychology, all boards are essentially 'vanity' boards. Which is to say that no state licensing board requires board certification and any practitioners seeking to distinguish themselves in such a manner are seemingly doing so for another reason. Among the reasons might be increased referrals, better reimbursement from insurers that deem the credential desirable, or a personal commitment to a higher standard of training and experience. In most respects, these issues are difficult, if not impossible, to resolve. A possible harmful consequence of competing boards is that it dilutes the potential for presenting a resolute voice for the field of clinical neuropsychology as a whole. On the other hand, competing boards may increase vigilance regarding standards of training and practice and have a positive effect on practice and quality in general.

Whither medical or mental health

A potentially divisive issue that confronts practicing neuropsychologists is that which requires them to label the services they provide as falling within the purview of *mental health* or *medical* services. The conflict is present on several different levels. The most straightforward of these concerns *reimbursement*. Namely, should neuropsychological assessment be billed as a medical or a mental health service? Generally speaking, the rate of reimbursement for medical services is higher than it is for mental health services. Thus, the question is really not that difficult to resolve for most practitioners. Nonetheless, the fact remains that we need to have ready justification of why our services qualify as a medical, and not mental health services. A growing body of materials and informative web sites now provide information that our colleagues have used to make such a case with reluctant or ill-informed insurers.

For some, this justification is a matter of simple fact. In the process of providing our service, we deftly address mental health issues (such as the presence or effects of depressive illness), because it is part of our training and part of the evaluation that we do. A potential conflict in this definitional struggle is revealed when we are asked to assist our medical colleagues in making decisions about issues that are more mental health related in nature. "Is this patient depressed? Does the patient have a somatization disorder? Is anxiety affecting the patient's cognitive functioning?" Clinically, the interface between medical and mental health is obvious and most of us would not shrink from characterizing a patient's mental or behavioral health concerns. Yet, it is often difficult for others to understand why a neuropsychologist might charge more for essentially the same service as a clinical psychologist who administers similar measures and comes to largely similar conclusions. Clinical psychologists and neuropsychologists who perform assessments of children with Attention Deficit Hyperactivity Disorder often find themselves in this situation. Again, many would argue that the neuropsychological aspects of such evaluations are built into the neuropsychologist. That is, a neuropsychologist can command a higher rate or use a different code (96117, neuropsychological testing versus 96100, psychological testing) because of their unique expertise and training. As with many professional endeavors, this will ultimately be determined by the perceived quality and value of the service rather than an intrinsic philosophical debate about the appropriateness of fees or code uses.

Some well-intended individuals exhort neuropsychologists to never use psychological assessment codes or allow reimbursement from mental health insurance coffers. While these recommendations are intent on improving the lot and status of practice in clinical neuropsychology, they would appear to be ignorant of the perils of such hard line policies. In other words, people need to be reimbursed for their services and many insurers have fairly inflexible procedures for determining what codes are paid, and through which funding mechanism (i.e., medical versus mental health). Perhaps the best and most relevant example of this problem is seen in the reimbursement policy of many regional Medicare administrators. Historically, the Health Care Financing Administration (HCFA), which is now known as the Centers for Medicare and Medicaid Services (CMS), is often seen as the lowest common denominator in the sense that their policies can easily be pointed to as a standard for other payors. For example, if Medicare regulations require that neuropsychological assessment be paid as a mental health benefit, and only psychiatric DSM or ICD codes can be reimbursed, Insurer A can adopt a substantially similar policy without appearing to be totally random and capricious. While it may be an honorable fight to only bill the neuropsychological testing code and to insist that the claim be routed through an insurer's medical benefit department, it might result in little or no payment, and/or significantly delayed payments. Most practitioners have little room in their budgets for such noble struggles. An approach taken by many resourceful and hard working practitioners has been to arrange meetings with medical directors of regional insurers to try and influence their decision making with persuasive information about the worth of neuropsychological services. This admittedly takes extra work and a good deal of confidence, and it can be very difficult for some — though it is certainly an important act of professional citizenship. While it may not be the most time and labor efficient model, a 'bottom up' approach to educating referral sources and the public is likely to effect the most long lasting change for the field.

Billing and coding practices

The *American Medical Association* developed the *Current Procedural Terminology* (CPT) system to serve as "a listing of descriptive terms and identifying codes for reporting medical services." The CPT is approved by the *Health Care Financing Administration* (HCFA) as the coding system to be used when billing for health care services. In the 1996 revision of the CPT system, Neuropsychological Testing (CPT code 96117) was moved from the Psychiatry section to the Neurology section and grouped with several other codes including Psychological Testing, Assessment of Aphasia, Developmental Testing, Neurobehavioral Status Exam and Cognitive Rehabilitation. Dr. Antonio Puente has played an integral part in helping to establish and define the "Central Nervous System Assessments/Tests" portion of the CPT codes, and he has presented thorough annual updates on how these codes are to be employed by practicing neuropsychologists. Much of this material can be found on the NAN website http://nanonline.org. I will not belabor the specifics of these recommendations, except to say that the process of billing for neuropsychological evaluations was, in its inception, designed to be simple and straightforward.

In theory, the typical neuropsychologist uses (or should use) very few CPT codes. In practice, of course, the clinical practitioner is confronted with a dizzying array of idiosyncratic guidelines promulgated by insurers who have had little or no experience with neuropsychological assessment. Again, this underscores the need for patient and reasoned interaction with varying strata of the insurance industry bureaucracy. Many of us have had maddening telephone conversations with prior authorization clerks and 'peer' reviewers that inspire thoughts of cabinet making and fast-food management positions as alternatives to making a living as a neuropsychologist. Debating the issue of *medical necessity* with such individuals generally does not fit into the description of what most of us thought we would be doing in the practice of our craft. It would seem that the system is not set up to maximize efficient authorization or payment, despite assurances from insurers to the contrary.

In a perfect world, neuropsychologists would conduct an evaluation, bill the appropriate number of units of Neuropsychological Testing (CPT 96117) and code a diagnosis that is factually accurate and descriptive of the patient's presenting problem. In the real world, every insurer faced with paying for health care services can have a different reimbursement policy. The worth of a given service is largely a market-driven issue, but the market has HCFA to essentially set the bar at its lowest point.

Since 1992, HCFA has employed a physician relative value unit (RVU) system for determining rates of reimbursement for a wide range of services as outlined by the American Medical Association's CPT guide. The RVU system was developed to pay "physicians based on the relative resources required to provide specific services to Medicare beneficiaries" (Dobson, Koenig, Sturm, & Cavanaugh, 2000). While an extensive review of this procedure is beyond the scope of this chapter, it is important for neuropsychologists to understand the process by which a given code is assigned relative value units (RVUs). Briefly, three basic components are considered when establishing a RVU value for a CPT code. First, there is physician work, or what is sometimes referred to as the 'professional component.' This is the most important and largest of the three components since it involves cognitive work. Second is the practice expense, or the 'technical component,' which is the assumed cost of providing the service. The third component has to do with the cost of malpractice insurance. In determining the RVU for neuropsychological assessment, the cognitive component value has not yet been assigned. The reasons for this are complex, but largely because under the Social Security Practice Act psychologists are not considered 'physicians' (though other non-medical doctorate and non-doctorate level providers are). Further, this code, together with other CNS assessment codes (e.g. 96100, Psychological Testing) are primarily used by psychologists. Hence, the service is considered essentially a technical (and not professional) service and it does not require a cognitive or professional component. Further complications have arisen in that all testing codes are being re-valued for the practice or technical component and the current methodology might not be favorable to testing by psychologists. The malpractice component for a psychologist is certainly negligible relative to the malpractice premiums paid by various physician specialists, and the fact that this does not enter the equation is not surprising or troubling. Whatever the truth might be regarding the process, the CNS assessment codes have been reimbursed based solely on the RVU number for the technical component.

At the time that this book was being prepared for publication, there was ongoing activity aimed at recognizing that CNS assessment codes did indeed involve a professional/cognitive component. Whether the codes will be split into a technical and professional component or whether the current testing code will be provided with a professional component is not yet known. However, these and related efforts are being lead by the American Psychological Association and representatives from the professional neuropsychological community. There has been confusion regarding what this might mean for neuropsychologists, though the movement is focused on getting recognition for the complexity and importance of the cognitive work product as opposed to simply being reimbursed for one's practice expenses. Certainly, this goal is not met for most practitioners with Medicare and Medicaid. That is, most practitioners cannot cover the cost of their office overhead when working for the reimbursement rates offered by these programs. The greatest unknown has to do with how this issue will be resolved in the seemingly very different circumstances of neuropsychologists who do their own test administration versus those who use technicians.

Given the foregoing, it is easy to understand how individual practitioners can become overwhelmed with the responsibilities of keeping up with required policies and procedures in order to be paid for their efforts. In general, professional neuropsychology organizations have fallen short in their efforts to inform and assist practitioners in these matters. The relatively small number of providers of these services has made it difficult to organize a coherent and effective advocacy program. Practicing NPs are often too busy to spend time tracking down such information, to say nothing of sharing it with colleagues and providing a clearinghouse for these useful data. While the APA through its Practice Directorate has made impressive strides in informing the public, consumers in healthcare, and payors, many of these efforts concern the more general practice of clinical psychology. As has been noted, clinical neuropsychology is distinct from general psychological practice. Fortunately, as this volume is going to press, there is a much stronger and concerted effort on the part of NANs newly formed Professional Affairs and Information Office (PAIO; http://nanonline.org/paio/index.shtm) and Division 40 of APA (http://www.div40.org). These groups have begun to produce materials, provide live support, and generally inform those in practice of resources that are available, as well as increasing advocacy efforts in a number of different environments. The internet has also made it convenient to keep abreast of these various developments by visiting the websites of Division 40, NAN, and APA, to name a few of the more active organizations. In fairness, it is easy to hold our professional organizations accountable for their lack of action and guidance, but without considering membership and a modest level of voluntary involvement as required acts of professional citizenship, it is impossible for these groups to make significant strides on behalf of practicing NPs.

Organization of this Volume

The Practice of Clinical Neuropsychology is organized into three parts. Part I, *Practice, Training and Evolution of Clinical Neuropsychology*, consists of the present offering, and two chapters that describe the evolution of training models in neuropsychology and trends in neuropsychology practice. In Chapter 2, Linas Bieliauskas and Brett Steinberg describe the process of change in defining standards for education and training in the field. While clinical neuropsychology has existed for forty or more years, formal guidelines were first promulgated just over twenty years ago. Chapter 2 provides a cogent historical description of this process up to the development of the Houston Conference guidelines.

In Chapter 3, Jerry Sweet and Paul Moberg provide an excellent, detailed review of several studies that have assessed the state of clinical neuropsychology practice. The chapter includes results from several of their own surveys and others that have examined critical aspects of neuropsychology practice including demographics, economics, and general practice parameters. The chapter also includes detailed data from the recent NAN/Division 40 survey distributed in 2001.

The book's second part, *Current Issues in the Practice of Clinical Neuropsychology*, includes several topical chapters that relate to the everyday conduct of practice. Chapter 4 by Ted Peck is a comprehensive treatment of the business aspects of practice in clinical neuropsychology. The chapter includes information gleaned from Dr. Peck's numerous workshops on this topic and provides the reader with valuable assistance on issues to consider when conducting a private neuropsychology practice.

Michael Schmidt provides a sweeping historical treatise on the rise of managed care and how this affects the practice of clinical neuropsychology in Chapter 5. The chapter includes excellent background to bring current changes in healthcare practice into focus, and assists the reader with understanding the basics of managed care and insurance terminology. It is outstanding background for beginning to understand how practitioners and insurance providers interact.

In Chapter 6, M. Frank Greiffenstein details how individuals might take advantage of their often sizable datasets in conducting valuable clinical research. He uses examples from his own practice and discusses traditional obstacles to the conduct of such work, as well as ways to facilitate a clinical research program within one's practice. The chapter is a fine illustration of how science and practice can be combined to produce high quality and relevant research worthy of peer-reviewed journals.

Anthony Risser's chapter (Chapter 7) completes the section with a wide-ranging discussion of Internet resources for practicing neuropsychologists. Dr. Risser discusses issues from the Internet's place in healthcare, to specific resources for neuropsychology practitioners. The chapter is a valuable primer for the novice and the well indoctrinated and underscores the versatility and volatility of the Internet as it relates to practice.

Finally, Part III, *A Survey of Settings and Practices in Clinical Neuropsychology*, provides detailed descriptions of several practice settings. As mentioned earlier in this chapter, the settings in which clinical neuropsychologist practice are richly varied. An effort was made to solicit chapters that represent common and perhaps not-so-common neuropsychology practices. While the selection of practices is obviously not all-inclusive, it should provide the reader with a sense of a range of important issues and considerations in practicing in such settings. For the newer neuropsychologist, the chapters will provide a glimpse of what it's like to practice in settings with which they might have little familiarity.

In Chapters 8 and 9, the co-editors of this volume provide detailed descriptions of their private practice settings. Robert Heilbronner describes his independent private practice with the various challenges and rewards encountered therein. John Courtney also gives an account of his pediatric neuropsychology practice in which he is closely affiliated with a physician colleague. As with all of the chapters in this section, these contributions offer insights that might not be readily apparent or available in other sources. It is the unique perspective of these neuropsychologists that we hope will be one of the true strengths of this volume. Such perspectives are typically not easily found outside informal gatherings at national and regional professional meetings.

Chapter 10 contains valuable insights into the conduct of forensic neuropsychology practice. David Bush discusses philosophical and practical issues in doing forensic neuropsychology and offers insights that should prove useful to anyone interested in practice in this arena. Many specific examples and helpful suggestions are provided to illustrate how different practice environs often call for different business and office practices.

The next three chapters (11–13) provide descriptions of neuropsychology practices within university settings. Ivan Torres and Neil Pliskin (Chapter 11) discuss the conduct of a neuropsychology practice in a large university medical center. Most such practices are fairly 'small fish' and need to be understood in terms of how they fit in with the traditional medical specialties. In comparison, Keith Yeates, Andrew Colvin, and John Beetar discuss the conduct of a pediatric neuropsychology practice within a university-affiliated department of pediatrics. The chapters underscore the size and complexity of such medical centers and describe how neuropsychologists fit into such settings and how they make the value of their services known to their medical colleagues. David Osmon and Yana Suchy describe a more focused kind of neuropsychology practice within a traditional psychology department. The issues and goals of such a program are typically quite different than those in the medical setting and this is clearly illustrated in Chapter 13.

Chapter 14 is a historical look back on a neuropsychology program/practice that evolved with changes in the VA healthcare system. Many of today's neuropsychologists received some manner of their training in VA settings and there is obviously great variability among the many VA neuropsychology programs. Dick Delaney was affiliated with one of the early and most successful neuropsychology training programs and he provides insights into neuropsychology practice in a system that has been a vital resource for neuropsychology.

In Chapter 15, Mike McCrea describes the building of a neuropsychology practice in a general medical center. Building a neuropsychology program or practice from 'scratch' in a hospital setting can obviously be a daunting task and one that requires considerable forethought and expeditious follow through. Dr. McCrea describes the development of his program when given an opportunity to establish a practice based on a perceived greater need for neuropsychological services.

Neuropsychology has long held a prominent role in medical rehabilitation programs since their inception. Joseph Ricker provides an account of the neuropsychologist's role in a large rehabilitation center (Chapter 16). In rehab settings, the neuropsychologist is often asked to provide a broader range of services than individuals in a typical clinical neuropsychology practice. This diversity in duties is captured in Dr. Ricker's chapter, as well as a range of current issues involved in providing services in this rapidly changing setting.

Kristie Nies and Bernice Marcopulos provide a thorough account of rural practice in Chapter 17. They discuss general issues in delivering healthcare services in such settings and talk about the various challenges inherent in working with rural and underserved populations. While their focus is on Appalachia, the relevance for practitioners in other rural settings is clear. The chapter provides examples of obstacles to providing quality services, in addition to more general issues in the conduct of their individual practices.

Finally, Norman Walker, Rudy Lorber and Kristie Nies discuss a range of issues relating to the practice of clinical neuropsychology in conjunction with school systems. This is an area of increasing importance as the expertise of neuropsychologists has come to be recognized as an important adjunct to traditional school psychology services. The authors' individual practices are described in addition to a comprehensive treatment of various issues involved in developing and maintaining a productive liaisons with school systems.

It is our hope that this volume provides a unique view to those interested in practice related issues in neuropsychology. While the topics and practice settings are by no means exhaustive, the reader will be afforded a good sense of the rich variability and opportunities available to practitioners in the field of clinical neuropsychology.

References

Ardila, A (2002). The Houston Conference: Need for more fundamental knowledge in neuropsychology, *Neuropsychology Review, 12,* 127–130.

Dobson, A., Koenig, L., Sturm, E., & Cavanaugh, J. (2000). *An evaluation of the Health Care Financing Administration's resource-based practice expense methodology.* Prepared for Health Care Financing Administration #500-95-0059 /TO#6.

Hannay, H.J., Bieliauskas, L.A., Crosson, B.A., Hammeke, T.A., Hamsher, K., & Koffler, S. (1998). Proceedings of the Houston Conference on Specialty Education and Training in Clinical Neuropsychology. *Archives of Clinical Neuropsychology, 13,* 157–250.

Lees-Haley, P.R., & Cohen, L.J. (1999). The neuropsychologist as expert witness: Toward credible science in the courtroom. In Sweet, J.J. (Ed.), *Forensic neuropsychology: fundamentals and practice* (pp. 443–468). Lisse, The Netherlands: Swets and Zeitlinger Publishers.

Chapter 2

THE EVOLUTION OF TRAINING IN CLINICAL NEUROPSYCHOLOGY: FROM HODGEPODGE TO HOUSTON

Linas A. Bieliauskas and Brett A. Steinberg

Historical Background

In 1984, the Joint American Psychological Association (APA) Division 40/ International Neuropsychological Society (INS) Task Force on Education, Accreditation and Credentialing in Clinical Neuropsychology issued a report describing training in clinical neuropsychology at that time (INS/APA, 1981, 1987). That report "came to the realization that training in clinical neuropsychology was far from standardized and that there was an increasing number of individuals who claimed competency in this area without indication of effective background or training" (p. 21, Bieliauskas & Matthews, 1987). The existence of multiple routes toward obtaining competence in clinical neuropsychology was part of the impetus for forming the American Board of Clinical Neuropsychology (ABCN) board certification procedures so that the public and other professionals would have a recognizable standard by which to judge the capabilities of those calling themselves clinical neuropsychologists.

The formation of the Task Force, was a preliminary step in formulating and organizing the nature of training in neuropsychology. Meier (1981) had already laid out a history of training in clinical neuropsychology, most of which will not be repeated here, but which demonstrated the rich partnership between clinical and experimental psychology and Neurosciences which the field of clinical neuropsychology represented. Meier then described four models for competency assurance in clinical neuropsychology, including a subspecialty in a traditional applied curriculum (such as for clinical psychology), an interdepartmental program in neuropsychology and clinical Neurosciences, an integrated scientist-practitioner curriculum for the Ph.D., and a coordinated graduate curriculum for separately credentialed Ph.D. and Psy.D. components. At the time, Meier attempted to devised a framework to encompass the variety of training approaches then in place and to emphasize that measurement of competence might perhaps be the best approach toward identifying specialist credentials rather than a review of the structure of the particular training model of which one was a product.

It should be emphasized that neither Meier (1981) nor the INS/APA Task Force were attempting to dictate the kind of training which should be employed in the training of clinical neuropsychologists. Rather, they were seeking to characterize the state-of-the-field at a time when it appeared that training efforts were coalescing and moving in some specific directions. The Task Force then issued a series of reports in order to further identify the essential components of training programs at various levels and to provide guidelines for the further development of such training programs. These reports were consolidated in the Guidelines report of INS/APA (1987), and included guidelines for doctoral training programs, internships, and postdoctoral training in clinical neuropsychology. Consideration was given to clinical and experimental psychology cores, training in Neurosciences, desirable didactic and experiential training, and exit criteria from each of the levels of training. These guidelines were eventually adopted as official documents by the Division of Clinical Neuropsychology (Division 40) of APA and were employed as a guide to formulate a training listing of those programs at each level which purported to be in compliance with these guidelines. It was the goal of Division 40 to provide a central listing of programs in response to increasing demand from students who wished to explore such training as well as to provide some guidance to programs which wanted to develop such training. The listing of programs which report that they are in compliance with the Division 40 guidelines can be found on the internet at www.Div40.org, and is updated annually. Division 40 also adopted a "Definition of a Clinical Neuropsychologist" in 1988 which broadly outlined training expectations for those wishing to identify themselves as specialists in the field (Definition, 1989; see Appendix A)

Another significant development as training became more organized, was the establishment of training organizations for each of the different levels of training in clinical neuropsychology. This would assure that the various training programs could come together and discuss areas of mutual interest and concern and lead to increased standardization of training experiences across the United States and Canada. The first of these organizations to form was the Midwest Consortium of Postdoctoral Programs in Clinical Neuropsychology in 1988, which eventually developed into the Association of Postdoctoral Programs in Clinical Neuropsychology (APPCN) in 1994. The Midwest Consortium, and then APPCN, developed formal bylaws, criteria for membership, and devised self-study forms to better identify a uniform training standard. Those programs which belong to APPCN can be found at their website: www.appcn.org. APPCN has been active in developing accreditation standards for specialty postdoctoral training while working closely with APA. At the time of this writing, APA had begun accrediting general postdoctoral training programs but had not yet engaged in strict specialty postdoctoral accreditation. APPCN is strongly encouraging this final development.

Though later in development, the doctoral and internship programs providing specialty training also began to become organized for the same purposes. The Association for Doctoral Education in Clinical Neuropsychology (ADECN) and the Association of Internship Training in Clinical Neuropsychology (AITCN) were in place by 1994, and continue to meet regularly. In 1995, the Clinical Neuropsychology Synarchy (CNS) was formed to provide a unified forum for all major organizations in clinical neuropsychology to discuss training and professional issues and the CNS continues to meet for this purpose on a regular basis as well. The members of the CNS include APPCN, ADECN, and AITCN as well as the National Academy of Neuropsychology (NAN), ABCN, and the American Academy of Clinical Neuropsychology (AACN).

Specialty Status and the Houston Conference

In 1996, after approximately a ten-year application process, Clinical Neuropsychology was formally recognized as a specialty in psychology by APA, joining the traditional specialties of Clinical, Counseling, School, and Industrial/Organizational Psychology. Incidentally, Clinical Neuropsychology was the first specialty to be recognized after such an application process and has since been followed by several others. With this recognition came the realization that Clinical Neuropsychology had now matured as a profession and that the model of training should be specified. Julia Hannay proposed a consensus conference and, with the support of the University of Houston, the conference was organized in the fall of 1997. A planning committee was formed by the CNS and the conference was organized with the co-sponsorship of the University of Houston, the board of Educational affairs of APA, AACN, ABCN, Division 40, APPCN, and NAN. All members of Division 40 and NAN and all training programs in the Division 40 listing were invited to submit applications to attend the conference. From these submissions, 40 delegates were chosen by the planning committee, bringing the total number of conference participants to 46 (including the planning committee). Delegates to the conference were chosen to be broadly representative of the field including the parameters of region of North America, practice setting, level of training, interest, gender, cultural diversity, subspecialization within the field, and seniority. Delegate selection and the format of the conference were modeled on earlier successful training conferences in psychology such as the Conference on Postdoctoral Training (Belar et al., 1993) and the Conference on Internship Training (Belar et al., 1989). That conference produced a policy statement formally recognizing training appropriate to the development of specialization in Clinical Neuropsychology. The statement is included as an appendix to this chapter, though the reader is encouraged to read the proceedings of the conference to achieve a full appreciation of the development of the document (Hannay et al., 1998). The conference statement can also be accessed at the website: http://nanonline.org/nan/subpages/general/houstn.html.

While there was considerable discussion and debate at the Houston Conference regarding training models, a consensual training model was developed which acknowledged the need for both specialized and generalized clinical training throughout a systematic program of doctoral studies, internship, and postdoctoral residency. Clinical Neuropsychology was acknowledged as a postdoctoral specialty with residency training as an integral part of the training background, leading to eligibility for specialty board certification through the American Board of Professional Psychology (ABPP), the parent board of ABCN. There was clear consensus that while continuing education was an expected activity for all specialists, continuing education was not seen as appropriate for acquiring core knowledge or skills or for primary career changes. Concern was raised at the time of the conference about whom the recommended training should affect and it was agreed that the policy developed was not intended to be retroactive, but to apply to future training in Clinical Neuropsychology, i.e., to those *entering* training after the document was to be implemented. All the member organizations of CNS, as well as CNS itself, endorsed the Houston Conference document within one year, so that effectively, the Houston Conference model of training is effective for those *beginning* their training in 1999 or later.

The Nature of the Specialty

Effectively, the Houston Conference produced a formal model for training in Clinical Neuropsychology which is essentially equivalent to models developed for specialties in medicine. The model really didn't create novel requirements but rather captured, in essence, the kind of training which the bulk of psychologists who were specialists in Clinical Neuropsychology had undergone. Basically, the model specified general and specific training at the doctoral level, internship, and postdoctoral residency. Board certification was identified as the desirable exit goal, again, making the specialty very similar to medical specialties. In essence, Clinical Neuropsychology had now become the first of psychology's specialties to forward such a detailed training model.

The vast majority of individuals who are now candidates for board certification through ABCN have completed training programs very much along the lines of the Houston Conference model, even though this is not yet be a formal requirement. Any training model is, by nature, a living entity and, thus, a work in progress. Nevertheless, the evolution of training for the specialty of Clinical Neuropsychology has been remarkable in terms of its exciting beginnings, gradual coalescence, and systematic development toward a formal model. There is a need to respect this such systematic development (Bieliauskas, 1999) and the aspirations it represents for the good of our patients and the health of our profession.

References

Belar, C.D., Bieliauskas, L.A., Klepac, R.K., Larsen, K.G., Stigall, T.T., & Zimet, C.N. (1993). National conference on postdoctoral training in professional psychology. *American Psychologist, 48*, 1284–1289.

Belar, C.D., Bieliauskas, L.A., Larsen, K.G., Mensh, I.N., Poey, K., & Roehlke, H.J. (1989). The national conference on internship training in psychology. *American Psychologist, 44*, 60–65.

Belar, C.D., & Perry, N.W. (1992). National Conference on Scientist-Practitioner Education and Training for the Professional Practice of Psychology. *American Psychologist, 47*, 71–75.

Bieliauskas, L.A. (1999). Mediocrity is no standard: Searching for self-respect in clinical neuropsychology. *The Clinical Neuropsychologist, 13*, 1–11.

Bieliauskas, L.A. & Matthews, C.G. (1987). American Board of Clinical Neuropsychology: Policies and procedures. *The Clinical Neuropsychologist, 1*, 21–28.

Cripe, L.L. (1995). Special Division 40 presentation: Listing of Training Programs in Clinical Neuropsychology — 1995. *The Clinical Neuropsychologist, 9*, 327–398.

Definition of a Clinical Neuropsychologist (1989). *The Clinical Neuropsychologist, 3*, 22.

Hannay, H.J., Bieliauskas, L., Crosson, B.A., Hammeke, T.A., Hamsher, K., & Koffler, S. (1998). Proceedings of The Houston Conference on Specialty Education and Training in Clinical Neuropsychology. *Archives of Clinical Neuropsychology, 13*, 157–250.

INS/APA (1981). Report of the Task Force on Education, Accreditation and Credentialing in Clinical Neuropsychology. *The INS Bulletin*, 5-10. *Newsletter 40*, 1984, *2*, 3–8.

INS/APA (1987). Reports of the INS-Division 40 Task Force on Education, Accreditation, and Credentialing. *The Clinical Neuropsychologist, 1*, 29–34.

Meier, M.J. (1981). Education for competency assurance in human neuropsychology: Antecedents, models, and directions. In S.B. Filskov & T.J. Boll (Eds.), *Handbook of clinical neuropsychology* (pp. 754–781). New York: Wiley.

APPENDIX A

Definition of a Clinical Neuropsychologist *The Clinical Neuropsychologist* 1989, Vol. 3, No. 1, p. 22

A Clinical Neuropsychologist is a professional psychologist who applies principles of assessment and intervention based upon the scientific study of human behavior as it relates to normal and abnormal functioning of the central nervous system. The Clinical Neuropsychologist is a doctoral-level psychology provider of diagnostic and intervention services who has demonstrated competence in the application of such principles for human welfare following:

A. Successful completion of systematic didactic and experiential training in neuropsychology and neuroscience at a regionally accredited university;
B. Two or more years of appropriate supervised training applying neuropsychological services in a clinical setting.
C. Licensing and certification to provide psychological services to the public by laws or the state or province in which he or she practices;
D. Review by one's peers as a test of these competencies.

Attainment of the ABCN/ABPP Diploma in Clinical Neuropsychology is the clearest evidence of competence as a Clinical Neuropsychologist, assuring that all of these criteria have been met.

This statement reflects the official position of the Division of Clinical Neuropsychology and should not be construed as either contrary to or superordinate to the policies of the APA at large.

APPENDIX B

The Houston Conference on Specialty Education and Training in Clinical Neuropsychology

Policy Statement

I. Preamble for Conference

Clinical neuropsychology is a specialty formally recognized by the American Psychological Association (APA) and the Canadian Psychological Association (CPA). Education and training in clinical neuropsychology has evolved along with the development of the specialty itself. Nevertheless, there has been no widely recognized and accepted description of integrated education and training in the specialty of clinical neuropsychology The aim of the Houston Conference was to advance an aspirational, integrated model of specialty training in clinical neuropsychology.

The Conference Planning Committee solicited participant applications by way of an announcement in the APA Monitor and letters to members of the Division of Clinical Neuropsychology (Division 40), the National Academy of Neuropsychology (NAN), and to the directors of training programs at the doctoral, internship, and postdoctoral levels as listed in *The Clinical Neuropsychologist* (Cripe, 1995). The committee selected a group of 37 clinical neuropsychologists to reflect diversity in practice settings, education and training models, specializations in the field of clinical neuropsychology, levels of seniority, culture, geographic location, and sex. Five additional delegates attended as representatives of the sponsoring neuropsychological organizations (NAN; Division 40; the American Board of Clinical Neuropsychology [ABCN]; the American Academy of Clinical Neuropsychology [AACN]; and the Association of Postdoctoral Programs in Clinical Neuropsychology [APPCN]). These delegates convened in Houston from September 3 through September 7, 1997. This document is the product of their deliberations. [Additional details may be found in the Proceedings of the Houston Conference.]

II. Introduction

The following document is a description of integrated education and training in the specialty of clinical neuropsychology. It is predicated on the view that the training of the specialist in clinical neuropsychology must be scientist-practitioner based, and may lead to a combined, primarily practice, or primarily academic career.

The scientist-practitioner model (Belar & Perry, 1992) as applied to clinical neuropsychology envisions that all aspects of general neuropsychology and professional education and training should be integrated; this is the 'horizontal' dimension of education and training. Integration should begin with doctoral education and should continue through internship and residency education and training; this is the 'vertical' dimension of education and training.

This document presents a model of integrated education and training in the specialty of clinical neuropsychology that is both programmatic and competency-based (see Section XV below). This model defines exit criteria and provides tracks and means for obtaining these criteria across all levels of education and training. Exit criteria for the completion of specialty training are met by the end of the residency program. The programmatic level at which these criteria are achieved may vary but not the content.

III. Who is a Clinical Neuropsychologist?

A clinical neuropsychologist is a professional psychologist trained in the science of brain–behavior relationships. The clinical neuropsychologist specializes in the application of assessment and intervention principles based on the scientific study of human behavior across the lifespan as it relates to normal and abnormal functioning of the central nervous system.

IV. Who should have Education and Training in the Specialty of Clinical Neuropsychology?

1. Persons who engage in the specialty practice of clinical neuropsychology or supervise the specialty practice of clinical neuropsychology.
2. Persons who call themselves 'clinical neuropsychologists' or otherwise designate themselves as engaging in the specialty practice of clinical neuropsychology.
3. Psychologists who engage in educating or supervising trainees in the specialty practice of clinical neuropsychology.

V. Professional and Scientific Activity

The clinical neuropsychologist's professional activities are included within the seven core domains delineated in the Petition for the Recognition of a Specialty in Professional Psychology submitted by Division 40 of the APA to the Commission for the Recognition of Specialties and Proficiencies in Professional Psychology (CRSPPP). These core domains are: assessment, intervention, consultation, supervision, research and inquiry, consumer protection, and professional development. The scientific activities of the specialist in clinical neuropsychology can vary widely. The specialist whose professional activities involve diverse cultural, ethnic, and linguistic populations has the knowledge and skills to perform those activities competently and ethically. The essential knowledge and skill competencies for these activities are outlined below.

VI. Knowledge Base

Clinical neuropsychologists possess the following knowledge. This core knowledge may be acquired through multiple pathways, not limited to courses, and may come through other documentable didactic methods.

1. Generic Psychology Core
   A. Statistics and methodology
   B. Learning, cognition and perception
   C. Social psychology and personality
   D. Biological basis of behavior
   E. Life span development
   F. History
   G. Cultural and individual differences and diversity
2. Generic Clinical Core
   A. Psychopathology
   B. Psychometric theory
   C. Interview and assessment techniques
   D. Intervention techniques
   E. Professional ethics
3. Foundations for the study of brain–behavior relationships
   A. Functional neuroanatomy
   B. Neurological and related disorders including their etiology, pathology, course and treatment
   C. Non-neurologic conditions affecting CNS functioning
   D. Neuroimaging and other neurodiagnostic techniques
   E. Neurochemistry of behavior (e.g., psychopharmacology)
   F. Neuropsychology of behavior
4. Foundations for the practice of clinical neuropsychology
   A. Specialized neuropsychological assessment techniques
   B. Specialized neuropsychological intervention techniques
   C. Research design and analysis in neuropsychology
   D. Professional issues and ethics in neuropsychology
   E. Practical implications of neuropsychological conditions

VII. Skills

Clinical neuropsychologists possess the following generic clinical skills and skills in clinical neuropsychology. These core skills may be acquired through multiple pathways, not limited to courses, and may come through other documentable didactic methods. Domains of skills and examples are:

1. Assessment
   - Information gathering
   - History taking
   - Selection of tests and measures
   - Administration of tests and measures
   - Interpretation and diagnosis
   - Treatment planning
   - Report writing
   - Provision of feedback
   - Recognition of multicultural issues
2. Treatment and Interventions
   - Identification of intervention targets
   - Specification of intervention needs
   - Formulation of an intervention plan
   - Implementation of the plan
   - Monitoring and adjustment to the plan as needed
   - Assessment of the outcome
   - Recognition of multicultural issues
3. Consultation (patients, families, medical colleagues, agencies, etc.)
   - Effective basic communication (e.g. listening, explaining, negotiating)
   - Determination and clarification of referral issues
   - Education of referral sources regarding neuropsychological services (strengths and limitations)
   - Communication of evaluation results and recommendations
   - Education of patients and families regarding services and disorder(s)
4. Research
   - Selection of appropriate research topics
   - Review of relevant literature
   - Design of research
   - Execution of research
   - Monitoring of progress
   - Evaluation of outcome
   - Communication of results
5. Teaching and Supervision
   - Methods of effective teaching
   - Plan and design of courses and curriculums
   - Use of effective educational technologies
   - Use of effective supervision methodologies (assessment, intervention, and research)

- It is recognized that the relative weightings of these dimensions may vary from one program to another

VIII. Doctoral Education in Clinical Neuropsychology

Specialization in clinical neuropsychology begins at the doctoral level which provides the generic psychology and clinical core. In addition, it includes foundations for the study of brain-behavior relations and the practice of clinical neuropsychology. All of these are specified above in Sections VI and VII.

Doctoral education in clinical neuropsychology occurs at a regionally accredited institution. All basic aspects of the generic psychology and generic clinical cores should be completed at the doctoral level. The foundation of brain–behavior relationships should be developed to a considerable degree at this level of training. Yet, variability may occur between doctoral programs in the degree to which foundations of brain-behavior relationships and clinical neuropsychology practice are emphasized.

Entry and exit criteria for this level are those specified by the doctoral program.

IX. Internship Training in Clinical Neuropsychology

The purpose of the internship is to complete training in the general practice of professional psychology and extend specialty preparation in science and professional practice in clinical neuropsychology. The percentage of time in clinical neuropsychology should be determined by the training needs of the individual intern.

Internships must be completed in an APA or CPA approved professional psychology training program. Internship entry requirements are the completion of all graduate education and training requirements including the completion of the doctoral dissertation.

X. Residency Education and Training in Clinical Neuropsychology

Residency education and training is designed to provide clinical, didactic and academic training to produce an advanced level of competence in the specialty of clinical neuropsychology and to complete the education and training necessary for independent practice in the specialty. The postdoctoral residency program is a required component in specialty education in clinical neuropsychology. The expected period of residency extends for the equivalent of two years of full-time education and training. The residency experience must occur on at least a half-time basis.

These programs will pursue accreditation supporting the following assurances.

1. The faculty is comprised of a board-certified clinical neuropsychologist and other professional psychologists.
2. Training is provided at a fixed site or on formally affiliated and geographically proximate training sites, with primarily on-site supervision.
3. There is access to clinical services and training programs in medical specialties and allied professions.
4. There are interactions with other residents in medical specialties and allied professions, if not other residents in clinical neuropsychology.
5. Each resident spends significant percentages of time in clinical service, and clinical research, and educational activities, appropriate to the individual resident's training needs.

Entry into a clinical neuropsychology residency program should be based upon completion of an APA or CPA accredited doctoral education and training program. Clinical neuropsychology residents will have successfully completed an APA or CPA accredited internship program which includes some training in clinical neuropsychology.

Exit criteria for the residency are as follows:

1. Advanced skill in the neuropsychological evaluation, treatment and consultation to patients and professionals sufficient to practice on an independent basis.
2. Advanced understanding of brain–behavior relationships.
3. Scholarly activity, e.g., submission of a study or literature review for publication, presentation, submission of a grant proposal or outcome assessment.
4. A formal evaluation of competency in the exit criteria 1 through 3 shall occur in the residency program.
5. Eligibility for state or provincial licensure or certification for the independent practice of psychology.
6. Eligibility for board certification in clinical neuropsychology by the American Board of Professional Psychology.

XI. Nature and Place of Subspecialties within Clinical Neuropsychology

In the future, subspecialties in clinical neuropsychology may be recognized (e.g., child, pediatric, geriatric, rehabilitation). In fact, many clinical neuropsychologists currently concentrate their professional and scientific activities in relatively focused areas of the clinical neuropsychology specialty. Thus, it is expected that some or all of these areas of concentration will eventually be seen as bona fide subspecialties. One implication of this view is that residencies may emerge that reflect concentrations in these subspecialties.

XII. Continuing Education in Clinical Neuropsychology

All specialists in clinical neuropsychology are expected to engage in annual continuing education. The goal of continuing education is to enhance or maintain the already established competence of clinical neuropsychologists by updating previously acquired knowledge and skills or by acquiring new knowledge or skills. Continuing education is not a method for acquiring core knowledge or skills to practice clinical neuropsychology or identify oneself as a clinical neuropsychologist. Continuing education also should not be the primary vehicle for career changes from another specialty area in psychology to clinical neuropsychology.

XIII. Diversity in Education and Training

The specialty of clinical neuropsychology should attempt to actively involve (enroll, recruit) individuals from diverse backgrounds at all levels of education and training in clinical neuropsychology.

XIV. Application of the Model

This document is not to be applied retroactively to individuals currently trained or in training in the specialty of clinical neuropsychology. Individuals entering the specialty or training for the specialty of clinical neuropsychology prior to the implementation of this document are governed by existing standards as to the appropriateness of identifying themselves as clinical neuropsychologists.

XV. Model of Integrated Education and Training in Clinical Neuropsychology

Figure 1 demonstrates how different degrees of specialty knowledge and skills (horizontal dimension) are acquired at various levels of training (vertical dimension). The model facilitates longitudinal integration and continuity in knowledge and skill acquisition with an emphasis that will vary according to level of training. The two charts show the education and training sequence for (A) an individual who acquires some of these areas primarily at the doctoral level and (B) an individual who acquires some of these areas to a lesser degree at the doctoral level and much greater degree at the internship and residency levels.

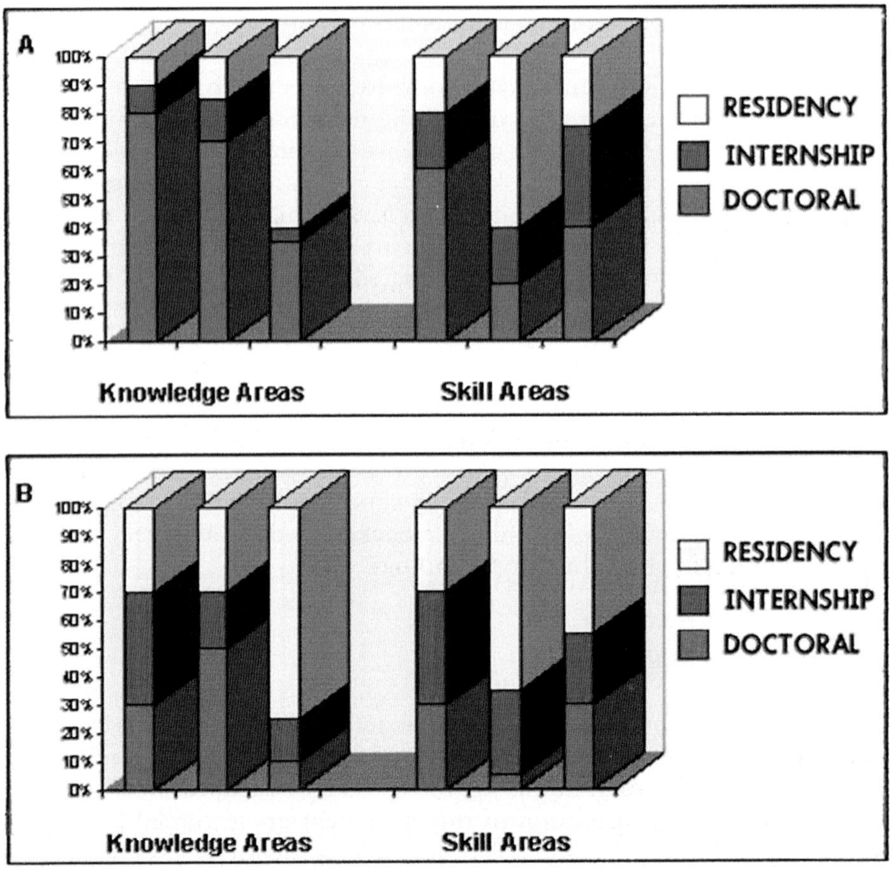

Figure 1. An illustration of an integrated model of education and training in clinical neuropsychology.
From: Hannay, H. J., Bieliauskas, L. A., Crosson, B. A., Hammeke, T. A., Hamsher, K. deS., & Koffler, S. P. (1998). Proceedings of The Houston Conference on Specialty Education and Training in Clinical Neuropsychology. *Archives of Clinical Neuropsychology, 13*, 157–250. Copyright by the National Academy of Neuropsychology. Reproduced with permission.

Chapter 3

THE PRACTICE OF CLINICAL NEUROPSYCHOLOGY: STATUS AND TRENDS

Jerry J. Sweet and Paul J. Moberg

Introduction

As the subspecialty of clinical neuropsychology evolves and matures, changes in beliefs and practices have been apparent. Within this chapter we will delineate these changes and attendant ramifications in an attempt to discern trends that might impact the future of clinical neuropsychology. This subject matter is both broad and detailed. When possible, we will attempt to document changes and trends within the field with data from multiple professional surveys (Sweet & Moberg, 1990; Sweet, Westergaard, & Moberg, 1995; Sweet, Moberg, & Westergaard, 1996; Sweet, Moberg, & Suchy, 2000a, 2000b; Sweet, Peck, Abramowitz, & Etzweiler, in press; Sweet, Peck, Abramowitz, & Etzweiler, in submission) and other sources, such as the American Psychological Association (APA) (Phelps, 1997). Additional primary source materials for the present chapter include APA membership directories and personal communications with Dr. Jessica Kohout and staff of APA's Office of Research.

To facilitate presentation of the most salient changes evident within the field, the chapter will be organized to consider the following topics: practice setting, practitioner characteristics, clinical practices, training, research, and economics. The reader will note that special consideration is given to private practice neuropsychology, which we believe has heretofore received little attention, even though having become the majority practice setting for clinical neuropsychologists during the mid-1990s.

Practice Setting

Traditionally, in medicine, dentistry, and other health care professions, the number of private practice clinicians has for many years been far greater than the number of clinicians employed in academia or institutional settings. However, unlike these other health care professions, the roots of clinical psychology are in philosophy and science and pertain to intellectual endeavors (i.e., theory-building, empirical research and teaching) (cf., Robinson, 1995; Bringmann, Luck, Miller, & Early, 1997), *not* service provision. For psychology's clinicians as a collective, both nationally and within the American Psychological Association (APA), majority status was achieved in the 1980s (Reisman, 1991). That is, considering the various types of psychologists who engage in clinical practice, which is a much larger group compared to clinical neuropsychologists, majority setting became private practice years ago. Subsequently, clinicians, especially private practitioners, have become an increasingly larger proportion of the membership of APA . In fact, in 1995 Division 42 (Independent Practice) had the largest divisional membership within APA. Given that clinical neuropsychology's cognate is primarily clinical psychology, a young specialty itself (Routh, 1996), which grew out of studies of human behavior in broad academic subfields of psychology (e.g., social, developmental, personality, learning), we should not be surprised at the relatively recent ascendancy of private practice.

In response to a request from the first author, Jessica Kohout, Ph.D., Director of the Research Office of APA provided data pertaining to the memberships of Division 40 (Clinical Neuropsychology) and Division 42 (Independent Practice) from 1985 to 1998. Table 1 shows the relative growth of Divisions 40 and 42 and the overlap of memberships between these divisions across this 13-year interval. Note that both divisions more than doubled in size and the percentage of joint memberships between the divisions increased between 1985 and 1995. Additional data from the APA Research Office indicates that

Table 1. Trends in APA divisional memberships relevant to private practice neuropsychology.

Year	Division 40 Members	Division 42 Members	% of Div 40 in Div 42	% of Div 42 in Div 40
1985	1785	5018	18.1	6.4
1989	2604	5290	14.6	7.2
1993	3449	8182	18.6	7.8
1995	3880	10558	21.3	7.8
1998	4349	6940	16.1	10.1

Data compiled by Jessica Kohout, Ph.D., Director, and staff at Research Office, American Psychological Association. Anecdotally, some of the rise and subsequent decline in Division 42 membership may relate to an enrollment campaign that offered membership free for one year.

from 1985 to 1995 the percentage of members of Division 40 who described their primary full-time work setting as 'independent practice' increased from 26.7% to 35.4%. Interestingly, whereas the percentage of Division 42 members joining Division 40 increased over the entire 13-year interval, from 1995 to 1998 the overall size of Division 42 and the percentage of members of Division 40 who also belonged to Division 42 declined dramatically. One conclusion from the changes in this APA membership data, although admittedly difficult to prove, would be that private practice neuropsychology has enjoyed relatively more growth in recent years than the remainder of private practice clinical psychology.

Within neuropsychology, which is considerably younger than clinical psychology (see histories of clinical neuropsychology by Jones & Butters, 1991; Benton, 1992; Meier, 1992, 1997), a shift to a private practice *majority* occurred between 1994 and 1999. For the moment, we will exclude those who are board-certified (who will be mentioned later) in favor of focusing on the largest number of clinical neuropsychologists, members of Division 40 who are not board-certified. In this group, we can see the private practice trend by comparing survey data collected in 1989 (Sweet & Moberg, 1990), 1994 (Sweet et al., 1996), and in 1999 (Sweet et al., 2000a). Among non-board-certified clinical neuropsychologists who belong to Division 40, the work setting designated as *private/group practice* increased from 39% in 1989 to 47% in 1994, and to 58% in 1999. By comparison, the second most common practice setting for Division 40 members was *medical* settings, which in 1999 was a distant 20%. The third most frequent work setting in 1999 was *rehabilitation* at 16%. From 1989 to 1999, *psychiatric* work settings decreased from 10% to 1%. The percent of respondents employed within universities and colleges has remained low, with 3% in 1989 and 2% in 1999.

Considered separately, as they represent only approximately 10–12% of neuropsychologists, those who are board-certified are more likely to work within medical settings (50% in 1989, 48% in 1994, 44% in 1999). However, among board-certified neuropsychologists there is also a trend toward increased private practice (25% in 1989, 32% in 1994, 34% in 1999).

Interestingly, with regard to employment setting, a 1995 survey by the Practice Directorate of APA (Phelps, 1997) found that among Division 40 members, approximately 36% reported solo or group private practice and 39% reported medical setting as their employment setting. Slight differences in findings between the Phelps and Sweet, Moberg et al. studies, and those from the Research Office of APA mentioned earlier, are probably due to use of different terminology and response options within survey questions.

In whatever manner one wishes to group clinical neuropsychologists with regard to work settings, it is apparent that private practice has become a primary employment category, and the numbers of neuropsychologists within this category appear to be growing in absolute numbers and proportionally across time. The impact of this shift of employment settings will be noted throughout the remainder of this chapter. Because of the importance of this work setting to clinical neuropsychology, an attempt will be made to understand apparent trends within healthcare and within clinical neuropsychology that may affect private practice in the future.

Practitioner Characteristics

Salient characteristics of practicing neuropsychologists can be found in Tables 2 and 3. Neuropsychology has been predominantly a male subspecialty since its inception. Not long after the founding of Division 40 of APA, the 1981 APA directory lists 78.9% males and 21.1% females in the divisional membership. In the 1997 APA directory, the Division 40 membership is listed as having 65.6% males and 34.4% females. At this more recent level, the percentage of females in Division 40 remains significantly less than the membership of the American Psychological Association at large, which in 1997 was 47% female. Across a ten-year interval from 1989 to 1999, there was *not* an increase in the proportion of women in Division 40 (Sweet et al., 2000a). This finding is especially noteworthy in that it occurs despite the apparently increasing feminization of psychology in general (e.g., Denmark, 1994; Metzner, Rajecki, & Lauer, 1994; Pion et al., 1998), which includes data from the National Research Council, compiled by the APA Research Office, showing that in 1997 women earned more than two-thirds of the doctorates awarded in psychology. The reasons for the disproportionately low representation of women in clinical neuropsychology, as compared to psychology in general, are not known. However, the most recent survey data from members of the National Academy of Neuropsychology (NAN) and Division 40 of APA strongly suggest that while the overall proportion of women in the field lags behind psychology in general, the proportion is definitely in flux (Sweet et al., in press). Basically, although women comprised only 38% of the total NAN and Division 40 sample, within those licensed less than ten years, 51% were women, and within those licensed less than five years, 63% were women. Clearly, these figures suggest that the gender composition of neuropsychology will be undergoing dramatic changes in years to come.

The average age of neuropsychologists increased from 42 in 1989 to 48 in 1999. The age increase of only six years across a ten-year interval is explained by the fact that the subspecialty continues to be popular and able to grow by attracting new young practitioners. Although board-certified neuropsychologists were significantly older in 1989 (46 versus 42), in 1999 they had become comparable in age to the rest of the Division 40 membership (49 versus 48). The fact that the average age of board-certified neuropsychologists increased only three years across a ten-year interval reflects the apparent importance and increasing frequency of pursuing board certification among young neuropsychologists. Lending support to the notion that clinical neuropsychology continues to be a popular choice among psychologists early in their career are data indicating that from 1989 to 1999 the average number of years since

Table 2. Select characteristics of clinical neuropsychologists and their practices by general work setting in 1999.

	Private Practice	Institution
Age	49	47
Years since degree	18	16
Percent with doctorate in clinical psychology	72	70
Percent of work time in clinical practice > 60%	91	70
Total *hours per week* of clinical practice	37	31
Percent of work time involving *neuropsychological* practice	70	61
Hours per week of *neuropsychological* practice	25	26
Hours per evaluation (includes report writing)	10	8
Use of an assistant in evaluation process	44	65
Percent of clinicians providing *treatment* to patients with brain dysfunction	77	61
Hours per week in forensic activities	8	3
Top three referral sources	Law Psychiatry Neurology	Psychiatry Neurology Internal Medicine
Hours per week providing supervision	2	4
Percent with involvement in research and teaching	66	86

Private Practice *n* = 193, Institution *n* = 208. Excerpted from Sweet, Moberg, & Suchy (2000b).

degree for Division 40 members has increased only four years (from 12 to 16) and for board-certified neuropsychologists has increased only two years (from 17 to 19). By implication, the field of clinical neuropsychology appears to be energetic and vital.

Adding to the appearance of neuropsychology as a growing and vibrant field is the substantial growth in memberships of neuropsychology organizations, which has been impressive in recent years. For example, Division 40 of APA had 636 members in 1981, 1785 members in 1985, 3880 members in 1995, and 4349 in 1998. NAN has also been a popular neuropsychological membership organization and has also seen notable growth. For example, impressive increase in the size of NAN occurred between 1993 and 1996, when membership grew from 1982 members to 3093.

The Ph.D. continues to be the doctoral degree of the vast majority of clinical neuropsychologists. In 1999, 95% of board-certified and 88% of non-board-certified neuropsychologists had Ph.D.s. These numbers have decreased only slightly from 1989 to 1999. Clinical psychology has been the identified field of the doctoral degree for the majority of clinical neuropsychologists since the beginning of the subspecialty. In 1999, approximately 72% of clinical neuropsychologists had a degree in clinical psychology, with 10% in counseling psychology, 6% in neuropsychology, 1% in neuroscience, and 1% in 'other'. It is noteworthy that across a ten-year interval there has been *no* proportional growth among Division 40 members holding a *specialty degree* specifically in neuropsychology. The data as a whole appear to suggest that the majority of practitioners have Ph.D. specialty training in clinical psychology with subspecialization in clinical neuropsychology.

Characteristics and Clinical Practice Associated with Board Certification

From 1989 to 1994, the number of hours per week of total clinical practice among Division 40 members increased from 28 to 33. From 1994 to 1999 the number of weekly clinical practice hours increased again, to 35. Across time, board-certified practitioners have devoted a greater percentage of their work each week to *neuropsychological* activities than their Division 40 colleagues (in 1989, 24 hours versus 15; in 1999, 28 versus 21), while putting in less overall time in clinical practice per week (in 1999, 32 hours versus 35). That is, *non*-board-certified neuropsychology practitioners engage in a greater number of clinical hours per week, of which a greater proportion pertains to *non*-neuropsychological activity. This difference can also be seen in percent of professional time spent engaged in neuropsychological evaluation and treatment (in 1999, 78% versus 53%). In keeping with this data, board-certified neuropsychologists carry out more evaluations per month and are more likely to use assistants or psychometricians (in 1999, 69% for board-certified versus 42% for non-board-certified). In general, the use of assistants declined from 1989 to 1999. Although different in previous years, in 1999 both groups spent approximately the same amount of time completing an evaluation (with report, 8.6 hours for board-certified versus 9.2 for non-board-certified).

With regard to philosophical approach toward test selection, in 1999, 65% of Division 40 members adhered to a *flexible battery* approach (i.e., variable, but routine groupings of tests for different types of patients), with the percentage of board-certified neuropsychologists even higher, at 74%. In contrast, 19% of Division 40 members endorsed a *standardized battery* approach for all patients, compared to 11% of those who are board-certified. Among Division 40 members, 17% prefer a *flexible* approach (i.e., based upon the needs of an individual case; not uniform across patients), which is comparable to the 15% of board-certified neuropsychologists who endorse this approach. Since 1989, trends regarding philosophical approach to test selection have been away from

Table 3. Select characteristics of clinical neuropsychologists and their practices by board certification status[1].

	Board-Certified	Not Board-Certified
Age	49	48
Years since degree	19	16
Percent whose work time involves total clinical practice of > 60%	70	86
Total *hours per week* of clinical practice	32	35
Hours per week of *neuropsychological* practice	28	21
Hours per evaluation (includes report writing)	8.6	9.2
Use of an assistant in evaluation process	69	42
Percent of clinicians providing *treatment* to patients with brain dysfunction	58	76
Hours per week in forensic activities	6	4
Top three referral sources	Psychiatry Neurology Law	Psychiatry Neurology Law
Hours per week providing supervision	4	2
Percent with involvement in research and teaching	90	65

1 In this table, board certification signifies passing credentials review, review of work samples, written examination, and oral examination under the auspices of the American Board of Clinical Neuropsychology, one of eleven specialty boards of the American Board of Professional Psychology. Board-certified $n = 215$, not board certified $n = 207$. Excerpted from Sweet, Moberg, & Suchy (2000a).

a flexible approach and toward a flexible battery approach, irrespective of board certification status. Among board-certified practitioners, there also has been a strong trend away from the standardized approach since 1989.

Although thought of by some as a field involving *assessment* only, a majority of neuropsychologists are also involved in treating patients with brain dysfunction. In fact, 76% of Division 40 members and 58% of board-certified neuropsychologists reported being involved in *treating* patients with brain dysfunction in 1999.

Referral Sources and Patient Populations

Board certification status does not appear to be associated with rankings of top referral sources. That is, board-certified and non-board-certified neuropsychologists have similar rankings of top referral sources, with the top three being psychiatry, neurology, and law (attorneys) for both groups. If primary care physicians (e.g., internal medicine, family/general medicine) are considered as a whole, it appears that this group is responsible for many referrals to neuropsychologists. This finding is not surprising in that primary care physicians have come to play an important 'gatekeeping' role in managed care and are also pivotal in the healthcare of a society that is on average aging. For different reasons, if rehabilitation professionals (e.g., rehabilitation nurse, rehabilitation specialist) and physiatry are combined, this group also represents a major referral source. Neurosurgery is a much more frequent referral source for board-certified neuropsychologists than those who are not board-certified.

Practicing neuropsychologists tend not to restrict themselves to patients within a narrow age range. Adult neuropsychologists have been greater in number than pediatric neuropsychologists, which has led in recent years to the latter being in greater demand in the health care marketplace. Relatively few neuropsychologists evaluate or treat young children (ages 6–11), and, even among those who work with children in this age range, such work constitutes less than 25% of practice for the vast majority. At the other end of the age range, neuropsychologists are much more likely to spend a considerable percentage of their work time with geriatric patients (age >65).

Training

As the field has evolved, training requirements and curricula have become more and more explicit. For example, the Houston Conference on Specialty Education and Training in Clinical Neuropsychology (Hannay et al., 1998) is the most comprehensive set of recommended standards at the graduate, internship, and postdoctoral levels. Additionally, the Association of Postdoctoral Programs in Clinical Neuropsychology (Hammeke, 1993) has promulgated standards that emphasize training at the postdoctoral level. However, for the general Division 40 membership there has not been much change in the last ten years with regard to where the "majority" of training in clinical neuropsychology has originated. That is, predoctoral (including internship), postdoctoral, and continuing education, respectively, have received the same rankings with nearly the same percentages in 1989 and 1999. In 1999, the percentages associated with each level of training were predoctoral = 43%, postdoctoral = 32%, and continuing education = 25%.

Research and Teaching

Clinical neuropsychology has often been viewed as well entrenched in the scientist-practitioner model of clinical psychology. It could be argued, cogently and relatively easily, that the strong scientific underpinnings of clinical neuropsychology are at the root of its rapid growth within psychology and its degree of acceptance in the healthcare community. Therefore, it is even more unfortunate than would otherwise be the case that involvement in research appears to be diminishing. In the Sweet, Moberg et al. surveys, respondents were asked to endorse the percent of professional time spent on "clinical research and teaching." In 1989, 19% of Division 40 members indicated zero involvement in research and teaching, whereas in 1999 the percentage had increased to 35%. At the same time, the numbers of individuals spending high percentages of time in clinical research and teaching have diminished. In 1989, approximately 6% of neuropsychologists invested 80% or greater of their time in research and teaching, whereas *none* were doing so in 1999. Among the board-certified neuropsychologists, who historically have had a greater degree of involvement in research and teaching, this trend is also evident. For example, in 1989 19% were involved at a level of 60% or more of their time, whereas in 1999 only 4% were involved at this level. The general trend in neuropsychology of decreasing involvement in research and teaching can be seen in other health care specialties as well, and has been viewed as a direct effect of pressures resulting from changes in health care economics.

Private Practitioners as the New Majority

Upon discovering in the 1999 data that private practice had become the work setting of the majority of North American clinical neuropsychologists, data from the previous 1989 and 1994 surveys were analyzed to allow comparison of private practice with the aggregate of clinical neuropsychologists practicing in other settings across ten years (Sweet et al., 2000a,b). For these analyses, the very small percentages of respondents who self-designated as working in "college/university" and "other" settings were eliminated from the original data sets. Those working in "medical", "psychiatric", and "rehabilitation" settings were combined into a category that was termed *institutional* and then compared to *private practice* (referring to either solo or group practice). Since the original samples were collected with an attempt to obtain approximately equal groups of board-certified and non-board-certified neuropsychologists, it was fortunate that the re-categorization by work setting still allowed reasonable size groups for statistical analyses.

Age is significantly different, with those in private practice averaging 49 years compared to 47 years in institutions. As one might expect from age, there is a significant difference of post-degree clinical experience between the groups (18 years for private practice; 16 years for institutions). The groups are comparable in terms of having attained Ph.D.s, the vast majority of which are in clinical psychology. Board-certified neuropsychologists are more likely to work in institutions, but approximately 34% were in private practice in 1999.

It should not be surprising that the number of private practitioners in clinical neuropsychology has increased substantially. Vaughn, D'Amato, and Dean (1998) examined trends in neuropsychological job offerings by looking at all the position announcements in the American Psychological Association's *Monitor* from 1976 to 1997. Position offerings in medical settings, such as hospitals, peaked in 1987 and were at their second lowest in the interval surveyed in 1997. As a percentage of all psychology positions offered in a year, neuropsychological positions hit a peak (12%) in 1993, but decreased to half that amount in 1996 and 1997. Meanwhile, the number of training programs for clinical neuropsychologists has been increasing and continues to produce a relatively high volume of new professionals annually. Unless healthcare economics that affect institutions improve significantly, it appears that most new neuropsychologists will be basing their practices in the private sector, rather than in institutions.

As might be expected, work setting has an effect on one's clinical and professional activities. For example, Sweet et al. (2000b) found that work setting was associated with percent of professional time spent on clinical practice, with private practitioners engaging in greater proportions of time on clinical practice (chi-square = 34.69, df = 4, $p < .001$) and greater numbers of clinical practice hours per week (37 hours vs. 29; $t = 4.2$, df = 245, $p < .001$). Nevertheless, institutional practice was associated with a greater number of neuropsychological evaluations per month (chi-square =13.47, df = 5, $p = .019$) *and* similar numbers of therapy patients per month (chi-square = 4.90, df = 5, $p = .429$). Such findings raise the possibility that private practice neuropsychologists may invest a greater proportion of clinical practice time in non-neuropsychological activities. In fact, this appears to be indicated in the greater percent of clinical practice time each week spent on *neuropsychological* assessment and treatment by institutional practitioners (69% vs. 55%; $t = 3.48$, df = 246, $p < .001$). The NAN/Division 40 survey results (Sweet et al., in press) reported similar findings, with those in private practice engaging in a greater number of clinical hours per week, but within their clinical time having a greater proportion pertaining to non-neuropsychological activities (e.g., four times the hours of psychotherapy with patients who do not have brain dysfunction and twice the hours of psychological assessment).

Also of interest is the finding that private practitioners spend more time per evaluation than institutional practitioners (9.7 hours vs. 7.7, $t = 3.82$, df = 246, $p < .001$). This is not a trivial time difference and would be associated with a meaningfully higher fee for service, as billing by the hour is universal. An explanation for this difference in time per evaluation is not readily apparent, particularly since healthcare reimbursement systems demand ever-greater efficiency. The answer is not to be found in differential preferences for standardized batteries, flexible batteries, or a flexible approach, as there are no associated frequency differences by group (chi-square = 2.23, df = 2, $p = .327$). Although there are differential preferences for use of technicians or assistants, with institutional practice associated with employment of a greater number (66% vs. 50%; chi-square = 6.24, df = 1, $p < .05$), it seems unlikely that this difference could contribute such a strong effect on time per evaluation. In fact, relevant data from Sweet et al. (in press) indicate that even if it did, the effect would be in the opposite direction. That is, institutional neuropsychologists are more likely than private practice neuropsychologists to utilize technicians or assistants and across settings those who do so actually average *more* hours of testing per case in non-forensic assessments. For example, when the purpose of an examination was to determine diagnosis, those using assistants reported significantly longer evaluations (With assistant $M = 6.6$ hours, $SD = 5.4$, No assistant $M = 5.9$, $SD = 6.2$; $F(1,1073) = 4.2$, $p = .04$). (Interestingly, although using assistants was associated with a lengthier examination, hours of billing per case were similar between those who use and those who do not use assistants.) Finally, comparing length of evaluations by work setting, only the forensic cases showed a statistically significant difference.

In the Sweet et al. (2000b) survey, private practice neuropsychologists were found to engage in a significantly greater number of forensic activities per week (8 hours vs. 3) and in the NAN/Division 40 survey private practitioners reported an approximately three times greater frequency of forensic activities than those in institutions (i.e., 27.3% vs. 9.5% forensic caseload). This difference between settings in the amount of forensic activity, which has been shown to be associated with lengthier evaluations, is likely to be one of the factors contributing to differences in evaluation length by work setting. Logically, it may also be the case that since private practitioners appear to engage in proportionately *less* neuropsychological activity per week (i.e., 25 of 37 clinical hours in private practice versus 26 of 31 clinical hours in institutions) and also engage in *more* forensic activity per week, the forensic activity of private practitioners may include more non-neuropsychological cases. Unfortunately, the phrasing of the survey questions of either survey does not allow more definitive delineation.

From a listing in the Sweet et al. (2000b) survey of ten types of information gathered in a neuropsychological evaluation, respondents were asked to rate their frequency from "never", "occasionally", "often", to "always". Only the category of "school or work records" was associated with work setting, with private practitioners more likely to investigate such information (chi-square = 10.5, df = 3, $p < .05$), no doubt related to the greater proportion of forensic cases. Other categories showing *no* association to group status (thus, comparable regardless of practice setting) were: psychological history, medical history, information from referral source, objective personality testing, projective personality testing, measures of mood and affect, mental status exam, achievement testing, and current neuropsychological data. Given that only one of ten categories was statistically significant, this finding may not be reliable. Also of interest is the fact that very few clinicians in either group collect projective personality test data "often" or "always". Gathering of this type of data has been decreasing in frequency in the last decade (Sweet et al.,

2000a) and now appears to be of *relatively* minor and infrequent interest for neuropsychologists.

Finally, as institutional employment settings (e.g., teaching hospitals) for neuropsychologists often have training components, it is not surprising that institutional practitioners are more likely to engage in research and teaching activities than their private practice colleagues (chi-square = 42.95, df = 5, $p < .001$). Supervisory responsibilities are also significantly greater ($p < .001$) within institutions, where the average is four hours per week, versus private practice, where the average is two hours per week. The NAN/Division 40 survey documented similar findings.

Economic Data

Of available recent surveys, four bear on the effects of managed care on neuropsychological practice. Sweet et al. (1995) reported that 54% of 259 clinical neuropsychologists had experienced decreases in hourly reimbursement and 35% reported decreased incomes within the prior five years that were attributed by the respondents to managed care. Exclusion from managed care provider panels was reported by 43% of survey respondents and 36% had experienced a decrease in referral sources. As a result of these negative effects of managed care, 25% had *increased* their patient load in an attempt to maintain their income. Of a smaller sample ($n = 77$) who offered specific concerns in response to an open-ended question at the end of the survey, 40% reported increased administrative and paperwork as a result of managed care.

Phelps (1997 Winter/Spring) found similar results in a larger sample of Division 40 members. In the Sweet et al. (1995) survey, 48% of 809 respondents reported difficulty obtaining reimbursement of services and 47% reported excessive precertification and utilization review (i.e., "administrative and paperwork") pertaining to managed care. Approximately 44% reported decreased income due to managed care fee structure. Importantly, 34% reported experiencing *ethical dilemmas* created by managed care.

In their 1999 survey, Sweet et al. (2000b) found that yearly income changes in the previous five years were associated with work setting and board certification status. For example, 56% of board-certified neuropsychologists working in institutions reported increased income versus 49% of board-certified neuropsychologists in private practice. For those *not* board-certified, income increases were reported less frequently, and were also affected by work setting; increases were reported by 47% in institutions and 41% in private practice. Decreases in yearly income demonstrated the reverse effect of these factors. That is, among those who were *not* board-certified decreases were more likely (38% in institutions and 48% in private practice) than for board-certified neuropsychologists (21% in institutions and 42% in private practice), and, as these percentages suggest, institutional setting appeared to act as a buffer to negative economic changes. Interestingly, among all those neuropsychologists who experienced increased annual income in the previous five years, this *positive change was attributed to voluntary professional changes* by more than 70% of respondents. However, when decreased annual income had been experienced, this *negative change was attributed to managed care* by more than 85% of respondents. These attributions were nearly identical across work setting.

In the most recent relevant national professional practice survey of clinical neuropsychologists sponsored by NAN and Division 40, (data collected in late 2000 and early 2001), Sweet et al. (in submission) found that 59% of NAN and Division 40 respondents had experienced increased earnings in the prior five years, while 10% reported no change, and 30% reported earning less. Among neuropsychology practitioners reporting increased income, those working in private practice reported an average increase of $30,216, whereas those in institutions reported an increase of only $12,502. Those with combined private practice and institutional employment reported an average increase of $22,423. Across the entire sample of full-time practitioners, a number of variables, such as years of licensed practice, work setting, percentage of forensic practice, percentage of self pay, and gender, were found to have significant, albeit modest correlations with income. Although associated with multiple factors, which tends to obscure causal analysis, clinical neuropsychologists working fulltime who reported zero percent of managed care patients in their practices reported an average income of $119,024, compared to those with a 76–100% managed care practice who reported an average income of $89,224. Similarly, individuals working fulltime with zero percent Medicare patients reported an average income of $109,251, compared to an average income of $85,236 with a practice of 76–100% Medicare patients. It is noteworthy that data from this same survey indicate that the average clinical neuropsychologist in the United States had 27.6% of the patients in their practices on managed care and approximately 18% on Medicare. Clearly, the combined impact of these reimbursement sources, which force practitioners to accept greatly discounted rates, on the income of neuropsychologists in the United States is very substantial. These factors are likely to be among the primary causes of the significant *decrease* in *average* income among neuropsychologists since 1993 (cf. Putnam & Anderson, 1994). These factors aside, the most recent salary data indicate that approximately 70% of clinical neuropsychologists have gross incomes between $60,000 and $160,000. Approximately 75% report incomes below $120,000, 95% of individuals report incomes at or below $240,000, and 98% report being at or below $296,000.

Although clear-cut in meaning for the most part, the above findings pertaining to the effects of major third party reimbursement sources, such as managed care and Medicare, have broader implications as well. It seems that one direct effect of managed care has been to increase clinical practice time, both because of greater demands administratively per case, and related to attempts of practitioners to offset potential income loss due to lower reimbursement and loss of business. As shown in 1994 and 1999 data from surveys by Sweet et al. (1996; 2000a) discussed above, there is a trend for clinical neuropsychologists in general to engage in *more* clinical practice and *less* education and research per week. Decline in these latter activities was present throughout the period of 1989 to 1999 and may continue in the future. It seems clear that beyond the effects on individuals, the field itself is being impacted negatively by the untoward economics of reimbursement in recent years. Less involvement in education and research has strong potential to detract from the evolution and improvement of the field through better training and expansion of the knowledge base that would normally take place across time.

Trends and Recommendations

During the 1980s the growth of clinical neuropsychology was tremendous. Memberships in relevant professional organizations multiplied and job sectors, such as rehabilitation, produced large numbers of new positions for neuropsychologists. Along with increased demand came a large increase in formal training programs or program tracks at the doctoral, internship, and postdoctoral levels. The subspecialty adopted a formal definition of individual practitioners (Division 40 Executive Committee, 1989), developed guidelines for training at the doctoral, internship, and postdoctoral levels (Report of the INS-Division 40 Task Force on Education, Accreditation, and Credentialing, 1987; Bornstein, 1988), began to identify programs that provided training (Cripe, 1991, 1995), and solidified expectations with regard to inclusion of postdoctoral training as an integral part of training to become a clinical neuropsychologist (Hammeke, 1993). At this point, numerous aspects of the field have been outlined and described (see Eubanks, 1997 for a summary of relevant citations). In other words, the field has grown tremendously and explicitly defined itself in recent years. There are several noteworthy implications of these professional developments.

The nature of the American health care systems of the 1980s that created enormous demand for production of high quality clinical neuropsychologists produced a large number of formal training programs. These programs have been continuing, for the most part, to turn out a large number of well-trained individuals, despite the fact that fewer neuropsychology practitioners are needed at present (see Johnstone et al., 1995 and Matthews, 1996 for relevant discussion). In general, the result is increased competition to obtain employment in general across all settings. Coupled with the apparent difficulty that practicing neuropsychologists have had in securing access to patients because of managed care, private practitioners may face increasing difficulty in initially setting up and maintaining their practices.

An equally important implication is that credentialing, already receiving increased emphasis due to the normal evolution of a relatively new field that better defines itself as it develops, has become even more important as a means of distinguishing oneself from a large and growing field of competitors. Board certification, in the past a less important distinction for clinical psychology generalists, has been deemed authoritatively within the subspecialty to be "...the clearest evidence of competence as a Clinical Neuropsychologist, assuring that all of these criteria have been met..." (referring to the definition of a clinical neuropsychologist) (Division 40 Executive Committee, 1989, p. 22). Although a variety of formats exist for acquiring board certification, the board certification process of the American Board of Professional Psychology (ABPP) is the most common for clinical neuropsychologists, which is also true of clinical psychologists with other specialties. Whether in a private practice or institutional setting, board certification has become more important to clinical neuropsychologists.

Although more difficult in the present healthcare environment, distinction as an expert within the field has been and remains attainable through the activities of the scientist-practitioner — namely, peer reviewed publication of clinical research. Within this text, perhaps the best example among private practitioners is that of chapter contributor Manfred Greiffenstein, a private practice neuropsychologist who has achieved distinction in the field through publication of research relevant to timely issues in the forensic arena. Although not common among private practitioners in any field, it *is* possible to achieve distinction through scientist-practitioner activities.

Forensic activities by neuropsychologists appear to be increasing, and have already become important for neuropsychology practitioners, especially those in private practice. Data from Division 40 members suggest that 7.4% of professional practice in 1995 was related to forensic activities (Phelps, 1997). In 1999, the forensic activity had increased to six hours per week for board-certified and four hours a week for non-board-certified clinical neuropsychologists. Further comparisons by work setting indicate that private practitioners engage in eight forensic hours per week compared to three per week for practitioners based in institutions. Moreover, attorneys are the number one referral source for private practitioners and are ranked fifth for institutional practitioners. The absence of managed care issues associated with such cases, plus the increasing demand, based upon greater recognition within the legal community that qualified neuropsychologists can make a distinctive contribution, may create continued growth in this area. Thorough coverage of practices and issues related to forensic neuropsychology can be found within the text edited by Sweet (1999).

Neuropsychology operates within a much larger health care context that contains forces powerful enough to affect all providers, regardless of discipline or specialty. Belar (1997) has provided a thorough discussion of emerging characteristics of the health care system that will affect the professional practice of psychology in health care, including the implications of the Pew Health Professions Commission report (O'Neil, 1993). Some aspects of this report seem pertinent to clinical neuropsychology. Specifically, among those related to neuropsychology, there appear to be health care trends in the direction of increased: (1) coordination of services across providers, disciplines, and settings, (2) focus on quality of life, (3) preservation of resources and explicit priority setting, as cost control gains importance, (4) individual accountability, and (5) integration of health care, education, and public safety. With regard to the ongoing influence of managed care, Belar (1997) states, "In summary, as the market matures, individuals and firms will increasingly purchase plans based on differences in value (not just cost), and the interests of health plans, public health systems, schools, and community agencies will increasingly converge." (p. 413) At this point, however, neuropsychologists are engaging in less research and teaching and a substantial number have experienced decreases in annual income, despite the fact that the average clinical number of hours increased substantially from 1989 to 1999.

The excellent discussion within Johnstone et al. (1995), a large collection of invited opinions regarding the future of health psychology, neuropsychology, and rehabilitation psychology, contains recommendations for coping with ongoing changes in the healthcare environment. Excerpting from one contribution to the Johnstone publication, the following points regarding independent practice for neuropsychologists can be considered as possible means of increasing professional survival:

> "*affiliate* with groups seeking participation in managed care; *join* hospital staffs, if possible; *adopt* flexible and negotiable fee schedules; *learn* specialized skills that will remain in competitive demand; *provide* focused, goal-specific services; *expect* clinical and fiscal accountability; *attend* to professional health care policy information; and *support* your state psychological association." (p. 349)

With regard to the latter recommendation, state psychological associations are not only the forum within which many practice issues can be addressed, but it is within such groups that private practitioners can accomplish important professional networking and gain local name recognition. State psychological associations also represent practitioners in their state with regard to state laws and policies that most directly affect clinical practice. For the future benefit of our field, all of the professional organizations that represent the interests of clinical neuropsychology, such as Division 40 of APA, the National Academy of Neuropsychology, and the International Neuropsychological Society may need to invest more time and resources into affecting relevant health-care policy (e.g., Medicare relative value units (RVUs), current procedural terminology (CPT) codes, and managed care coverage benefits and practice guidelines).

Summary

Private practice has grown significantly in recent years and compared to institutional work settings (e.g., medical, psychiatric and rehabilitation), is now the largest employment setting for clinical neuropsychologists in the United States. Despite strenuous health care economic conditions, and perhaps because of the large number of clinical neuropsychologists that continue to be trained despite less demand compared to the 1980s, private practice neuropsychology is also growing at a faster rate than other employment settings.

Private practitioners resemble their peers in institutional settings in many ways. For example, both groups have: comparable views toward test selection and type of information gathered, similar age and gender of clinicians with comparable levels of experience, and similar referral sources. Private practitioners also have distinctive characteristics. They are less likely to be board-certified (although this appears among clinical neuropsychologists to be increasing at a rate much greater than private clinical psychologists in general), more clinically active — but less so in neuropsychology, more involved in forensic activity, less involved in research and education, and more likely to invest more time per evaluation.

With continued increases in supply of clinical neuropsychologists, but less demand in the current health care marketplace, private practitioners need to be proactive in positioning themselves for access to the growing numbers of managed care patients and increased competition in general. Experts in the field have offered advice regarding steps that may increase access to patients. As partial remedies for increased competition, earning credentialing distinction through board certification, or professional peer distinction through involvement in scientist-practitioner activities and peer review publication, and participation in state psychological associations may be helpful to practitioners. The major professional organizations that represent clinical neuropsychology will need to emphasize the needs and interests of the new majority of private practitioners if the field as a whole is to remain vital and effective.

Acknowledgment

The author gratefully acknowledges Jessica Kohout, Ph.D. and staff at the Research Office of the American Psychological Association for provision of relevant data discussed within this chapter.

References

Belar, C. (1997). Clinical health psychology: A specialty for the 21st century. *Health Psychology, 16*, 411–416.

Benton, A. (1992). Clinical neuropsychology: 1960-1990. *Journal of Clinical and Experimental Neuropsychology, 14*, 407–417.

Bornstein, R. (1988). Entry into clinical neuropsychology: Graduate, undergraduate, and beyond. *The Clinical Neuropsychologist, 2*, 213–220.
Bringmann, W., Luck, H., Miller, R., & Early, C. (1997). *A pictorial history of psychology*. Chicago: Quintessence Publishing.
Cripe, L. (1991). Listing of training programs in clinical neuropsychology — 1991. *The Clinical Neuropsychologist, 5*, 226-237.
Cripe, L. (1995). Listing of training programs in clinical neuropsychology — 1995. *The Clinical Neuropsychologist, 9*, 327-398.
Denmark, F. (1994). Engendering psychology. *American Psychologist, 49*, 329–334.
Division 40 Executive Committee (1989). Definition of a clinical neuropsychologist. *The Clinical Neuropsychologist, 3*, 22.
Eubanks, J. (1997). Clinical neuropsychology summary information prepared by Division 40, Clinical Neuropsychology, American Psychological Information. *The Clinical Neuropsychologist, 11*, 77–80.
Hammeke, T. (1993). The Association of Postdoctoral Programs in Clinical Neuropsychology (APPCN). *The Clinical Neuropsychologist, 7*, 197–204.
Hannay, H.J., Bieliauskas, L.A., Crosson, B.A., Hammeke, T.A., Hamsher, K. deS., & Koffler, S.P. (1998). Proceedings: The Houston Conference on Specialty Education and Training in Clinical Neuropsychology. *Archives of Clinical Neuropsychology, 13*, 157–249.
Johnstone, B. et al. (1995). Psychology in health care: Future directions. *Professional Psychology: Research and Practice, 26*, 341–365.
Jones, B.P., & Butters, N. (1991). Neuropsychological assessment. In M. Hersen, A. Kazdin, & A. Bellack (Eds.), *The clinical psychology handbook*, 2nd ed. New York: Pergamon.
Matthews, C. (1996). Slouching toward the millennium: Some survival prescriptions for neuropsychology. *Archives of Clinical Neuropsychology, 11*, 261–269.
Meier, M. (1992). Modern clinical neuropsychology in historical perspective. *American Psychologist, 47*, 550–558.
Meier, M. (1997). The establishment of clinical neuropsychology as a psychological specialty. In M. Maruish, & J. Moses (Eds.), *Clinical neuropsychology: Theoretical foundations for practitioners*. Hillsdale, NJ: Lawrence Erlbaum Associates.
Metzner, B., Rajecki, D., & Lauer, J. (1994). New majors and the feminization of psychology: Testing and extending the Rajecki–Metzner model. *Teaching of Psychology, 21*, 5–11.
O'Neil, E. (1993). *Health professions education for the future: Schools in service to the nation*. San Francisco, CA: Pew Health Professions Commission.
Phelps, R. (1997, Winter/Spring). Profiling Division 40 members: CAPP practitioner survey. *(Division of Clinical Neuropsychology) Newsletter 40, 15*, 5–7.
Pion, G., Mednick, M., Astin, J., Hall, C., Kenkel, M., Keita, G., Kohout, J., & Kelleher, J. (1998). The shifting gender composition of psychology. *American Psychologist, 51*, 509–528.
Putnam, S., & Anderson, C. (1994). The second *TCN* Salary survey: A survey of neuropsychologists, Part I. *The Clinical Neuropsychologist, 8*, 3–37.
Reisman, J. (1991). *A history of clinical psychology*, 2nd ed. New York: Hemisphere.
Report of the INS-Division 40 Task Force on Education, Accreditation, and Credentialing (1987). Guidelines for doctoral, internship, and postdoctoral training in clinical neuropsychology. *The Clinical Neuropsychologist, 1*, 29–34.
Robinson, D., (1995). *An intellectual history of psychology*, 3rd ed. Madison, Wisconsin: University of Minnesota Press.
Routh, D. (1996). Lightner Witmer and the first 100 years of clinical psychology. *American Psychologist, 51*, 244–247.

Sweet, J. (Ed.) (1999). *Forensic neuropsychology: Fundamentals and practice.* Lisse, Netherlands: Swets & Zeitlinger.

Sweet, J. & Moberg, P. (1990). A survey of practices and beliefs among ABPP and non-ABPP clinical neuropsychologists. *The Clinical Neuropsychologist, 4,* 101–120.

Sweet, J., Moberg, P., & Suchy, Y. (2000a). Ten-year follow-up survey of clinical neuropsychologists: Part I. Practices and beliefs. *The Clinical Neuropsychologist, 14,* 18–37.

Sweet, J., Moberg, P., & Suchy, Y. (2000b). Ten-year follow-up survey of clinical neuropsychologists: Part II. Private practice and economics. *The Clinical Neuropsychologist, 14,* 479–495.

Sweet, J., Moberg, P., & Westergaard, C. (1996). Five year follow-up survey of practices and beliefs of clinical neuropsychologists. *The Clinical Neuropsychologist, 10,* 202–221.

Sweet, J., Peck, E., Abramowitz, C., & Etzweiler, S. (2002). National Academy of Neuropsychology/Division 40 of the American Psychological Association practice survey of clinical neuropsychology in the United States, Part I: Practitioner and practice characteristics, professional activities, and time requirements. *The Clinical Neuropsychologist, 16,* 109–127.

Sweet, J., Peck, E., Abramowitz, C., & Etzweiler, S. (in press). National Academy of Neuropsychology/Division 40 (American Psychological Association) practice survey of clinical neuropsychology in the United States, Part II: Reimbursement experiences, practice economics, billing practices, and incomes. *Archives of Clinical Neuropsychology, 18.*

Sweet, J., Westergaard, C., & Moberg, P. (1995). Managed care experiences of clinical neuropsychologists. *The Clinical Neuropsychologist, 9,* 214–218.

Vaughn, E., D'Amato, R., & Dean, R. (1998, November). *Two decades of employment in neuropsychology: Neuropsychology had a great fall.* Presented at the annual meeting of the National Academy of Neuropsychology, Washington, DC.

PART II

CURRENT ISSUES IN THE PRACTICE OF CLINICAL NEUROPSYCHOLOGY

Chapter 4

BUSINESS ASPECTS OF PRIVATE PRACTICE IN CLINICAL NEUROPSYCHOLOGY

Edward A. Peck, III

In the mid-1980's, there were relatively few clinical neuropsychologists in private practice. Today, many neuropsychologists engage in either full or part-time private practice. In turn, many things about private practice have changed in the past fifteen to twenty years. The most obvious and dramatic changes which have occurred since I went into private practice in neuropsychology revolve around the time and service limits the US healthcare insurance industry has placed on our capability to provide professional care to patients and the associated reductions in funding for those services which they do authorize.

When I first began lecturing on business issues in clinical practice, I found that many individuals in the audience would rather have a root canal than deal with the business side of their professional activities. Some of the reasons given for their avoidance type behaviors were as follows:

1. I am a professional, not a bookkeeper.
2. It is beneath me to focus on money with my patients.
3. I can't do my job if I have to worry about who pays the bills, or if the bills even get paid.
4. I am a salaried employee. I don't have to think about costs.
5. I didn't study that in school.
6. If I had wanted to deal with the business end of things, I would have gotten an MBA.
7. It scares me and upsets me too much.

8. I would prefer not to think about it.
9. It will give me a *Professional* Traumatic Stress Disorder.
10. I am a clinician — not an administrator.

My reaction to the above comments is simple. Do you think that Broca, Wernicke and Freud avoided asking for payment from those patients who could *afford* to pay for their services?

During the past decade, as the restrictions on funding for clinical services have increased, so has the apparent level of interest expressed by colleagues about the business of running a practice in clinical neuropsychology. It really doesn't matter whether you are in a solo or group practice, single or multi-specialty practice, medical school or for profit or nonprofit hospital. If your practice pays its bills and salaries from the revenue generated through clinical efforts and your practice involves billing insurance companies and other similar sources for this revenue, then any change in the funding for your services becomes a critical issue. This book chapter is designed to provide information concerning the business aspects of running a private practice in Clinical Neuropsychology. The information I have gained in my years of experience *and especially in the business mistakes I have made*, serve as the underpinnings to this chapter (Peck, 1990; Neblett, Peck, Hylton, & Isner, 1999).

There is an ongoing change in how the American health care system reimburses for mental health services. This, of course, includes how we as neuropsychologists are reimbursed for our professional services. In response to these significant changes in reimbursement, neuropsychologists have begun to make changes in terms of how we deliver our professional services. I frequently hear remarks from neuropsychologists about how they spend 8, 10 or 12 hours carrying out a comprehensive neuropsychological assessment, followed by several more hours of report preparation, only to later discover that they have been paid only for one or two hours of their time, if at all. One neuropsychologist told me that he had to fire his office manager and secretary because he could no longer afford to pay their salaries. When I inquired about how he managed his time, it became clear that he was being paid for many fewer hours than he was spending on each clinical case. His lament was "How can I spend less time and still be ethical?"

It's a pressing question. How do we make accommodations to reduced service funding and still sleep at night? How do we make these accommodations and not get sued for malpractice? How do we make accommodations and still stay within the ethical boundaries of the American Psychological Association and our state psychological associations. This chapter has been written with the purpose of providing the practicing clinical neuropsychologist with information about how to survive in the current mental health marketplace.[1] I will emphasize a proactive response to the management of

[1] For the record, most of the information contained in this book chapter is directed toward the patient who is *not* receiving pro bono care due to their financial limi-

your professional practice. I believe that, if you are proactive in your business planning, you can avoid a lot of problems, rather than always trying to play catch up with a situation which has already gotten out of control.

Establishing Your Office Cost of Practice

Let's start with a basic question. *Do you actually know how much it costs you to run your practice, or your portion of your practice, on a per hour basis?* It is a fundamental question. If you don't know how much it costs to pay all of your fixed office expenses, i.e. your basic office overhead before you pay the first penny of your salary, then how can you know when you are signing on with an insurance carrier which is paying 'X' per hour for psychotherapy and 'Y' per hour for testing, whether you are (a) going to operate at a loss, (b) break even with zero profit, or (c) make enough money to pay your overhead and have something left over to go toward your salary? How would you know, when you are negotiating a fee with a client, that you are not losing money in the arrangement? It is time to think about the basic cost of delivering your professional service to the public from a business management point of view. In truth, without having a better understanding of such things, we are at a loss as to how to make some of the business decisions that we have to make on a daily basis.

Please examine Table 1. What you see in this table is a standard list of itemized, office cost categories. For simplicity, this table is organized with cost categories that are most relevant to a solo form of private practice. Your particular situation may require additional cost items. Hypothetical financial data has been entered so as to demonstrate the impact of expenses on the relevant cost per hour data. For ease in calculating the basic office expenses, personal salary information is not included. What this table provides is the type of information your accountant should give you on a monthly basis as a result of your expenditures and practice income. This information is critical to how you establish your cost of practice.

---

tations. Psychologists are directed by the APA to provide a reasonable amount of pro bono care. I am not aware of any position by the APA which requires the psychologist to provide pro bono care to a financially able person because of insurance based, contractual limitations. Instead, some service restrictions may be the result of a contractual issue between the patient's insurance company and the participating psychologist who is also under a contract with the patient's insurance company.

Each clinical situation needs to be critically evaluated by the psychologist for both professional and ethical issues as well as for insurance contractual issues. When there is a question by the psychologist regarding ethical and professional behavior being in conflict with contractual issues, the psychologist should be encouraged to seek appropriate steps to clarify the situation and to behave in a professionally appropriate manner.

Table 1. Sample financial report.

Revenues	Current Month October	Current Year To Date 10 Months	Prior Year To Date 10 Months
Fees Received	46484.87	350875	320897.50
Other Income	2490	30115	18737
Interest Earsed	30.39	429	190
Total Revenue	49005.26	381419	339824.50
Cost of Practice			
Accounting	300	3000	2800
Advertising	50	500	425
Bank Charges	17.81	581.79	500
Co. Car Loan	350	3500	0
Co. Car Expenses	65	650	639
Charity Contributions	100	225	200
Continuing Education	120	250	250
Dues & Subscriptions	400	2805	3000
Employee Benefits	660	6660	5000
Equipment — Capital	0	2000	1000
Equipment — Other	125	300	500
Insurance — Malpractice	100	900	900
Insurance — Co. Car	90	900	860
Insurance — Other	140	1140	1000
Interest — Loans	43.49	825.74	0
Legal Fees	125	350	675
Licenses	100	450	450
Maintenance — Equipment	475	2900	2500
Miscellaneous	50	2400	700
Office Expense	239	3100	3000
Postage	135	1650	250
Refunds	50.50	1117	1750
Registration — Meeting	180	450	400
Rent — Office	2000	20000	17000
Repairs	0	1000	800
Supplies — Office	54	1334.75	1000
Supplies — Test	125.25	375	350
Taxes — Payroll	4800	48000	39000
Taxes — Other	0	375	375
Telephone	210.24	2848.90	2500
Telephone Ans .Service	90	900	800
Travel	616	3300	1000
Meals & Entertainment	75	590	200
Wages	8711.52	77810.64	74508.97
Total Expenses	20597.81	193188.82	164332.97
Net Income/Loss	28407.45	188230.18	175491.53
Total Billable Hours (173)	173	1730	1730
Total Billable Hours (245)	245	2450	2450
Cost of Practice Per Hour for 173 Hours Per Month	119.06	111.67	94.99
Cost of Practice Per Hour for 245 Hours Per Month	84.07	78.85	67.07

When you look at the line items and their estimated costs in Table 1, please personalize the line items to your own situation. You may need to add or delete items, depending upon advice from your accountant. [What do you mean, you don't have an accountant! Who coordinates all of the payroll and tax information?] After personalizing this information, you need to calculate how many hours a week your office is actually open for business. I am not referring to the nights and weekends that you work at home. I am talking about your office hours when there are billable time slots available for appointments. For example, suppose your office is open for 40 hours a week or 2080 hours a year. That works out to a rounded figure of 173 hours a month. Your office may be open for more or less hours per week. Please ignore CEU days, vacation time or sick days etc., where you are out of the office, as the overhead still has to be paid, even though you are not present in the office and generating revenue.

Now look at the various expenses that have to be paid. Be certain to consider that some cost categories, e.g. malpractice insurance, are billed only once or twice a year. Divide your total month end costs by 173 hours (or by the correct number of available hours for your situation) and you will obtain your actual office overhead cost per hour for that month. You can redo the math and compute your hourly cost of practice for the year. If you use a technician and you are able to bill for more than one patient charge per hour (e.g. you see a psychotherapy patient while your technician is simultaneously testing a patient), then you need to add in those additional hours. Similarly, if there are other professionals in your practice who also generate billable income, then include their available hours in the formula. Of course, having additional employees also creates more overhead per hour, but the point is that a busy technician or fellow professional should be able to generate more income to the practice than the overhead incurred.

Don't forget, the cost of practice figures generated in Table 1 do not include your salary or the salary for other professionals in your practice. You will need to add your monthly salary information to the salary line item in order to calculate your actual hourly cost of practice.

Why do we need to know this information? The obvious reason is that if your revenues are in excess of your expenses then your practice is making a profit. If your revenues are less than your expenses, then your practice is operating at a loss. Basically, we are talking about having enough in your office bank account to pay the bills and, maybe, even your salary! Any excess left over from the prior month goes into your reserve to help pay the next month's bills.

After you have determined your actual cost of practice per hour, you can ask other questions concerning how you run your practice. For example, does signing an agreement where you are paid $51.50 per hour from that managed care company help you to stay in business? Does spending an additional five hours beyond the preauthorized number of hours, with no reimbursement for the extra time, help you to pay your bills? How you decide to spend your time is your personal and professional business. The real question, though, is whether you can stay in business with how you actually spend your professional time. Having an accurate picture of your office finances helps you to make better business decisions.

You should be able to examine the fluctuations in your expenses (and your monies received) on a month-to-month basis, as well as how these things look across the entire year and how the current figures compare with those from the prior year. For example, if your last year's rent from the beginning of January through the end of October was $17,000 and this year it is $18,000, obviously your rent has gone up. Now, ask whether you have been able to reduce expenses in one or more other categories to compensate for this increase. The point is, where is that extra $1,000 coming from to pay the increased rent? When your secretary asks for a 5% raise, or when you want to buy that new computer, those expenses have to come out of the work that you are generating and the fees you are collecting. If the insurance company reduces its hourly rate of payment, that means that you will need to replace that lost money from somewhere else — or pay it out of your salary.

You can look at each of the line items in Table 1 in terms of the cost of your practice on a per hour basis. As mentioned above, you can figure your cost per hour both with and without your salary. It just depends on how you want to run the calculations. Let's offer another example, look at your capital expenses for equipment. If you buy a computer this month, it is going to change your equipment expense costs and, as a result, your total cost per hour. Can you afford a new computer?

When I applied this analysis to my actual business costs, I realized that I needed to find out what each insurance company actually paid my company on an hourly basis for each relevant CPT code. Table 2 presents a sample form that my office has generated in order to track each insurance company's actual payments for individual CPT codes. We currently use a set office charge of $275.00 per hour for all in-office services. This includes both assessment and psychotherapy and whether the case is clinical or medical legal in nature. In this manner, we cannot stand accused by an attorney of billing at a different rate for clinical versus medical legal cases. In most insurance contract situations, we have to adjust off the balance of the fee beyond the established contractual rate.

In reviewing Table 2 and comparing the established fees, it is clear that (a) the insurance based payment for a specific CPT code will vary across insurance companies and (b) some of the fees are paid at hourly rates which are below our established cost of practice per hour. Thus, there is a clear disincentive to see patients with those lower payment rates. When a company pays less per hour than it costs my office to provide the service, then there is a financial problem and I have to make up that financial loss somewhere else. In other words, if you agree to see a patient where you will be paid less per hour than what will cost you to provide the professional service then you have to find some way to make up that difference. Hopefully, you will see enough

Table 2. Office charges and reimbursement schedule for selected CPT codes.

CPT codes	Procedure	Charges per Hour			
		Carrier # 1	Carrier #2	Carrier #3	Carrier #4
90801	Diagnostic Interview	275	275	275	275
	Ins. Payment per Hour	95.50	60	51	25
	Co-payment per Hour	15	30	25	25
96100	Psychological Testing	275	275	275	275
	Ins. Payment per Hour	75	60	49	25
	Co-payment per Hour	15	30	10	25
96117	Neuropsychological Testing per Hour	275	275	275	275
	Ins. Payment per Hour	76	60	49	25
	Co-payment per Hour	15	30	10	25
90844	Individual Therapy	275	275	275	275
	Ins. Payment per Hour	75	55	51	25
	Co-payment per Hour	15	30	15	25

cases with insurance plans that pay more than your hourly cost of practice. Similarly, if you are going to do a pro bono case, you are still going to have to pay your fixed cost per hour in order to meet your overhead expenses. One way to make up the difference is to use several technicians and to have multiple patients seen for testing or other services in your laboratory at the same time. Another way is to do medical legal work at your full fee charge.

Now, let's look at some individual cost of practice items. We will begin with postage, because it seems to be a small expense at face value but can become a rather large expense if it is not effectively controlled. People who don't have to worry about office expenses may try to tell you that you should not worry about "little things such as the cost of a stamp." Well, using current postal rates, it costs 55 cents to send a five page, single-sided report through the mail. If the patient wants their report sent to fifteen different doctors, that's an $8.25 expense before you add in ancillary costs such as copying the report fifteen times, the cost of your the paper (75 pages), fifteen envelopes and the cost in salary for someone to complete the task and mail out the material. You should not have to underwrite this expense out of what the insurance company will pay for the testing service! Yes, you may be required to send a report to the referral source and to make a copy available to the patient (unless it is not in their interest, according to APA and certain state standards) but you should not have to underwrite supplemental postal costs. Similarly, it is not uncommon for a patient to receive a copy of their report and then several months later to ask for another copy because they 'lost' the first one. The replacement copy should be charged to the patient.

Thus, we have an office policy where, with the appropriate written release, we will send a copy to the referral source, the primary care physician and to the patient (unless it is contraindicated). After that, the patient can take personal responsibility for sending a copy of *their* copy of the report to whomever they choose. In turn, if we are asked to mail out additional copies, we charge the patient an advance fee of $5.00 to $10.00 *per copy* (depending on the length of the report and whether there is a supplementary form which has to be enclosed) for copying and postage/handling. I don't think there is any legal or ethical situation in which you should refuse to send a report if the patient legitimately cannot pay the fee and if there is a medical necessity[2] issue. By the same token, you do not have to assume the financial burden each time the patient 'wants' you to send out another copy of their report.

Suppose it costs a total of $5.00 in staff salary and other overhead items to pay your secretary to pull the chart, copy the report, buy the envelope (even in bulk, you still had to buy the envelope), type the address, apply the correct postage and mail the item. Now, suppose that you are asked to do this 500 times a year. That is another $2,500.00 in costs that can be reimbursed as opposed to being listed as a non-reimbursable, cost of practice expense.

Similarly, my office saves postage costs by faxing reports. At this time, almost 90–95% of our local reports are being faxed. That is one reason why the postage costs in Table 1 are relatively low. When a local referral call is taken, my secretary always asks for their fax number and explains that we will fax the report directly to them as soon as the report is completed. By using a fax method of distributing your report, you are getting your reports to your referral sources a day or so faster and you have saved the postage fee. You have also saved on the associated hidden costs of copy toner and paper supplies. I can't wait until more offices can accept e-mail reports in a secure manner. You have to decide when to copy and mail a document versus paying the long distance fax charge.

Let's consider the costs involved in carrying out a neuropsychological consultation. You may ask why does it cost money to do a consultation? Well, take a look at any of the test supply catalogues. How much it costs to purchase the Halstead–Reitan Neuropsychological Test Battery equipment. Itemize the cost of purchasing an MMPI-2 booklet and answer sheets and also the cost of the MMPI-2 scoring software. Now itemize each patient's per use fee for the computer scoring of an MMPI-2 report. Itemize the purchase cost of the WAIS-III and Wechsler Memory Scale-III kits, their computer software (don't forget to include the per page cost of your printer for printing the WAIS-III/WMS-III/MMPI-2 etc. reports) as well as the cost of a single

[2] "Medical Necessity" is defined by Medicare as "covered services that are reasonable and necessary for the diagnosis or treatment of an illness or injury or to improve the functioning of a malformed body member." Many insurance companies either use the Medicare definition or have developed definitions which are similar to this definition.

WAIS-III/Wechsler Memory Scale-III set of answer sheet booklets. Itemize the purchase cost of other test supplies and computer software. Without going into further detail, by the time you have set up a fully functioning neuropsychological testing laboratory, you have spent at least $4,000.00. Those equipment costs are included as an expense based cost of practice. Given the relatively short life span of tests such the Wechsler Adult Intelligence Scale-III, Wechsler Memory Scale-III and Minnesota Multiphasic Personality Inventory-2, these expenses have to be absorbed by relatively few patient assessment fees. Similarly, the per use fees for computer software and the use of copyrighted answer sheets drives up the cost of testing each patient. These costs have to be considered along with the other overhead costs in calculating your profit/loss for each patient assessment.

Now, you have just given a comprehensive battery of neuropsychological tests and psychological questionnaires and an insurance company pays you the whopping sum of $312 dollars (co-pay included) for a case with the actual reimbursement at $52 dollars an hour for six hours. Remember, that is what you receive whether you spend six hours or 20 hours on the case. Now, suppose that you have to allocate $52.00 in equipment and test scoring costs to this case. Once you actually analyze your time and equipment cost expenses for this case, does spending a large number of additional (and unpaid) hours providing professional service in further testing and in writing an extensive report continue to be justified from a business perspective? Of course, the issue of staying in business has to be balanced with other professional and ethics concerns.

You also have to factor in other cost items when seeing that patient. Have you ever calculated how much your malpractice insurance costs per patient seen per year? Just divide the total cost of the insurance by the number of individual patient cases seen that year. Surprised at how much it is? That per patient cost, for example, also has to be added to the cost of completing that $312.00 consultation. How much does it cost per year for other forms of insurance, your advertisement in the telephone book, all of those dues and subscriptions, CEU costs, employee salaries, and benefits, the new copy machine your staff are bugging you to buy and the service contracts on your equipment, and there is postage again. Don't forget your salary and benefits. Also, maybe there are a couple of long distance calls to get the patient scheduled and confirmed. All of these are costs that have to be considered versus the fee you collect for the consultation. Then you have to consider the salaries of your technical assistant and your clerical staff. How much time did this case cost you in terms of their salaries? These are overhead costs as well. Where will you make up the money to cover your overhead? Cutting your expenses is the main means of reducing your overhead. To repeat my point: If your costs, when broken down in a very simplistic but forthright manner, exceed the funds received, then you are operating at a financial loss.

Management of Office Overhead

Fixed and variable expenses

Most accountants will tell you that fixed costs are the items which, once contracted for, do not change during a set period of time. Examples of fixed costs include rent, maintenance contracts for equipment, employee base salaries and fringe benefits, the base cost for the telephone. Variable costs, as the term implies, are those expenses that may change each month and whose changes may result from increases or decreases in use. The long distance phone bill is a good example of a variable expense. Other variable expenses are postage and copy costs, disposable office supplies and transcription costs.

What are some of your variable costs that are also hidden or indirect costs? These are costs that are not obvious upon examining a financial spreadsheet but that, nevertheless, are actual expenses.

In my opinion, the largest variable and hidden cost for our profession is lost earning capacity related to the actual amount of time spent on a clinical neuropsychological assessment beyond an insurance company's actual authorization time limit. Let's face it, whether we do it because we want to do it the 'right' way or we are fascinated with the case or any other set of reasons which we want to offer, most neuropsychologists spend more time on patient cases then is covered by reimbursement. So, if you are in a managed care situation and you have a contract that says you cannot bill for anything after three hours and you want to spend a total of eight hours, go right ahead. However, you must realize that, if you are paying $115 an hour to stay open and you take that extra five hours, you've just spent $575.00 in non-reimbursable overhead expenses on that case! That is five hours where you could have carried out other billable patient activity or gone home early and spent the time with your family.

What about reports? How much time are you actually spending in terms of writing or dictating reports? How long should the report be? If you are writing a 10–12 page report in a clinical situation that is wonderful, but it is also expensive in terms of overhead. In truth, does anyone else appreciate how wonderful you are because you spent your entire Sunday afternoon preparing some tome of a report? Do your referral sources make jokes about "how many trees died so that you could print your report?" Have you ever asked your referral sources how much detail they want in your reports?

I remember when I wrote what I believed were very detailed and very lengthy reports, only to have a neurologist tell me that he was going to stop referring patients to me unless I sent him shorter reports! He explained that it was costing him too much money to convert my long reports into microfilm! At that moment, I learned to be selective regarding the intended audience of my reports and to determine what the referral source typically desires in terms of actual report detail. I have discovered that many of my referral sources want only a brief report of one to three pages. In turn, generating such a short report can be an art form in terms of the difficulty involved in being so concise, but it can also result in your saving a considerable amount of overhead expense. With appropriate care, a short report can still meet all of the required documentation standards required in our field. I recommend that you generate a lengthy report (and take the time to do so and incur the costs in doing so, etc.) only when it is truly necessary. My main post-doctoral supervisor typically wrote one-page neuropsychological reports using the S.O.A.P method. His hospital-based physician referrals loved them.

What about the costs associated with report preparation? In addition to your time allocated costs, how much money are you spending with a transcription service? Are they charging you by the line? If you are paying a transcriptionist 10 cents a line to type a report, how much money are you actually spending on that report? Should you write a shorter report to help keep overhead costs under control? Let's assume that there are 40 lines per page and you want to have a 10-page report typed. Remember that you may be paid as little as $312.00 for the entire evaluation and that you need to cover all of your overhead. In this regard, you have to consider the cost of the transcriptionist preparing a short versus long report as a variable amount of overhead.

If you type your own reports, you have the flexibility of reducing the actual page length of a report by doing such things as using smaller fonts, making the margins narrower and changing to single or one-and-a-half spacing between lines. Suddenly, that five-page report is now down on four pages. What about two-sided printing? It is still going to take as long for you to prepare, but maybe you are getting the 55 cents postage down to 34 cents. It may sound silly and penny pinching, but it all adds up.

What about voice-activated dictation software? I no longer needed a transcriptionist after I started using voice-activated software. This change alone saved $20,000.00 a year in direct employee overhead. The reports are completed as soon as *you* dictate them, as there is no turn around time in waiting for the transcriptionist to prepare the report. The result is that the report typically goes out at least one day faster than when you use a transcriptionist. How much time does it take to become highly efficient with voice activated software and templates? It took me a couple of months to really get up to speed, but I think the extra time that I put in getting to the point has paid off in the long run. Voice-activated software for dictation is not for everybody, but the potential is there for you to greatly reduce transcription costs and shorten turn-around time using this kind of software. Currently, I also use a number of template style reports that I have prepared for general patient use. In a template style report, the structure of the report is already prepared and I merely fill in the individual history, facts, scores, and impressions as I go along.

What about the costs associated with the long-term storage of archived patient charts? Do you have an attic or basement that is full of archived charts in cardboard boxes? Are you supporting a well-fed army of crickets who dine on the stored material? Do you pay a facility for offsite storage of archived patient charts? Have you considered standard paper versus, microfilm versus electronic storage? Which is the best choice for your practice? Several years ago, I realized that archived patient record storage was costing my practice approximately $150.00 a month or $1800.00 a year. Shortly thereafter, I decided to move my old patient records to CD-ROM. As of the present time, we have moved over 5,600 complete patient charts (reports, raw data, registration forms, billing information and correspondence) onto 18 CD-ROM disks. Each disk is backed-up for safety purposes and the second copy is stored in an off-site location. The files can be password protected for additional patient confidentiality and protection.

In 2001, we upgraded our office copier to a 40 page a minute digital copier and scanner with network capability. We can put a 50-page chart on the machine, set up a coding system for file numbering, hit the button, walk away, and the machine scans the complete chart in only a few moments. It saves the file on a built in zip drive and we later move the files to the CD-ROM (write-once storage format), and make back-up copies of the CD for additional protection of the records. The files are image based and are not OCR treated. My legal advisor had determined that our storage process meets the Virginia state code for record retention. A psychologist consultant has determined that our storage process meets APA guidelines for record retention and patient confidentiality. In the long run, this technique has reduced our storage and retrieval costs dramatically while not significantly increasing other aspects of our practice overhead.

As an aside, moving these records to a computer medium has actually generated additional revenue. In Virginia, the Subpoena Duces Tecum cost for copying is .50 a page for the first fifty pages and .25 a page for additional pages. However, the charge is 1.00 a page if the record is retrieved from a computer medium. How many of your old records are subject to Subpoena Duces Tecum requests each year?

What about telephone costs? Who is the patient calling when they are borrowing your phone? Do you use the most cost effective long distance calling plan? Are you spending a lot of time returning local and/or long distance calls from patients in non-emergency situations? If it is appropriate, are you charging the patient (not the insurance company) for your time on the phone?

When a patient wants to speak to me about a non-emergency issue and I am not available, my secretary sets up a return call appointment time for the patient to call me back. This way, I don't spend my office time chasing down a patient, getting their voice mail (which may not be secure) and possibly running up a long-distance bill in the process. Things like that save you time and overhead costs in the long run. It also gives the patient a confirmed time when they know that they can reach me. If they fail to call, they cannot blame me for not following through and contacting them. We have also purchased a telephone call account tracking software program and use it to log the length of all calls made and received as well as tracking all received call based caller ID. It is basically the same kind of software used by lawyers for billing purposes. In our office, it also serves as a documentation record if there is any disagreement about charges for time spent on a call or whether someone says they called and there is no record of such a call, and so forth.

What about insurance fees and maintenance contracts? Make it a practice to compare rates from the APA Trust and other leading medical malpractice insurers *prior* to each renewal. Similarly, ask that companies bid on your equipment maintenance contracts. Hopefully, you will be pleased with the money saved.

Information-Based Decision Making and Professional Service Delivery

One of the most frequent pairs of practice based questions expressed by other clinical neuropsychologists concerns (a) how does one monitor and manage the insurance information for each patient to determine when a preauthorization is needed (and then obtained) and (2) how can we train office staff to collect and manage this information? Figure 1 presents an organizational flow chart which describes the steps for your staff to collect information prior to the initial appointment and then to use that information to determine whether or not a preauthorization will be needed prior to actual service delivery.

First of all, you must realize that you, as the professional, cannot handle every telephone call and collect every bit of patient preregistration data by yourself. You cannot afford to spend the large amount of time 'on hold' waiting to speak with an insurance case manager. You *must* hire and train one or more individuals to carry out this type of activity for you.

In my solo practice office, I have found that it is cost effective to have two full-time clerical staff. One handles the general duties of the office receptionist, collects the patient preregistration information and makes all appointments. This person also collects the patient's insurance information and contacts the insurance company when necessary and thus knows when to schedule the patient after the appropriate preauthorization has been obtained. The second individual works in patient billing and accounts. This person checks diagnoses versus approved services before a report is sent out, makes certain that the account is billed correctly for the pre-authorized service and 'fights' with the insurance carrier when the insurance company does not live up to their contract with our practice in terms of generating a correct payment. Each person has many years of experience and we have developed a highly trained, team approach to handling the administrative aspects of patient services and insurance billing/payment.

Training your office staff to collect the insurance preregistration information and then to follow-up with obtaining the appropriate insurance preauthorization is one of the critical elements to the successful management of your practice. Figure 1 addresses a 'flow chart' type of organizational pathway to some of the more critical aspects of collecting appropriate patient and insurance information prior to scheduling the patient.

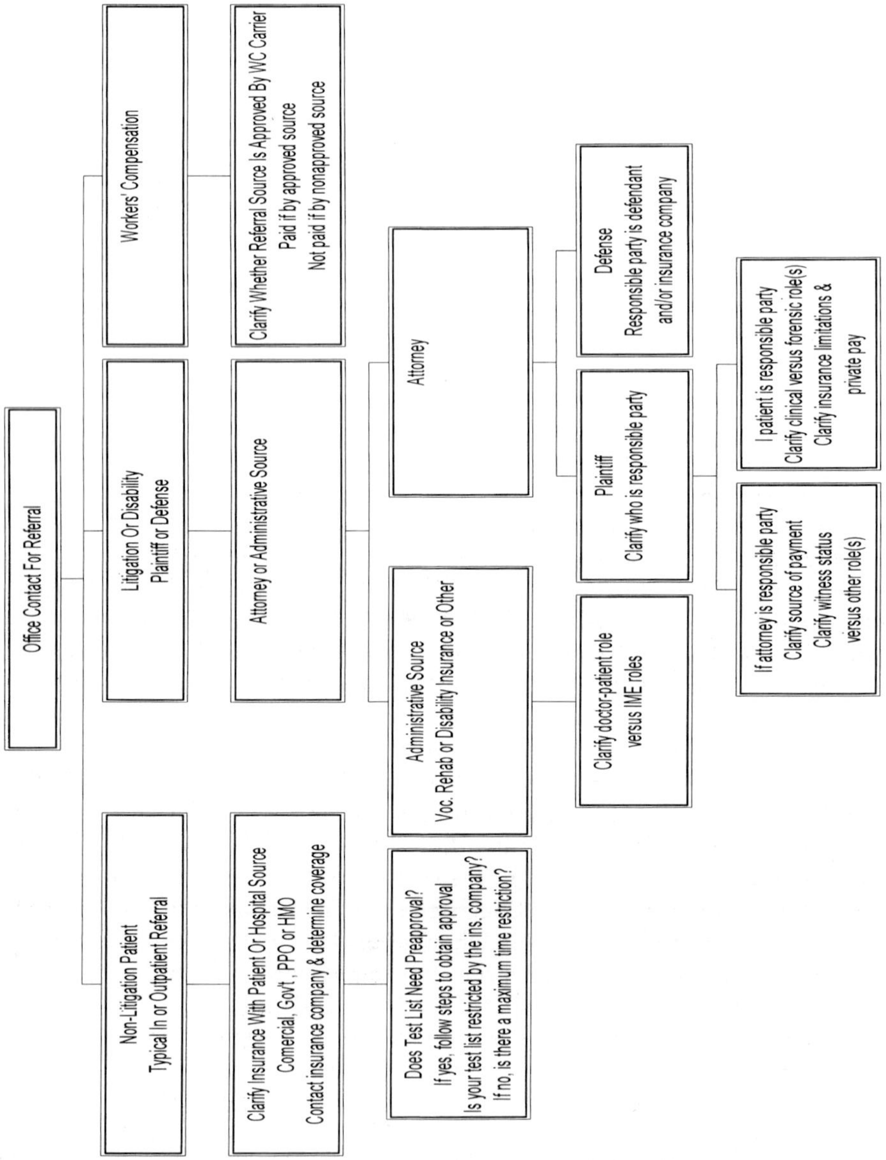

Figure 1. Flow chart of the steps necessary to collect insurance information.

Step 1

At the time of the initial telephone referral and before the patient comes in for the first appointment, the receptionist must determine the type of referral. This may be a typical outpatient or inpatient referral, medical legal or Workers' Compensation case. For simplicity sake, I have not listed the many other types of potential referral types.

In scenario A, consider the referral as a typical inpatient or outpatient referral. Your receptionist determines that there is no medical legal or Workers' Compensation element identified as part of the referral component. The correct insurance company name, plan type (e.g., commercial, HMO, PPO), patient name and insurance ID has to be collected prior to seeing the patient in the office. After this information is collected, the insurance company is contacted and the actual insurance plan is (a) verified as to current coverage being in effect and (b) the insurance carrier verifies whether or not a preauthorization is needed for an initial Diagnostic Interview appointment. At this point, the insurance carrier may allow only an initial, one-hour interview. Typically, the managed care insurance patient has to return for a second appointment to complete the testing as that service requires a separate authorization and will not be approved until a Diagnostic Interview/Neurobehavioral Interview is completed and additional paper work is submitted to the insurance company which establishes the medical necessity for the requested testing based time units. Other issues to be addressed with the insurance carrier include, for example, whether this is an inpatient and is the hospital billing this patient on a per diem basis. If the hospital is billing on a per diem basis, is neuropsychological testing part of the per diem fee? If so, then the neuropsychologist has to negotiate with the hospital for fees as the insurance carrier is not responsible for payments to anyone other than the hospital. If it is not a per diem basis, then proceed with negotiations for obtaining preauthorization for neuropsychological related services.

Step 2

Once the responsible party is clarified and a determination as to whether preauthorization is or is not necessary, the patient should be informed about the planned services, the cost of the services and any risks involved as well as any limitations on service which may be imposed by their insurance carrier. In a non-emergency situation, the patient can be examined only after the contractual issues with their insurance company have been satisfied. This may involve obtaining a pre-approval for a specified test list and/or a specified number of hour based units of testing/psychotherapy.

What can the neuropsychologist do about the following situation? After carrying out a diagnostic interview, you determine that the patient, who is not someone who is financially limited in a manner, which would suggest a need for pro bono services, has a legitimate referral question that can be best assessed by 8.0 hours of neuropsychological testing. However, the insurance carrier, in its infinite wisdom, determines that only 4.0 hours of testing, scoring and report preparation are to be approved for this case. Your responses may include the following:

a. Refuse the case. Unfortunately, in Virginia, more than 60% of the insured are covered under some form of managed care. To keep refusing to provide services typically means that the patient will never be evaluated or that the referral source will go elsewhere. In either scenario, your practice will suffer financially.

b. Carry out the 8.0 hours and 'eat' the 3.0 lost hours. This means that you are definitely going to operate at a loss. Continually, working under this type of financial loss will likely lead to the bankruptcy of your practice.
c. Discuss the insurance limitation on services with the patient. Educate the patient regarding their right to appeal. This scenario often works better than you might surmise, as the carrier also knows that the patient can complain to their employer's human resources division about such treatment. Contract renewal issues may be pending and the carrier may not want an angry client at that time. Also, the carrier knows that they will likely send out a patient satisfaction survey each year. Unless corrected, this situation will typically result in low ratings for that insurance company.
d. If option c does not result in the appropriate number of hours of authorized testing, then offer to allow the patient to purchase the needed remaining hours on a priori agreement basis. Appendix V presents a form that we use to address such a situation. The patient is allowed to negotiate the hourly rate and we frequently permit the patient to purchase the additional hours at the contractual rate that my company, Neuropsychological Services of Virginia, has already agreed to accept from the insurance company. At that point, if the patient has been educated about the situation, is financially able to afford the additional services and still chooses to refuse to purchase the additional testing hours, then so be it. The form documents that there may be limitations on diagnostic accuracy, etc and that they have been informed of these limitations in advance of the service delivery and that they still agree to participate under these restricted circumstances.

When in doubt about a situational ethics issue, I again recommend that you seek appropriate discussion and clarification from relevant sources.

Step 3

This step involves submitting the insurance claim and collecting the money owed to your practice. This issue is addressed in the next section of this chapter.

Scenario B involves medical-legal referrals. In each situation, there needs to be a clear and unequivocal understanding regarding who is the responsible party. Under no circumstances should a situation be permitted where a contingency fee relationship is agreed to as part of a medical legal situation.

First, let us consider civil based medical legal referrals. Is this a referral by the plaintiff's attorney or from the defense attorney? If it is from the plaintiff's attorney, then the secretary must clarify who is to be the responsible party. Typically, the plaintiff's attorney is the responsible party and will retain the neuropsychologist directly. This is the same situation if the defense desires to retain the neuropsychologist.

In a criminal case, the responsible party may be the court who agrees to pay for the professional services, or the defendant (or their attorney).

As a general rule, the neuropsychologist should not accept a medical legal referral where the patient's insurance company is to be billed, as medical legal referrals are not viewed as meeting the written criteria for 'medically necessity.' This does not prevent the neuropsychologist from performing a clinically necessary work-up but such a clinical work-up will not usually be extensive to the point where all relevant forensic opinions can be developed and clarified.

In Scenario C, the referral relates to a Workers' Compensation injury. The rules regarding this type of referral vary from state to state. In Virginia, where I practice, the WC carrier is legally responsible for payment if it is a valid WC claim and if the referral source to the neuropsychologist is already approved by the WC carrier to provide services to this patient. Thus, if a patient goes out of the approved treating pathway and, for example, sees a doctor recommended by their attorney and that doctor refers the patient to you for neuropsychological related services, you will not be paid by the WC carrier because you are not part of the WC approved service providers for this case. Depending upon individual state laws, there may be a prohibition upon your collecting the fee from the patient in the case where you cannot legally collect from the WC carrier. Thus, a predetermination of an authorization from the WC carrier is critical to collecting for the services rendered.

Insurance Claim Submission and Dealing with Post-Submission Claim Problems

If you have collected the appropriate patient and insurance information prior to providing your professional service, then you might think that submitting your bill to the insurance company will result in both prompt and accurate payment. You are naive if you believe this to be true. My full-time billing person has more than twenty years of hospital and medical/mental health practice billing experience. She uses one of the latest and efficient computer billing programs commercially available. Yet, she spends a great deal of her time resolving billing and claims based errors that originate at the hands of the various insurance companies receiving our claims. One of the more common excuses that we hear from insurance carriers when the claim is submitted correctly but is not paid appropriately is "Oh, that must be a random key punch error."

In 1998, my postdoctoral fellow at the time, Julie Neblett, and I carried out a prospective study of the 'random keypunch error' phenomenon. We analyzed every testing based claim that my practice submitted to an insurance company during a several month time period in 1998–1999. Figure 2 presents summary data from this analysis. As can be seen, our data shows that 18.5% of the 146 claims submitted were initially paid incorrectly by the insurance

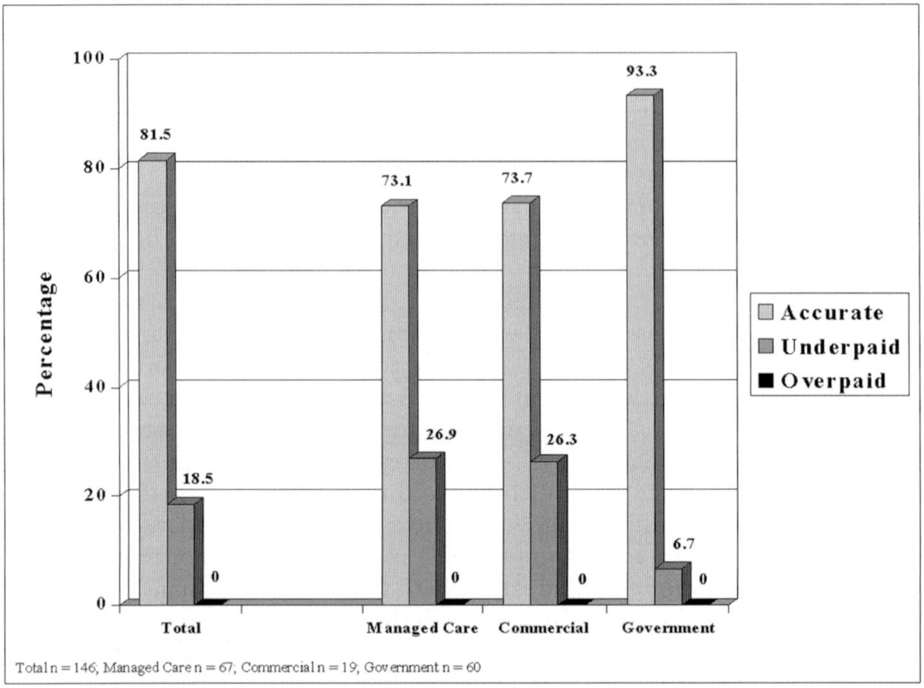

Figure 2. The 'random keypunch error.' Managed Care n = 67; Commercial n = 19; Government n = 60; Total n = 146.

carries. Each of these 18.5% claims was subsequently reprocessed and paid at 100% of the allowed amount. The breakdown of insurance company subtypes reveals that both managed care and commercial insurers underpaid these claims at virtually identical error rates while Medicare and Virginia Medicaid underpaid far less frequently. The most common error pattern was for underpayment of time units billed. For example, if the insurance company preapproved 6.0 units hours and we billed 6.0 hours, the insurance company subsequently paid for fewer than 6.0 units. No claims were paid for more units of services than were submitted. Thus, this error pattern does not seem to reflect 'random key punch error.'

What can your office do to minimize the 'random key punch error' problem? What can your office do to minimize the many other reasons why your submitted insurance claims are not processed and paid correctly? Is the decision not to pay your claim correctly, or at all, based upon something an insurance company executive read in a John Grisham novel? It may interest you to realize that the easiest way to minimize this problem is for you to (a) realize that the issue *is* there in your patient accounts and (b) that *you* need to take direct responsibility for communicating frequently with your billing staff and

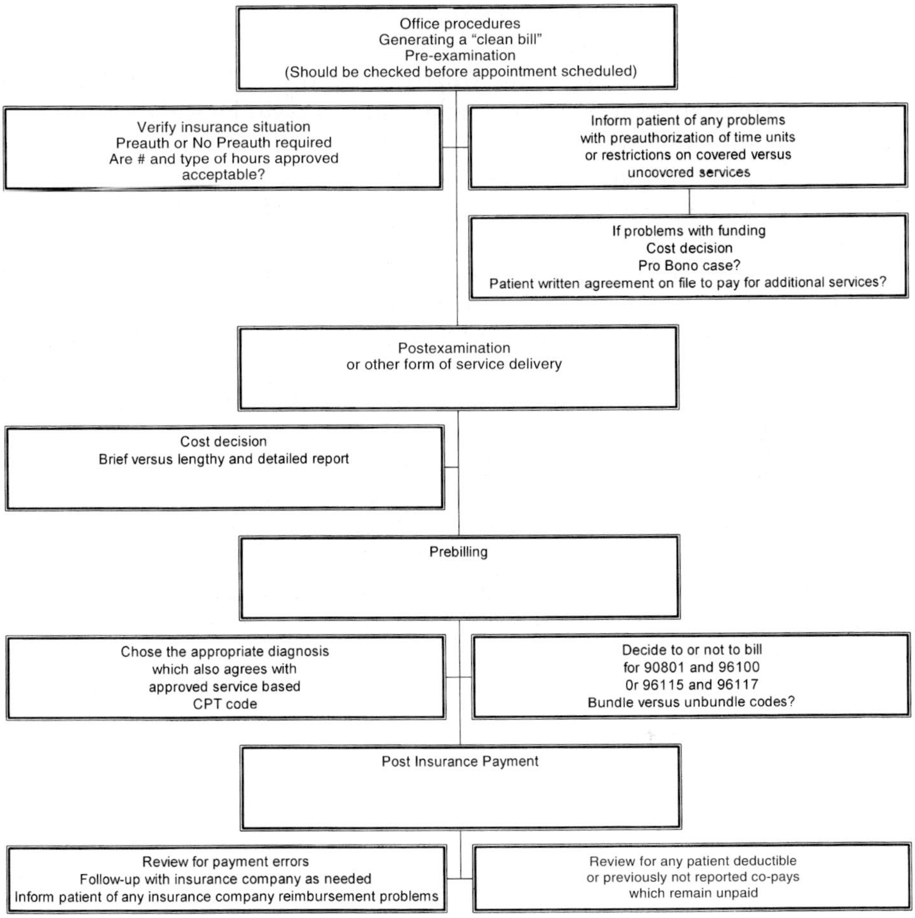

Figure 3. Flow chart of the steps involved in tracking the billing process.

requesting specific billing type tracking information on every account submitted for payment. Make certain to let your billing staff know that this is an issue in which you are *very* interested and that you desire a two-way dialogue with them concerning the management of this aspect of your practice.

Figure 3 presents a flow chart for the steps involved in tracking the billing process from preauthorization to claim submission and then a review of claim payment status. As can be seen, each set involves a selected set of actions that are relevant to the claims process. For example, the lead or first diagnosis used on the report should be the lead diagnosis on the insurance claim form. Furthermore, this lead diagnosis should be consistent with the service provided. In other words, many insurance companies will reject a claim for

CPT 96117 (Neuropsychological Testing) if the lead diagnosis is DSM-IV or ICD-9-296.20 Major Depression.

Some insurance companies allow you to 'unbundle' a Diagnostic Interview or Neurobehavioral Status Exam procedure and a Psychological or Neuropsychological Testing procedure on the same day. Other insurance companies do not allow the two procedures to be billed on the same day. Thus, they must be 'bundled' under the testing code or be billed separately on different dates.

In conducting a post payment review, your staff must look for errors that have led to a reduced payment. Some of the most common errors that we noted in our 'random keypunch' study were:

a. Automatic reduction of multiple unit charges to only one unit for payment.
b. Stating that a documented, preauthorized service was never preauthorized.
c. Changing the preauthorized and appropriate CPT based procedure, e.g., 96117, Neuropsychological Testing, to any other procedure code which, of course, was either not preauthorized and/or is paid at a lower dollar amount per time unit.
d. Pend your claim for 'medical review' when the procedure was already reviewed and authorized. We were also told to send in a copy of the exam report, when the report has already been sent in with the original insurance paperwork claim.

Many of these individual error patterns tend to be consistent for a specific insurance company. Your trained staff should be able to develop a sense of what each insurance company tends to do to slow down the payment process or avoid it all together. By the way, we typically demand (and receive) that the insurance company pay interest whenever a claim is denied or underpaid due to insurance company error. Figure 4 below provides an additional level of detail that should be employed in reviewing the actual insurance company EOB or Explanation of Benefits form.

Some Common Business Related Patient Requests; What is the Appropriate Response?

These responses are based upon a review of the current APA ethics code as well as my years of clinical and business related experience. My responses should be viewed as guidelines to be considered by the reader. You may develop other responses to these situations that are also appropriate or, perhaps, even more appropriate than what is noted below. The main thrust of each response deals with (a) making a priori service delivery decisions about the contractual arrangements you set up with the patient and (b) using your understanding of how the patient's insurance approval and reimbursement system works.

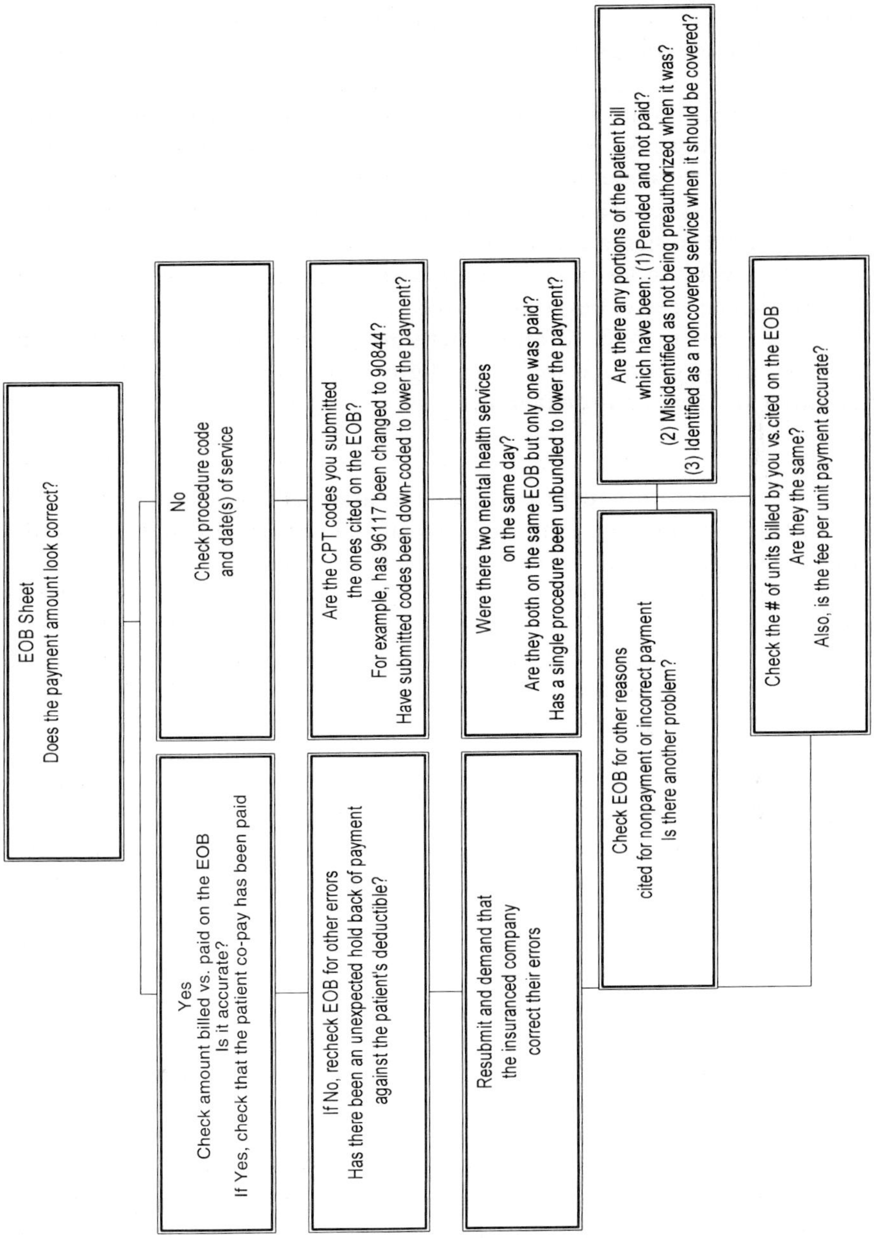

Figure 4. Checks that should be made on the actual insurance company Explanation of Benefits form.

Situation A

The patient who wants to be seen but you are 'out of network' for their insurance plan.

Response: If you are not in their insurance company's network, you can see them but you are not necessarily obligated to follow the contractual obligations for that plan. You should educate the patient about paying privately or arranging a 'self pay' contract for 100% of the services to be rendered. You may choose to try to negotiate a 'single case agreement' with the insurance company where they agree to pay you a specified amount for the agreed upon service and the patient is responsible for their specified co-pay. You may choose to try to refer them to an 'in network' provider. You should never agree to "see the patient first and then 'fight' with the insurance carrier for payment after the service is delivered."

Situation B

The patient who wants you to carry out a comprehensive, *court ordered*, forensic examination which is to be billed in its entirety to their insurance company and/or the patient wants you to accept a contingency fee arrangement where you are paid only after the legal case is resolved and there is money recovered.

Response: Don't accept either type of referral. You may be in violation of several ethical rules as well as run the risk of committing fraud in terms of your contractual relationship with the insurance company. Ask yourself the questions, "Is the referral question and the resultant testing medically necessary as they relate to the making of a diagnosis and/or alleviating a medical or mental problem?" "Would the testing be necessary if there was no active litigation?" Can you be neutral in your opinion if you agree that the only way to be paid for your services is to help improve the chance of a legally derived financial recovery?

Situation C

The patient wants educational testing, e.g., a Woodcock Johnson PsychoEducational Test Battery-III and related measures, to identify a diagnosis of a learning disability and the patient wants you to bill the services to their insurance company. They are not complaining of any other form of medical, neurologic illness or injury or mental health problem.

Response: This issue has several overlapping components. First, it is my understanding that most insurance carriers do not consider testing for educational purposes, such as to identify a learning disability, either a covered service or as meeting the criteria for medical necessity. Many insurance carriers also do not accept most academic related, LD diagnoses as covered diagnoses. Certainly, there may be exceptions to this generalization, but this is otherwise the situation as I have confronted this frequent type of referral. I usually recommend a referral to the local school system or have the patient agree to a self-pay arrangement for this type of service.

Situation D

The patient demands to be tested without waiting for the standard preauthorization process to be completed, as is required by their particular insurance company. You do have a contract for the requested services with this insurance company and your contract with this company specifies that a preauthorization is required prior to service delivery. The patient tells you that, "We are not going to wait. It will be fine. The insurance company will pay you. I'll take care of it if they give you a problem." The referral context does not involve an emergency situation.

Response: Aside from the probability that you are already considering certain diagnoses for this individual, let's analyze what is actually going on in this situation. First, what this patient is demanding of you is, in point of fact, likely to be a violation of the patient's contract with their insurance carrier. In turn, if you actually do what is demanded and not wait and go through the preauthorization process, *as it is written in your contract with this insurance company,* then it is likely that you will be in violation of your contract with this company. The insurance company would likely be within their contractual duty to not pay for the service.

There is a second issue present in this scenario. The patient has never agreed to be legally responsible (to you or to your practice) for payment of these services in the event that the insurance company does not pay your claim. All he has said is that he will work on the insurance company to pay the bill. He has not given you a written contract in which it is specified that he will pay the bill if the company does not pay. In some situations, entering into a contingency arrangement where the patient agrees to pay if the insurance company will not pay for the service may be a violation of your contract with the insurance carrier and it may also raise certain APA ethical issues associated with professional practice relationships.

I recommend that you do not agree to provide the demanded services under the above set of circumstances. Instead, I recommend that you educate the patient about their need to follow their contract with the insurance company and go through the preauthorization process.

A Review of Some Sample Forms for a Private Practice in Clinical Neuropsychology

I am frequently asked about the forms used in my office to help with day-to-day patient care issues. The items that follow are examples of the types of forms that we have developed to address common situations that occur in management of my practice. Please feel free to adapt them to your practice as needed. However, please note the following caveats. Many of the forms have been reviewed by our company attorney for acceptable legal standards according to the laws of the Commonwealth of Virginia. You will need to determine whether the wording in these forms is legally valid in your jurisdiction. Also, I feel that these forms and the situations in which they are used reflect an appropriate professional standard of practice according to the relevant APA ethics standards. Please do not try to interpret these documents out of context and please remember that the APA ethics rules are currently in flux. I take no position that these forms will always be viewed as representing an acceptable standard of practice according to the APA Ethics Code and I note that my office will change these forms whenever it is deemed necessary so as to maintain acceptable legal and ethical standards. Finally, each of these forms is designed to be completed on an *a priori* service delivery basis. This issue is critical in many of the circumstances relevant to these forms.

A. Referral Form: (Appendix I)
This intake form is typically completed a telephone call from either the referral source, the patient or a third party. Page one of this three page form asks for the usual information regarding the patient. Page two addresses insurance information. Please note that it also prompts for secondary and tertiary insurance information. It is common that a patient may have a non-preauthorization type primary insurance (e.g., Medicare) but that the secondary insurance is a managed care plan and that the preauthorization process has to be addressed. You do not want this issue to come up for the first time when the patient is already in the waiting room for their appointment. The third page is used if the referral involves a litigation or WC type of referral.

B. Registration Form: (Appendix II)
Page 1 asks for the typical information. Page 2 addresses a number of specific issues. Without going into a line by line annotation, please note several items of particular interest: first, that the issue of not accepting contingency fee arrangements is noted; second, that the time for testing includes administration, scoring and report preparation as well as report discussion; third, that the costs of responding to medical legal matters requires time and that fees will be charges for these services; fourth, I have had insurance carriers withdraw monies already paid to my practice, for no apparent reason, after extended time delays. The form makes it clear that the patient/responsible party is liable and responsible for paying any such withdrawn sums to my company. This means that the insurance company is really going to have to deal with their enrollee and the enrollee's company who holds the contract with the insurance carrier.

C. Waiver of Insurance: (Appendix III)
This form is an adaptation of the standard Medicare "Advance Notice for Medically Unnecessary Services — Waiver of Medical Necessity" form. This type of form should be used in those situations where you have a Medicare enrollee who is requesting services that, in their specific situation, are not likely to be deemed medically necessary by Medicare. This might include professional contact situations involving referrals for assessment involving

civil or criminal type legal matters, educational testing leading to a diagnosis of a learning disability or administrative related testing only to determine whether the beneficiary meets the criteria for a private disability insurance award. In many situations, Federal rules still require the provider to submit the claim, even though they have good reason to believe in advance that the service (e.g. forensic issues) are not going to meet the accepted standard of medical necessity. This signed waiver allows the provider to bill the enrollee for the service instead of having to write-off the claim. For further information regarding this complex issue, please refer to the Virginia Medicare Part B Provider Services Manual (1997) or Medicare Newsletters (1994, 1995) for additional information.

What follows is Medicare's published position on the use of such a form. Due to the technical language in this public document, the reader is requested to refer directly to the original source as cited. For the record, this information is either taken verbatim or is closely paraphrased from Medicare, 1997.

1. The provider should obtain a signed Advance Notice whenever he/she believes Medicare is likely to deny a service as not medically necessary.
2. In order to be acceptable to Medicare, an Advance Notice must be provided in writing and must clearly identify the particular service(s) to be provided and why the provider does believe Medicare is likely to deny payment for these specified services. Furthermore, a provider should not give an Advance Notice to a Medicare beneficiary unless the provider has genuine doubt regarding the likelihood of Medicare payment.
3. The provider still needs to bill Medicare under this situation. However, the form itself does not need to be sent along with the claim but should be kept in the patient's chart until such time that Medicare requests to see the signed form. Instead, the provider should bill the service with the modifier 'GA' to indicate that a Medicare approved Advance Notice has been signed. Without the 'GA' modifier, Medicare may well determine that the claim should not be paid and that the beneficiary is not financially responsible to the provider for the specified service.

Appendix IV is a related form is actually designed to address similar issues with patients who are enrolled in other types of insurance that are not covered by Medicare. This form might be used to address a non-covered service such as an educational evaluation leading to the diagnosis of a learning disability, or for forensic or purely administrative services.

D. Insurance Coverage Limitation On Service: (Appendix IV)

I see this form as both controversial and relevant to the current health care situation. It is designed to be given to individuals who are financially able to pay for services which have otherwise been denied or severely limited by their insurance plan. It is not to be used as an 'opt out' with pro bono cases. The thrust of this form is to educate the patient/responsible party that there is a clear discrepancy between what the professional has determined to be an appropriate level of service and what the insurance company has determined to be medically necessary and appropriate. Even with an a priori arrangement, you may not be permitted to use such a form with every commercial or managed care insurance plan. You should clarify which insurance companies will permit this type of arrangement with a patient.

A good example of this type of situation is the insurance company that will not authorize more than 1.0 hour of testing for a child with a referral for a potential ADHD diagnosis. Their position seems to be is that we should base our professional diagnosis on a few questionnaires and nothing else. My expressed concerns about other differential diagnosis issues and assessment techniques are not viewed by this insurance company as reflecting medically necessary or appropriate services. Another good example is the situation cited earlier in this chapter where 8.0 hours of neuropsychological testing (CPT code 96117) are deemed appropriate for the particular referral question, but only 4.0 hours of 96117 is approved. In each case, the psychologist and patient/responsible party have already exhausted the appeals process and the request for the additional time based service has been denied. In situations such as these, the form is designed to provide a written document wherein it is shown that the psychologist has given the patient/responsible party the option of purchasing the additional time to appropriately complete the consultation or to document that they are refusing to be held financially responsible for the additional services. However, in the situation where they refuse financial responsibility, they are also made aware of and sign an acknowledgment of the following (from Appendix V):

> "...I have been informed that the restricted professional services resulting from my decision not to accept financial responsibility for the additional recommended service may very well restrict the accuracy of any diagnosis to be offered as well as limit the accuracy of any treatment recommendations. I hereby release and absolve Dr. Peck and NSV from any and all professional responsibility and legal liability for any inaccuracy and/or limitation in professional care which may result from my instruction to Dr. Peck and NSV to deliver only those services which I contract with him through my insurance carrier."

Certainly, you can always choose to provide the free service to this person, who may have far more financial resources than you, but the choice is yours to make. I am merely trying to educate the reader about the real cost of working without generating revenue for your business.

Some Summary Thoughts and Guidelines Regarding the Business Aspects of Clinical Neuropsychology

I enjoy helping people or I wouldn't work in this field. I feel that my time has value and that the business arrangements that I make regarding renting office space, etc, are both reasonable and appropriate to providing care to my patients. I believe in employing good staff people who are willing to "give an honest day's labor for an honest and fair day's pay." I cannot continue to provide quality services if I cannot meet my business related financial obligations. I will not be able to maintain my practice. In other words, I will be out of business.

One cannot provide "Cadillac quality care at Pinto rates of reimbursement." Sadly, it is necessary to have to restrict services in certain situations, or face significant financial losses that could well result in the loss of one's business — and result in the situation where you are unable to help other patients. I am reminded of a lecture I once gave involving situation ethics and the business of service delivery in clinical neuropsychology. I asked the class of clinical interns and postdoctoral residents to imagine the following scenario.

> "You are employed by a hospital and you have been asked to carry out a 'comprehensive' neuropsychological consultation regarding a 34-year-old CVA patient. After reviewing the chart and interviewing the patient, you prepare a list of tests that you consider to reflect an appropriate means of addressing the referral question. Your test list totals 9.0 hours of testing, scoring, and report preparation. The patient is a participant in a managed care company and the case reviewer allows you a total of 3.0 hours of testing units. What do you do in this situation?"

Approximately 50% of the class said that they would give all of the tests and take the full nine hours, even if the insurance company was not going to cover any service beyond the 3.0 hours authorized. Several members of the class took the position that to do anything less than what they had already determined to be necessary would be unprofessional and unethical. After listening to their comments, I added the following information.

> "Before you continue with the consultation, you inform your supervisor of the insurance situation and your plan to do all of the testing. The supervisor's response is "While the hospital respects your professionalism, it does not have to support you financially in this decision. Thus, for every hour that you spend on this case beyond the 3.0 hours approved by the insurance company, twenty-five dollars will be deducted from your next paycheck.""

The class was then asked whether the personal loss of one hundred and fifty dollars of their own money would change their decision regarding whether they would provide the additional 5.0 hours of professional service. Of course, pandemonium reigned for a few minutes as the class personalized the ethical dilemma they now found facing them. This ethical dilemma is what we now face on a daily basis.

It is easier to make business decisions regarding service delivery when you (or your business and its' employees) do not suffer the financial consequences of your choices. However, if you continue to operate you business at a loss, you will not stay in the business of helping others.

When you go to the dentist, you are asked to pay your bill. When take your child to the pediatrician, or you visit your own doctor, you are asked to pay your co-pay then and there. Look at the sign on the your family doctor's waiting room and personalize what the sign means to you. Typically, it will state that the doctor cannot see you without your HMO authorization number — unless you are willing to pay the entire bill yourself. It will also state that your co-pay is due at the time of service. Don't feel that it is evil to live up to a contract that *you* signed with the insurance company so that you could see their enrollees. Please understand that the patient also signed a contract where they agreed to give the insurance company the authority to make decisions about the extent of medically necessary services that will be granted to them. If you don't wish to operate under the contractual obligations of an insurance company, then don't sign a contract with them which binds you to terms which you cannot tolerate and/or under which you cannot survive.

Here is my version of the Facts Of Managed Care Life:

1. Always follow the rules.
2. Always check for the requirement of preauthorization.
3. Always collect the co-pay; it may be a violation of your contract with the carrier not to do so.
4. Always communicate your plan of care to both the patient and the insurance company.
5. Always explain to the patient what you asked the insurance company for in the preauthorization request and what they have authorized you to provide to the patient.
6. Do not forget that the rules change so fast that what worked yesterday with an insurance company may not work today.
7. Always remember that there are no rules.

What Will our Business Management Practices Look Like in the Future

a. General Reimbursement:

I see reimbursement stabilizing at or slightly above the standard for regional Medicare payments. I also see more services, e.g. per use computer software administration/scoring fees being 'carved out' of the assessment fee. This will result in an even greater reliance on forensic and other professional services where fee structures are less regulated. I also envision more and more psychologists choosing to 'opt out' of insurance company contracts in their entirety and working solely on individualized and private contract arrangements with patients.

b. Reimbursement for Technician Services:
I see a bifurcation of charges/payments for technical assistant services and the professional service component. This will make it more difficult for the neuropsychologist, who does not employ a testing technician, to bill/collect for testing at the 'professional' rate.
c. Paperless Office:
Now that it is legal to utilize computer based storage of documents and to use computer based signatures on legal documents, I see less need for traditional based paper retention of records. Several major hospitals have gone to the 'paperless' system where no papers are generated. In turn, I see the neuropsychologist's office becoming paperless. Testing will be increasingly dependent upon Internet-based, interactive computer administration/scoring and the resulting reports and other records will be totally computer based as well. Records will be faxed from one computer to another or will be sent by means of encrypted Internet files.

d. Internet-Based Assessment:
Internet based assessment will become common. Once Medicare and other insurance companies allow for services where the professional is not actually physically present on site with the patient, the entire question of in office testing will become moot. The patient will not have to come to the neuropsychologist's office if they can go to another site such as the PCP's office and be interviewed and then assessed via internet based audio video communication. For the Internet connected patient with a video camera, testing can take place at home. Will Internet based, video interactive forms of psychotherapy and cognitive rehabilitation be next?

Acknowledgment

I would like to acknowledge the significant technical assistance provided by my postdoctoral fellow, Laura B. Jaycox, PsyD in the preparation of this book chapter.

References

Medicare News (1994, June) (The Travelers Companies). *Medically Unnecessary Services—Limitation Of Liability*, (No. 13) 21–23.
Medicare News (1995, September), (The MetraHealth Insurance Company). *Advance Notice For Medically Unnecessary Services*, (No. 19) 3.
Medicare Part B Provider Services Manual, Virginia Medicare Part B Carrier. (1997, January) Section 10 — Waiver of Liability.
Neblett, J.C., Peck, E.A., Hylton, V.H., & Isner, A.B. (1999, August). *Insurance reimbursement patterns for psychological and neuropsychological evaluations.* Paper presented at the annual meeting of the American Psychological Association, Boston, MA.

Peck, E.A. (1990) Developing A Private Practice In Neuropsychology. In Keller, P.A. & Heyman S.R. (Eds.), *Innovations in clinical practice*, Vol. 9. Professional Resource Exchange, Sarasota, FL.

Peck, E.A. & Jaycox, L.B. (2001, April). *Current business aspects of clinical psychology with particular reference to insurance issues.* Workshop presented at the meeting of the Virginia Psychological Association, Roanoke, VA.

APPENDIX 1

PATIENT REFERRAL FORM

Referred by ______________________________ Date Referral Received ____________

Street Address
____

Referral called in by ______________________________ Phone
No.____________________

PATIENT NAME ______________________________ DOB ____________ Age _______

____
Responsible party, if other than patient Relationship to patient

Address ______________________________ City/State ______________ ZIP _________
Home Phone ____________________ Work Phone ______________________________

MVA? [ ]Yes [ ]No **If Yes,** DOA ______________ **Head Injured?** [ ]Yes [ ]No - **If Yes,** LOC? [ ]Yes [ ]No [ ]Don't know

Are you represented by an attorney? [ ]Yes [ ]No If YES, see other form.

Sending us medical records? [ ]Yes [ ]No Do we send directions to our office location? [ ]No [ ]Yes ___Verbal
___Mailed

Current Problems/Reason for Referral
____

____

____

____

____

____

____

____

____

Testing hours requested: ____________________ Testing hours authorized: ____________________

______________/______________/__________ Confirmed appt with ______________ on ______________
Appt day **date** **time**

PATIENT INFORMED: BRING $__________ COPAY 48-HR NOTICE____ GLASSES/etc.____ MEDS LIST____

Payment Plan $________ down/$________/month
____

IF IN LITIGATION or WORKERS' COMP, 6 6 6

INSURANCE INFORMATION

Primary Ins. ______________________________________ Telephone # ______________________

Policy is in the name of (if other than patient) ____

ID # __________________________________ Group # ____________________ Eff. Date:

Yearly deductible $_________________ **Has deductible been met?** ____ Yes _____No

Copay: $____________ per hr/unit **-or-** per visit - **Preauthorization No. DIINT** ____________________

PSYCH _______________ hr/unit _____ **NEUROPSYCH** _________________hr/unit
Psychotherapy _________ hr/unit

Employer (if applicable) ____

Notes ____

____

____

File under Mental Health Benefits? _____ No _____Yes File under Medical Benefits? ______No ______Yes

SEND CLAIM TO: DIINT:____

____ TESTING (if different):_____________________

____

Telephone # if different from above: ____

Is there a SECONDARY insurance? _____No _____Yes - **If Yes, get the following information**:

Company name ______________________________________ Telephone #____________________

Policy is in the name of ____

ID # _________________________________ Group # ________________________

CLAIM TO: ____

Is there a TERTIARY Insurance? ____No _____Yes - If yes, get the following information:
Company Name_____________________________________Telephone #_____________________________
Policy is in the name of ______________________ ID#___________________________ Group #_______________
Claim TO: ____

IF IN LITIGATION:

PATIENT ______________________ Type of Litigation: ______________________

ATTY NAME ______________________ PHONE NO. ______________

FIRM NAME ____

ADDRESS ____

CITY/STATE ______________________________ ZIP ______________

IS MEDPAY COVERING? [ ]Yes [ ]No - **If yes**, send medpay agreement form - Date form sent ____________

NOTES____

____

NEED "LTR OF REPRESENTATION" FROM ATTY (STATING THAT THEY REPRESENT THIS PERSON, REQUESTING COPY OF REPORT, IF DESIRED, ETC.)

Ltr in file ________ Called atty requesting ltr ____________________
(date)

NOTES____

____

____

IF WORKERS' COMP:

REFERRAL SOURCE (must be **Primary Care** Physician, WC Approved Referral Source or representative from carrier):

EMPLOYER ____

STREET ____

CITY/STATE____

TELEPHONE NO. ______________________________

(Call before appt to confirm coverage)

Claim No. ______________________ Case Worker ______________________

____

SEND CLAIM TO (if other than Employer):

____

____

____

____

APPENDIX 2

PATIENT REGISTRATION

First Name:________________ Middle:________ Last Name:________________

Address:____________________ City:__________ State:____ ZIP:______

Home Phone: (____)____-_______ SSN:____/____/____ Sex: [ ] Male [ ] Female

DOB:____/____/____ AGE:____ Referred by:____________________

Were you injured while working? (Workers' Comp) [ ] NO [ ] YES-->Date of Injury: ____/____/____

Accident? [ ] NO [ ] YES-->Motor Vehicle? [ ] YES [ ] Other ________ Date of Accident ____/____/____

Are you represented by an attorney? [ ] NO [ ] YES-->Attorney Name ____________________

Have you been treated before for these symptoms? [ ] YES [ ] NO Are you here on an emergency basis? [ ] YES [ ] NO

Are you covered by insurance health plan(s)? [ ] YES [ ] NO If YES, we need to make a copy of your insurance card(s).

Primary Ins. ____________________ Secondary Ins. ____________________

Vocational Status:

- [ ] full-time student
- [ ] part-time student
- [ ] homemaker
- [ ] retired
- [ ] full-time employed
- [ ] part-time employed
- [ ] limited employment
- [ ] unemployed
- [ ] disabled
- [ ] other ________

Education:______Years Completed Degree:______

Handedness: [ ] right [ ] left [ ] ambidextrous

Occupation:____________________

Employer:____________________

Work Phone:____________________

Marital Status: [ ] Single [ ] Separated [ ] Divorced [ ] Married [ ] Widowed

Medication	Dosage (mg)	# per day	Medication	Dosage (mg)	# per day
1)			4)		
2)			5)		
3)			6)		

Responsible Party, if other than patient: (who is responsible for payment of all costs incurred)

First Name:______________ Middle:______ Last Name:________________

Address:____________________ City:__________ State:____ ZIP:______

Home Phone: (____)____-_______ SSN:____/____/____

Employer:____________________ Work Phone: (____)____-_______

Responsible party's relationship to patient: [ ] Spouse [ ] Child [ ] Parent Other ________________

Note: Fees are posted at the receptionist's window.

PAGE 1 OF 2

GUARANTEE OF PAYMENT AND ASSIGNMENT OF INSURANCE BENEFITS: For value received, the undersigned guarantor and/or patient (hereinafter the "Responsible Party") promises to pay to Neuropsychological Services of Virginia, Inc. (hereinafter "NSV") all charges incurred for services rendered to the Responsible Party. The Responsible Party understands that NSV will process the paperwork to complete insurance claim(s) but only as a courtesy to the Responsible Party, and the Responsible Party authorizes NSV to release any and all medical information necessary to complete insurance claim(s) and assigns any monies due and owing under the insurance contract to NSV. **It is, however, understood and agreed that the Responsible Party is responsible for all monies due and owing for services rendered by NSV in the event insurance does not pay for these services.** It is acknowledged that the ultimate completing and following-up of any insurance claims is the responsibility of the Responsible Party. It is further agreed by the Responsible Party, that in the event any monies received by NSV from the insurance carrier which are at any time after their receipt withdrawn from NSV by the insurance carrier, the Responsible Party will be responsible for those monies then due and owing, and waives any defense for payment the Responsible Party may have against NSV. In the event this account is turned over to an attorney for collection, the Responsible Party hereby agrees to pay all costs of collection including, but not limited to, court costs and 33 1/3% attorney's fees. The Responsible Party authorizes use of this form on all insurance claim submissions. Release of records to referral sources is also authorized. The Responsible Party agrees to be bound by the terms and conditions of this account with NSV.

A minimum of 48 hours' notice is required for cancellation of appointments. If this notice is not received, the Responsible Party may be charged for the full amount of time which was reserved for the appointment at the rates posted in the office of NSV. This may include legal fees for the time associated with subpoenas, depositions, and other court-related activities. Insurance will not be billed for missed/canceled appointments. Your copay is expected at the time of service. We will file the Responsible Party's initial insurance claim(s) and provide documentation necessary for insurance reimbursement. We do not, however, guarantee that each service will be covered or what percentage will be covered. The Responsible Party may incur extra charges for refiling of insurance claims.

In the event that the Patient's/Responsible Party's insurance does not cover our services (or any portion thereof), NSV will work with the Responsible Party regarding payment (e.g., setting up a payment plan). NSV expects full payment within thirty (30) days of the date of service. **The Responsible Party hereby agrees that accounts not paid within thirty (30) days will be charged a late fee of $15.00 and will accrue interest at the rate of 1.5% per month (18% A.P.R. - a minimum of $1.00 will apply).** The Responsible Party bears ultimate financial responsibility for all services rendered to the Patient/Responsible Party, including workers' compensation claims and personal injury cases, regardless of the outcome of litigation. In the event that coverage is denied under workers' compensation, the Responsible Party will pay any unpaid balance, notwithstanding any appeal of such denial. With respect to personal injury cases, the Responsible Party is responsible for fees incurred, NSV may not be able to seek payment from third parties, and NSV cannot wait on the outcome of pending litigation for payments. NSV does not accept contingency fee arrangements, as that is prohibited in Dr. Peck's profession. If there is any remaining balance(s) due at the time of settlement, the Responsible Party hereby authorizes their attorney to clear the Responsible Party's outstanding accounts. In the event the Responsible Party has **"medpay"** available and health insurance, NSV considers medpay to be the primary insurer. The Responsible Party's signature also constitutes the irrevocable agreement to a waiver permitting payment of medpay insurance claims directly to NSV prior to claimant receiving such funds.

Responding to Forensic/Medical Legal requests, conferences and telephone calls with attorneys involve additional time and record keeping. The Responsible Party is responsible for all direct costs and expenses associated with NSV and its attorney responding to discovery requests (including depositions and subpoena duces tecum time and labor costs) and with conferences including, but not limited to court appearances, preparation of reports, photocopying, faxes, long-distance telephone calls, out of office travel, overnight delivery and courier services. These expenses are billed to the Responsible Party and to the Patient's/Responsible Party's Attorney. The Responsible party, however, remains responsible for payment of these charges if not paid in full within sixty (60) days.

NOTE: Testing includes time for (1) administering and (2) scoring the tests, (3) preparing the report, and (4) discussion of the results (feedback). In nonforensic/nonmedical-legal cases, this will typically add 1-4 hours to the actual testing time. Forensic/medical-legal cases typically require even more time and may include record review and consultation(s) with attorney(s), etc. In certain cases (such as, but not limited to, medical-legal cases), a more comprehensive and time-consuming assessment may be needed than what may be approved under your insurance plan [for example, when an insurance plan covers up to 3 hours of testing/report preparation but Dr. Peck feels that your case requires additional hours of testing/record review/report preparation/etc]. The responsible party as noted below accepts responsibility for these charges.

If you have any questions, please speak with our Secretary, our Office Manager, or **Dr. Peck**. Your signature indicates that you have read the above and agree to the terms contained therein. These agreements are irrevocable.

Patient Signature: ______________________________ Responsible Party: ____
Date: _____________ Date: _____________

Parent/Guardian Signature (if patient is a minor or unable to sign**): ______________________________ Date: ___________

****If patient is a minor, are you her/his legal guardian?** [ ]YES [ ]NO If **NO**, please see Dr. Peck regarding this matter.

PAGE 2 OF 2

APPENDIX 3

Neuropsychological Services of Virginia, Inc.
2010 Bremo Road, Suite 127, Richmond, Virginia 23226-2444

Edward A. Peck III, PhD
Diplomate in Clinical Neuropsychology/ABPP-ABCN
Diplomate in Medical Psychotherapy/ABMT

Telephone
804/285-2555
Fax 804/282-0314

Provider/Supplier Notice to Beneficiary Regarding Service(s) That Are Likely to Be Denied Payment by Medicare Part B as "Not Reasonable and Necessary"

Physician/Supplier Notice to Beneficiary:

Medicare will pay only for services that it determines to be "reasonable and necessary" under section 1862(a)(1) of the Medicare law. If Medicare determines that a particular service, although it would otherwise be covered, is "not reasonable and necessary" under Medicare program standards, Medicare will deny payment for that service. I believe that, in your case, Medicare is likely to deny payment for the following services(s) for the reason(s) noted below:

Description of Service(s): ______________________________

____

____

Reason(s) for Medicare's Denial: ______________________________

____

____

______________________________ ______________
Provider's Signature Date

Beneficiary's Acknowledgment and Agreement to Pay:

I have been notified by my physician/psychologist/supplier that he or she believes that, in my case, Medicare is likely to deny payment for the services identified above, for the reasons stated. If Medicare denies payment, I agree to be personally and fully responsible for payment.

______________________________ ______________
Beneficiary's Signature Date

______________________________ ______________
Witness Date

APPENDIX 4

Neuropsychological Services of Virginia, Inc.
2010 Bremo Road, Suite 127, Richmond, Virginia 23226-2444

Edward A. Peck III, PhD
Diplomate in Clinical Neuropsychology/ABPP-ABCN
Diplomate in Medical Psychotherapy/ABMT

Telephone
804/285-2555
Fax 804/282-0314

Provider/Supplier Notice to Beneficiary Regarding Service(s) That Are Likely to Be Denied Payment by Your Insurance Carrier as "Not Reasonable and Necessary"

Physician/Psychologist/Supplier Notice to Beneficiary:

Your insurance company: ______________________________ will pay only for services that it determines to be "reasonable and necessary" under their contract with you/the enrolled individual and Dr. Peck/Neuropsychological Services of Virginia. If your insurance company determines that a particular service, is "not reasonable and necessary" or viewed as a covered service or lead to a covered diagnosis, your insurances company will deny payment for that service. I believe that your insurance company is likely to deny payment for the following services(s) for the reason(s) noted below:

Description of Service(s): ____

____

____

Anticipated Reason(s) for Insurance Company Denial: ______________________

____

____

____

______________________________ ______________
Provider's Signature Date

Beneficiary's Acknowledgment and Agreement to Pay:

I have been notified by my physician/psychologist/supplier that he or she believes that, in my case, my insurance company is likely to deny payment for the services identified above, for the reasons stated. If my insurance company denies payment, I agree to be personally and fully responsible for payment.

______________________________ ______________
Beneficiary's Signature Date

______________________________ ______________
Witness Date

APPENDIX 5

Neuropsychological Services of Virginia, Inc.
2010 Bremo Road, Suite 127, Richmond, Virginia 23226-2444

Edward A. Peck III, Ph.D.
Diplomate in Clinical Neuropsychology/ABPP-ABCN
Diplomate in Medical Psychotherapy/ABMT

804/285-2555
Fax 804/282-0314

Insurance Coverage Limitation On Professional Service

Patient Name: ________________________________

Responsible Party: ____________________________

Insurance Carrier: ____________________________

Dr. Edward A. Peck and Neuropsychological Services of Virginia (NSV) have informed me that they requested ______ hourly units of Psychological or Neuropsychological Testing (which includes the time to test, score and prepare the report) from my above named insurance carrier in planning to address the referral question(s) at hand. It is Dr. Peck's professional opinion that such an amount of professional testing service is necessary to attempt to properly address the referral question(s) at hand. I understand that the above named insurance carrier has preapproved only ______ hours of the total requested testing service. Dr. Peck and NSV have given me the opportunity to purchase the remaining ______ hour units at the standard hourly rate ($275.00) for this office unless otherwise agreed upon in advance. I am not asking for indigent care services. I have been offered the option of a payment plan versus lump sum payment due at the time of service.

Please initial, in the space provided, either of the following two options.

______ Yes, I *do* accept financial responsibility for the payment of the above remaining ______ hour testing units. I understand that these additional testing services, beyond what has been approved by the above noted insurance carrier, will be provided on a self pay/private pay basis.

______ No, I *do not* accept financial responsibility for the payment of the above remaining ______hour testing units. I understand and accept that the additional recommended testing services, beyond what has been approved by the above noted insurance carrier, will not be provided at this time. I have been informed that the restricted professional services resulting from my decision not to accept financial responsibility for the additional recommended service may very well restrict the accuracy of any diagnosis to be offered as well as limit the accuracy of any treatment recommendations. I hereby release and absolve Dr. Peck and NSV from any and all professional responsibility and legal liability for any inaccuracy and/or limitation in professional care which may result from my instruction to Dr. Peck and NSV to deliver only those services which I contract with him through my insurance carrier.

I understand that I may appeal my insurance carrier's decision regarding the above decision to approve fewer testing hour units than requested and that such an appeal may delay Dr. Peck's and NSV's ability to deliver professional services within my insurance carrier's contractual limits and provisions.

______________ Date	______________________________ Responsible Party
______________ Date	______________________________ Witness

Chapter 5

INDEPENDENT PRACTICE AND MANAGED CARE

Michael Schmidt

Throughout my years of clinical practice, I have often thought that if our health care system would just stand still for a minute I could get a handle on it. My wishes have not only been ignored — they have been mocked. The past 20 years have seen changes in health care that are of a revolutionary magnitude. The changes are not over, as insurers continue to develop and try out new reimbursement models that allow them to sell their products, control costs, and maintain profitability.

The modern-day neuropsychologist must be aware of these changes and understand the processes that are taking place in the health care delivery system. The aim of this chapter is to provide the neuropsychology practitioner with a useful understanding of the current health care delivery system, starting with a brief overview of managed health care, including definitions of major terms. The next section contains a historical overview to explain how the present system evolved. This is followed by a discussion of current developments, the impact of managed health care on providers, and some suggestions for both the field of neuropsychology and the individual practitioner.

An Overview of Managed Care

A formal definition of 'managed health care' has not been adopted, but the *Passkey for Health Insurance Licensing* (1993) offered the following: "A system of delivering health care that involves agreements with selected providers, utilization review, quality standards, and incentives for members to use selected providers" (pp. 200-201). This contrasts with a traditional indemnity plan, in which the insurer only has a contractual obligation to the insured. When the insured party incurs a loss that is specified by the contract, the insurer is obligated to pay certain benefits. The insurer has no relationship, contractual or otherwise, with the service provider.

Managed health care differs importantly from indemnity plans in that the provider *does* have a relationship, either contractual or statutory, with the insurer. The provider may not simply treat the patient as he or she deems appropriate and bill the insurer for the usual and customary charges for these services. The provider also might not be free to make referrals to other providers as she or he feels appropriate. Examples of statutory restrictions are seen in Worker's Compensation (WC), CHAMPUS, and Medicaid/Medicare, where reimbursement is based on a fee schedule, not the provider's charges. Statutory requirements may also apply to services billed to private insurers. In Colorado, when a patient is seen for personal injury (e.g., an automobile accident), the Personal Injury Protection (PIP) insurer must be notified within 30 days of the initial consult. In Illinois Worker's Compensation, 'daisy chain' referral patterns (where a provider refers to another provider, who then refers to a different provider who, in turn may refer to another provider, and so on) are strictly limited.

Although these statutory limitations significantly impact the manner in which providers practice, it is probably more common to think of 'managed health care' in terms of providers having contractual relationships with private insurers. These insurers are often referred to as Managed Care Organizations (MCOs) or Organized Systems of Care (OSCs). In this chapter, the term 'MCO' will be used.

Within this basic concept of managed care, insurers have developed an almost bewildering assortment of plans (or products) that they market to employers and the public, along with an array of acronyms and initials that nearly rival those in psychology. A brief description of these models will provide the neuropsychologist with some essential vocabulary.

The Preferred Provider Organization (PPO) has become very popular and in this model the insurer contracts with various independent practitioners or clinics to provide services for its members. It is not unusual for these plans to include contingencies that allow members to receive services from providers who are not on the PPO panel under specified circumstances. The Exclusive Provider Organization (EPO) is similar to a PPO, except that the member *must* be treated by providers on the panel. To the member, this plan appears similar to a closed panel HMO (described later).

Commercial insurance companies sell these plans to companies or individuals, the terms of which are governed by a contractual relationship. The insurance company then assumes the financial risk associated with fulfilling its contractual obligations and if all goes well, the company turns a profit. Alternatively, large companies or organizations with sufficient financial resources may meet the legal requirements for self-insuring. In this situation, the company assumes the financial risk but may contract with an insurance company to oversee the health plan. These are deemed Administrative Services Only (ASO) arrangements.

A somewhat different approach is the Health Maintenance Organization (HMO), a term coined by the Nixon administration. In this system, the providers are either partners in or employees of a multispecialty HMO clinic. Only services provided by the HMO are covered, except for medical emergencies. Kaiser Permanente is a good example of this type of plan. Kaiser Permanente is a multispecialty clinic that sells health coverage directly to the public for a set fee. Providers within Kaiser Permanente are salaried, which provides a means of controlling costs. The clinic assumes financial risk for providing the contracted services, which creates an incentive to emphasize prevention and an outcome-oriented approach to treatment. Insurance companies have also established HMOs, either through ownership or contractual arrangements.

The Independent Practice Association (IPA) model is closely related to the HMO. Like the HMO, providers receive a set fee per member to provide whatever services are needed. However, the IPA providers may maintain their own private practices and may not be employees of the IPA. HMOs like Kaiser Permanente are sometimes referred to as Closed Panel HMOs, while IPAs are sometimes termed Open Panel HMOs.

The Point of Service (POS) plan is a hybrid between a PPO and indemnity plan. Members may receive services from an HMO provider, a PPO provider, or from any other provider of their choosing. The plan includes a gradient of financial incentives (lower deductible, lower co-pay) that makes it cheapest for the member to receive treatment from an HMO provider, somewhat more expensive to be treated by a PPO provider, and generally quite a bit more expensive to seek services from other practitioners.

Other variations continue to be developed and tried. One issue that is currently being addressed is coordination of benefits. Traditionally, health benefits and Worker's Compensation benefits have been kept separate. Problems can arise with this arrangement, such as when there is controversy about whether care is related to a work-related injury or whether it should be covered by health benefits. The 24-Hour plan is an effort to address this problem, integrating health and disability (Worker's Compensation) benefits (Hughey, 1997). The insurance company contracts with the employer for both services, with potential cost and administrative overhead savings. The member receives treatment from the insurance company panel of providers for both work-related injuries and other health problems, and there is no need to sort out whether the treatment is for a work-related injury.

Historical Perspective

Insight into the current status of health care delivery can be gained by reviewing relevant history. The two major issues are: 1) Where did modern health care delivery concepts come from? and 2) What forces led to the dramatic changes that have taken place over the past 25 years?

Managed health care is not a modern phenomenon. In fact, its roots can be traced back to the development of the multispecialty group practice, which is often attributed to the Mayo Clinic in Rochester, Minnesota in the late 1800s. Dr. William Mayo moved to Rochester in 1863 and was joined by his two physician sons in the 1880s. The first partner was added to their clinic in 1892, and from there other physicians joined the practice. Important logistical issues were worked out, such as coordination of care, development of a central clinical chart for each patient, and means to transport the chart through the clinic as patients were seen by various specialists. The first patient was formally registered at the Mayo Clinic in 1907. Their model of care has been quite successful, and the Mayo Clinic enjoys a reputation of providing world-class quality care at competitive prices. In fact, within the era of managed health care, the Mayo Clinic successfully opened satellite operations in Jacksonville, Florida and Scottsdale, Arizona. In 1992, well after managed care became common, the Mayo Clinic began forming regional networks of clinics and hospitals.

Early managed care concepts are also seen in WC. The first constitutional WC act was passed in Wisconsin in 1911. The goal of WC was to provide health care to workers who were injured on the job while at the same time controlling costs for employers, who paid for the coverage. The exact nature of WC benefits varies from state to state, and statutes are revised frequently. Typically, treatment providers have to go through an application process to be qualified to treat WC patients, and reimbursement is based on a fee schedule set by statute rather than the rates set for services by each provider, known as his or her usual and customary charges. The injured worker has very little control over selecting treatment providers, and referral patterns among providers are also often regulated.

By combining the multispecialty clinic model, originated by the Mayo Clinic, with a novel concept of prepayment, the Health Maintenance Organization (HMO) was born. One of the pioneering HMO efforts began in California, in the context of WC benefits. As the Los Angeles Aqueduct was being built across the desert during the Great Depression, Dr. Sidney Garfield established Contractors General Hospital near Desert Center to treat the thousands of workers involved in the project. This hospital was struggling financially when Harold Hatch became involved and suggested insurance companies pay the hospital a fixed rate per day per worker. The fee was 5¢ per day, and for an additional 5¢ per day the worker would be covered for non-work-related medical problems (presaging the modern 24-hour care model). After this, Dr. Garfield established a similar model for workers building the Grand Coulee Dam. As this project wound down in 1941, he was asked to establish a similar clinic in the San Francisco Bay area, to provide treatment for shipyard workers who were building ships for World War II. At the end of the war, there were fewer employees at the shipyards and the clinic became a private health plan, eventually known as Kaiser Permanente. Whereas an HMO model within the context of WC seems to be a fairly natural fit (because the WC system is strongly regulated and emphasizes cost control), transitioning Kaiser Permanente to a private insurer was a major step. Although the HMO model is cost-effective in terms of health care delivery, start up costs are high.

Similar steps in prepaid health care were developed in the Pacific Northwest, again within the context of WC. In Tacoma in 1917, employers contracted with a group of physicians to provide care for injured workers for a set fee per month, which led to the Blue Shield plan. Blue Cross began at Baylor University in Texas in 1929. Noting that schoolteachers had difficulty paying medical bills, a plan was developed where they could obtain up to 21 days of inpatient care for a $6 per year premium. This was the initial Blue Cross plan. The Blue Cross concept grew and was strongly affiliated with the American Hospital Association (AHA) until 1960. These programs united and became the largest and oldest health insurer in the U.S. (Cunningham & Cunningham, 1997). The AHA strongly supported such prepayment plans for financial reasons (Kiesler, 1992).

Managed care concepts were gradually endorsed by a number of different elements in American society. Kaiser Permanente is an example of industry adopting an HMO model. Labor unions, such as the Teamsters in St. Louis, also adopted this model of delivering health care. Government (e.g., the Health Insurance Plan of Greater New York) and consumer groups (e.g., Group Health Cooperative of Puget Sound) also developed HMO models (Bennett, 1992).

These early efforts at managing health care had limited impact through the 1970s for several reasons. HMO clinics were available in only a few markets, and the American Medical Association (AMA) was strongly opposed to this model of care delivery (DeLeon, Uyeda, & Welch, 1985). Both the AMA and AHA opposed government regulation and any efforts that might diminish profitability, such as the Social Security act of 1935 (Stevens, 1989). The restrictions imposed by WC plans applied only to work-related injuries. Therefore, health care was funded primarily by indemnity plans, which paid the usual and customary fees of any qualified provider who delivered reasonable and necessary services. Starting around World War II, the cost of health insurance was borne increasingly by employers, as health insurance became a common component of employee benefit packages (VandenBos, 1993).

Two other important developments occurred in Congress. First, the Medicaid and Medicare plans were enacted in 1965. By getting into the business of public health care, the federal government had a vested interest in health care costs, and the ability to back this interest up with legislation. Annual cost increases for the Medicaid program have typically been 10% or more (Frank & VandenBos, 1994), and enrollment had risen to 31 million by 1992 (Merlis, 1993). In 1992, 40% of health care spending in the U.S. was by the federal government (Kerry & Hofschire, 1993).

The second development in Congress was passage of the Employee Retirement Income and Security Act (ERISA) in 1974, in response to the failure of retirement plans because of problems such as mismanagement, companies going bankrupt, and theft (Pedulla & Rocke, 1999). The intent of ERISA was to provide federal regulation of employee benefits, mostly to avoid further pension fund failures, and to make this regulation consistent across all states. The law contains a clause that preempts state regulations, with the exception of those state laws that regulate insurance, banking, and securities. Churches and government entities are exempt from ERISA. Hawaii has been granted a waiver from ERISA and several other states are seeking ERISA waivers (Frank & VandenBos, 1994).

Modern Health Care: the Dilemma

Over the years, health care became big business. By 1930, hospitals had become the fifth largest industry in the U.S. Health costs increased steadily and in recent years they seemed to be spiraling out of control. From 1960 through the early 1990s, increases in health costs were four times the rate of general inflation (Hall & Ellman, 1990; Letsch, 1993). In 1983, health care was the third largest industry in the U.S. (Hager, 1983). Health care comprised 6% of the Gross Domestic Product (GDP) in 1965 (Kiesler & Morton, 1988). Commonly cited statistics from the Health Insurance Association of America indicate that cost inflation in health care exceeded 20% in 1988 and 1989, at which point health costs comprised about 12% of the GDP. By 1993, health care accounted for over 14% of the GDP (Congressional Budget Office, 1993).

Some began to question whether these increases in cost were justified. Kiesler (1992) noted "the United States pays more than any other country for health care, has arguably the best hospital care in the world, and as a nation has mediocre health" (p. 1079). Hospitals emphasized expensive services, especially surgery, and catered to paying patients (Stevens, 1989) and health care costs were 40% more in the U.S. than in any other developed country (Schieber & Poullier, 1991).

A number of factors have been cited as contributing to increasing health costs. These factors included inefficiencies in health care delivery, improved and expanded medical technology, defensive medicine, the aging of the U.S. population, increased use of more expensive medications, cost shifting, increased utilization of child and adolescent inpatient mental health care, saving and prolonging lives of seriously ill individuals who will then require increased medical services, and increased numbers of providers (Binner, 1986; Goran, 1992; Frank & VandenBos, 1994).

Several authors (Kiesler & Morton, 1988; Drum, 1995) also pointed out that under indemnity reimbursement, competitive market forces do not seem to work normally in health care. They cite evidence that hospitals that have nearby competition actually charge more than those without such competition. In part, this may be that to remain competitive these hospitals have to keep up with the other hospitals and offer extras whenever possible. For example, when one hospital acquires a new piece of equipment, other nearby hospitals generally need to follow suit. Similarly, provider fees continued to rise despite increasing numbers of providers. Health care providers were in a position to set fees as they saw fit and, unless they were deemed to be not 'reasonable and customary', they would be paid. Also, when new health benefits were made available, they were used and health costs increased.

While it may seem the mark of a truly civilized society to spend over 10% of its GDP on health care (as compared to such endeavors as waging war), those who were footing the bill found it to be an increasingly difficult burden. It was clear that American health care was in trouble. Something was going to be done, either through government regulation or a drastic change in the health care delivery system. These trends led Feldman (1992a) to write that because providers did not adequately control costs " . . . they killed or at least seriously wounded the goose that laid the golden egg, a goose that for them is not likely ever to be as prolific." (p. xii). However, it should also be kept in mind that insurance companies designed, marketed, and made profits selling indemnity plans, and thus should share some of the blame.

Modern Health Care: the Solution

A major problem with indemnity insurance plans is that they are passive risk sharing mechanisms with no incentives for cost containment. Increases in health care costs were passed along to the consumer as increases in insurance premiums, and nobody had any real financial accountability (Drum, 1995). Early efforts to manage health care costs within indemnity plans were straightforward but unsophisticated. Cost savings were obtained by reducing benefits (e.g., 20 outpatient therapy sessions per year), capping lifetime benefits (e.g., a $100,000 lifetime benefit for mental health care), and increasing patient costs (e.g., deductibles and co-pays). Some of these methods do not create excessive burden but can reduce utilization of services. For example, relatively small co-pays can reduce insurance company costs for each office visit, but more importantly serve to reduce number of office visits (Manning et al., 1984).

However, some of these cost-shifting methods (e.g., deductibles, lifetime benefit limits) could create significant financial burden for patients and thus callously restrict access to care. The consequences can be fairly serious and widespread (Kunnes, 1992). For employers the fallout may include employee dissatisfaction, higher absenteeism, increased employee turnover with resultant higher costs for recruitment and training, and increases in disability or WC benefits when untreated disorders result in disability. For the insurer, ultimate treatment costs may be increased when early interventions are delayed. For providers, there may be a temptation to 'play the insurance game,' to tailor diagnosis and treatment to the insurance company's reimbursement policies. It goes without saying that patients suffer the most.

New approaches to health care delivery were sought. Congress passed the HMO Act in 1973, thus legitimizing and providing some initial guidelines for HMOs as a means of trying to control spiraling health care costs. After this legislation, HMOs grew steadily, with a peak in the mid 1980s (Gabel, DiCarlo, Fink, & deLissovoy, 1989). Enrollment in HMOs grew steadily from 14 million in 1983 to over 30 million in 1988, at which point the majority of individuals with employer-sponsored health care were enrolled in MCOs. By 1997, 85% of employee benefit health insurance was provided through MCOs (Pedulla & Rocke, 1999). Whereas indemnity plans could control costs only by reducing benefits and shifting costs to the patient, MCOs can employ these methods in conjunction with additional mechanisms, such as contracting for lower rates with providers and case management. These procedures can be very effective. For example, costs at Kaiser Permanente increased only about 10% per year from 1980 through 1990 (Goran, 1992).

In addition to comparing HMO and indemnity plan costs, some demonstration projects have been done to determine if health care costs could be contained via managed care mechanisms, and to determine if quality of care suffered. For example, the Hawaii Medicaid demonstration program was done from 1984 through 1987 (Pallak, Cummings, Dorken, & Henke, 1993). This program demonstrated that managed mental health care produced significant reductions in patient *medical* costs, whereas unmanaged mental health services did not. Also, managed care patients used about one-third of the outpatient visits that their unmanaged care counterparts used. The Fort Bragg Study (Bickman, Guthrie, Foster, Lambert, Summerfelt, Breda, & Heflinger, 1995) is another commonly cited example. This study demonstrated that a costly, coordinated approach to mental health care was no more effective than ad lib treatment provided in similar communities. Thus, more was not necessarily better.

Similar to the private sector, the federal government was feeling the impact of increased health costs and began making efforts to control these costs. Peer reviews began in the early 1970s for Medicare/Medicaid and in 1979 for CHAMPUS (Frank & Lave, 1992). These were initial efforts to reimburse only those services that were deemed reasonable and necessary. In 1983, the federal government significantly modified the reimbursement system for Medicare/Medicaid through the Prospective Payment System (PPS), a concept previously used in New Jersey. The goal was to control hospital costs along with creating incentives for hospitals to function more efficiently (Hall & Ellman, 1990). The mechanism for accomplishing this was the Diagnostic-Related Group (DRG), which set reimbursement rates for hospitalization expenses based on the patient's diagnosis. DRGs were not applied to physician payments, but in 1992 the Medicare fee schedule included a different mechanism for determining provider reimbursement rates known as the relative value scale (RVS). This scaling method for rates attempts to take into account the time, mental effort, technical skill, specialty training, and differential costs of malpractice insurance in setting the reimbursement rate for a particular service. For example, the RVS for neuropsychological evaluation may differ from the RVS for developmental testing, and thus these two services would be reimbursed at different rates. CHAMPUS reform initiatives were begun in 1988 as a series of demonstration projects. The CHAMPUS TRICARE managed care system was legislated with the 1994 Defense Authorization Act.

In combination, these efforts have led to managed care models being used in all major aspects of health care, including government benefits (Medicaid/ Medicare and CHAMPUS), WC, and private health care. In 1991, Colorado became the first state to enact legislation also allowing MCO plan auto insurance (PIP) to be offered.

In the same sense that health care has been big business for many years, managed health care is now poised to become big business. Early MCOs were primarily under the guidance of physicians, but in recent years business interests have become prominent and corporations own an increasing number of MCOs. As a result, profitability and investor value have become driving forces in modern health care delivery, and more or less aggressive business practices have become an integral part of MCO operations (Cummings, 1998). In fact, Drum (1995) suggested that a major move towards managed health care occurred when 'corporate America' found that the health care industry could be turned into a competitive market, and that profits could be made. Then, like any industry, market forces such as supply and demand took over, health care companies competed, and some have risen to a position of dominance. Providers have not been in a good position to prosper in this reformed marketplace, perhaps in part because there has been a large increase in the number (i.e., supply) of providers in recent years. The number of physicians per capita increased 50% from 1970 through 1990 (Physician Payment Review Commission, 1994) and from 1974 through 1992 the number of licensed psychologists increased threefold, from 20,168 to 63,500 (Shapiro & Wiggins, 1994). As a result, providers have experienced reduced fees, additional layers of administrative overhead needed to cope with the business demands of the MCOs, and competition for finite positions on MCO panels. The health care system continues to be in flux. Consumer dissatisfaction with managed care has become more vocal, and companies are taking steps to address this. In 1990, the National Committee for Quality Assurance was formed and this non-profit organization assesses the quality of managed care plans. It appears that NCQA develops standards carefully, and the APA has had some input into proposed Managed Behavioral Health Organization standards (Vein & Cullen, 1996). NCQA accreditation is becoming an increasingly important credential for MCOs, and will likely be a certification that businesses seek out when they buy insurance plans for their employees. Market dynamics are also changing. In some states, small employers are allowed to group together to purchase health insurance for their employees (Frank & VandenBos, 1994).

On the legislative front, health care reform was a major focus early in the Clinton administration, one that was vigorously resisted on multiple fronts. At present, patient bill of rights legislation is being considered and it appears this legislation will pass in some form. In the absence of significant changes in federal policies, most states are proceeding with various health care reforms independently, Frank and VandenBos (1994) reported that 21 states had passed health care reform bills and legislation was pending in an additional 25 states. Twenty-nine states allowed mental health services to be delivered by managed care, but only 11 states included freedom of choice principles and only three require admission of 'any willing provider' to MCO panels. Sixteen regulate Quality Assurance and four regulate Utilization Review activities, which will be discussed later.

A major legal concern at present is the preemptive nature of ERISA (Pedulla & Rocke, 1999). Health insurance plans provided by employers must conform to state insurance, banking, and securities regulations. For example, states may mandate minimum standards for health insurance plans. However, employee benefits (including health insurance) are exempted from other state regulations by ERISA. Self-insured plans also benefit from ERISA exemption and, additionally, may be exempt from state insurance regulations. Because of these exemptions, patients who are denied health benefits may have very little legal recourse. Typically, damages may be sought for actions such as breach of contract or malpractice through civil litigation, but ERISA prevents the insurance carrier from being subject to the state statutes enabling these remedies. Only violations of the state insurance code (and, less relevant, the banking and securities codes) are actionable. If reparation is sought in federal court, the legal issue is limited to appropriateness of benefits administration, and unless the insurance company's decisions are 'arbitrary and capricious,' they will be upheld. Compensatory and punitive damages are not allowed. In recent years, some limitations to ERISA exemption have been made. For example, MCOs can be held vicariously responsible for negligence resulting in injury to members. Needless to say, ERISA reform is a high priority for many consumer and provider groups.

Providers have reacted to managed health care in various ways. Some have begun actively marketing their services, and all of the media contain substantial numbers of advertisements for medications, hospitals, clinics, and individual practitioners. Psychiatric hospitals began extending privileges to nonphysician providers and developed "under utilization" reviews. The American Psychological Association adopted a somewhat cautionary position paper regarding managed care (Tanney, 1989) and is supporting a carefully selected series of lawsuits against MCOs (Cullen, 1997; Rocke, 1999; *Virginia lawsuit propels legal initiative to curb MCO abuses*, 1999). In a major change of policy, the AMA voted in June 1999 to support physicians unionizing.

Mental Health Care

Until recently, the fortunes of neuropsychology have been strongly tied to those of mental health, making it important to briefly review the history of mental health services in the U.S. and the unique aspects of the interplay between these services and managed care. Kiesler (1992) suggested that mental health services were part of social welfare policy, but in recent years they are increasingly under the purview of health care policy. The passing of the Community Mental Health Centers Act in 1963 marked the first significant federal recognition of mental health issues, and was aimed at improving access to mental health services. Despite this increased emphasis on mental health, MCOs were initially reluctant to include mental health services in their plans. Although the first prepaid mental health treatment was made available by the Community Health Association in Detroit in the 1950's (Bennett, 1992), few other plans were developed until studies by Avnet (1962) and others demonstrated that limited mental health coverage was financially feasible. Following this, MCOs began gradually including these services. The HMO Act of 1973 required some minimal benefit levels for mental health care, and many states also passed legislation requiring that some mental health benefits be included in health insurance policies. There was an increased need for mental health practitioners, and psychologists became an important part of this movement. An early struggle for psychologists was obtaining recognition and reimbursement as independent practitioners (Cummings, 1988; Drum, 1995). Although these efforts established and expanded the profession of clinical psychology, they also resulted in the survival of clinical psychologists being strongly dependent on insurance payments.

Mental health benefits have accounted for about 8% of total health care costs, and about half of this for HMOs (Martinson, 1988). However, several trends in mental health care caused these costs to increase in the early 1980s. These included increases in psychiatric inpatient care and residential treatment for children, more psychiatric treatment being done in general hospital programs that were not formal psychiatric units, and increased ownership of psychiatric hospitals by large corporations (Kiesler & Simpkins, 1991). Inpatient care accounted for over 70% of mental health costs and 23% of all hospital days (Kiesler & Sibulkin, 1987), and psychological testing was considered a profit center by many hospitals. Mental health care costs began rising disproportionately and in recent years mental health and substance abuse treatment accounted for about 20% of health care costs (American Psychiatric Association, 1988; Goran, 1992). In the late 1980s, estimates of annual increases in mental health and substance abuse costs ranged from 18% to 47% (Pearson, 1992). Costs for treating mental disorders ranked third among diagnostic categories (Mechanic, 1987). As a result, many insurance companies developed mental health 'carve outs', in which particularly strong cost control measures were placed on mental health benefits (Altman & Price, 1993). This was primarily through different levels of benefits (e.g., higher co-pays), and specialized case management efforts. However, a positive point for members is that many companies found that costs could be contained while still allowing members direct access to mental health services, without referral from their Primary Care Physician (PCP). Medicaid has also moved to control mental health costs in recent years through capitating mental health benefits (Dangerfield & Betit, 1993).

The restrictions in mental health carve outs include limited benefits for psychotherapy and psychological testing, and increased levels of control of these services. In the past few years, steps have been taken to remove neuropsychology from these restrictions by classifying it as a medical assessment rather than as a mental health service (Puente, 1994). These efforts have succeeded in classifying neuropsychology CPT codes under neurology rather than under psychiatry. However, despite this some MCOs continue to consider neuropsychology to be essentially a mental health service and attempt to apply their more restrictive mental health carve out policies to neuropsychological assessment and treatment.

Utilization Review

Cost containment necessarily requires some type of rationing of health care services, but this rationing can be done in many different ways. It is important for providers to understand the differences between benefit limitation versus case management approaches to treatment rationing. Also, a basic appreciation of managed care principles and procedures is helpful for the provider because MCOs place great emphasis on these methods as they develop increasingly sophisticated approaches to managing costs.

Early efforts to control health costs consisted of limiting benefits and shifting costs to patients, but in doing so, this system did not discriminate between 'good' and 'bad' or 'necessary' and 'unnecessary' care. More recent efforts have involved case management using quality assurance principals. The stated goal of this type of case management is not to restrict access to care, but rather to dole out treatment carefully in an effort to avoid unnecessary expenditure. This model of controlling benefits requires the MCO to be involved in treatment decisions to some degree. The vehicle by which this is implemented is Utilization Review (UR).

UR is defined as "a set of techniques used by or on behalf of purchasers of health benefits to manage health care costs by influencing patient care decision making through case-by-case assessments of the appropriateness of care prior to its provision" (Institute of Medicine, 1989). MCOs use UR to determine if services are necessary, and therefore whether these will be reimbursed. Concordant with this definition, the American Board of Quality Assurance & Utilization Review Physicians (1997) stated that UR may occur prior to service delivery (i.e., preauthorization of services), but also that UR can occur concurrently to monitor care as well as retrospectively. Initially, there appeared to be quite a bit of inconsistency in UR procedures, and providers expressed great frustration. Legislation was planned, and the managed care industry feared this would seriously impact UR activity, which was seen as an essential element of cost savings. In response to these issues, the American

Managed Care and Review Association established the Utilization Review Accreditation Association in 1990. This organization set standards aimed at making UR more consistent. Despite these accreditation efforts, 24 of the states had passed laws regulating UR activities by 1992. These laws set standards for UR organization employee qualifications, time limits for the review process, and means for appealing denial of care. Many of these issues are at the heart of the patient bill of rights bill currently being considered by Congress. Because standards vary from state to state, it is important for providers, MCO members, and advocacy groups to know the UR standards in their state (American Psychological Association Practice Directorate, 1993a).

UR requires a set of protocols and procedures for guiding decisions about treatment (Frank & Lave, 1992). Some states require that treatment denials be done by UR personnel whose degree is the same as the treatment provider. Other states do not require this, and individuals with various levels of training and expertise conduct UR. Case managers are often nurses, social workers, or psychologists by training. Case managers may have extensive expertise or even specialty credentialing in UR methods, but relatively less knowledge about the specialty services they are reviewing. The case manager may look to set procedures and guidelines for making decisions. Some of these are promulgated within the company and others may come from external sources. Some companies have protocols for treating certain disorders, such as depression, or for evaluating specific disorders, such as ADHD. To this point, few guidelines are available for utilization of neuropsychological services. The American Academy of Neurology (1996) has published indications for neuropsychological assessment in the care of neurological patients, and DSM-IV (American Psychiatric Association, 1994) mentioned that neuropsychological evaluation was necessary for diagnosing post-concussive disorder. Despite this, case managers do make decisions regarding neuropsychological evaluation, and often these proceed on a test-by-test basis, with certain tests being allowed and others being denied.

Another aspect of case management is the identification of specialists and subspecialists for referring patients. In a mental health carve out, therapists may be identified as specializing in grief issues, counseling for chronic illness, or sexual abuse therapy. Neuropsychology is often difficult to characterize; some case managers think of neuropsychology as part of mental health and others understand it as being more part of medical diagnosis and care. To make matters worse, relatively few patients are referred for neuropsychological services, so case managers may not have a lot of experience handling these cases.

'Quality Assurance' (QA) is a term that is used increasingly by MCOs in relation to UR efforts. Although practitioners may think of 'quality care' as being above average or optimal, MCOs may apply different definitions (Berlant, 1992). Quality may refer to 'standard practice' or the level of care afforded by the average practitioner, it may refer to scientifically validated care, or it may be used to mean 'not substandard' care. Quality may also be tied to outcomes, and may be minimally defined as treatment that avoids adverse outcomes, or a higher standard such as treatment that is effective. Consumer satisfaction and risk management may also be QA standards. It is important to know which definition of QA is being used when evaluating the QA principals and efforts of MCOs. Typically, three types of information enter into QA (Donabedian, 1980). Structural aspects include staff qualifications and credentials, and the adequacy of the organizational structure to provision of care. Process aspects refer to the manner in which care is delivered, such as standards of practice. Outcome issues relate to indicators of patient improvement or satisfaction.

In the same sense that there are board certifications for treatment providers, case managers may also obtain specialty credentials. The American Board of Quality Assurance & Utilization Review Physicians (ABQAURP) was initiated in 1977. In 1998 subspecialty recognition became available for case management, managed care, risk management, and worker's compensation.

Legal Issues

A number of legal issues may confront practitioners as they attempt to adjust to the managed care environment. One example is the increasingly frequent dilemma that occurs when an MCO denies services that the clinician feels are necessary (Appelbaum, 1993). The clinician may have a legal responsibility to appeal the decision (Stout, 1997). In psychotherapy, it might be necessary for clinicians to inform the patient that payment for treatment could be terminated before either the clinician or the patient feels that therapeutic goals have been achieved. In some circumstances it could be incumbent on the therapist to continue treatment after payment has been terminated. MCOs have an obligation to review cases with reasonable care in reaching decisions to disallow care, and to disclose appeals procedures when care is denied. They also may have a duty to select appropriate providers for their panels and may incur vicarious liability for the actions of their paneled providers.

Other issues are at an administrative level. Organizing providers into MCOs can run afoul of antitrust statutes, 'creative' approaches to collecting fees can be seen as fraud, and some UR activities can lead to civil action. Interested readers will find *A practical guide to legal issues in utilization and risk management* (ABQAURP, 1997) and *Health care law and ethics* (Hall & Ellman, 1990) to be useful references regarding the details of legal issues.

The Impact of Managed Care on Practice

Market Forces

There is no doubt that managed health care has impacted the independent practice of neuropsychology. In a 1994 survey, 75% of neuropsychologists were concerned that health care reform would negatively impact their practices (Sweet, Westergaard, & Moberg, 1995). Sixty-four percent felt that patient evaluation time would be diminished by health care reforms. Many (36%) had already experienced reduced referral sources, reduced patient referrals (39%), and increased administrative time (40%). A large number (43%) had been excluded from managed care panels. Sixteen percent noted that neuropsychology had been included in mental health rather than medical benefits by MCOs.

These results can be compared with a recent national survey of practicing psychologists (Phelps, Eisman, & Kohout, 1998), 79% of which reported that managed health care had negatively impacted their professional work. Concerns voiced by independent practitioners included increased administrative load (e.g., treatment precertifications), mentioned by 62% of the sample, fewer patients (50%), being excluded from managed care panels (40%), problems getting reimbursed (33%), and losing market share to less trained providers (32%).

The practices of MCOs have also been criticized. A recent study by the American Psychological Association Practice Directorate (1994a) found that psychologists were concerned that cost containment was emphasized at the expense of quality of care. Knapp and Bowers (1996) found large percentages of psychologists felt that MCOs did not appear concerned about patients' access to care (76%) or patient choice (82%). Sixty-one percent noted that being rejected by a panel had disrupted patient care and 40% found that MCO rule changes negatively affected patient care. Most felt MCO policies were not clear (55%), that issues related to provider choice were poorly defined (66%), or that MCOs did not responded promptly to inquiries (61%). Few (31%) felt that the MCOs flexibly met the patient's treatment needs. About half felt patients did not understand how to appeal MCO decisions. However, although 50% of providers were concerned that they would experience negative consequences if extension of services were requested, only 5% had actually experienced such consequences.

The changes produced by managed health care have caused some to be concerned about whether independent practice will survive, and the difficulties caused by managed care have caused some psychologists to consider a career change (APAPD, 1994a). However, survey data to date are optimistic. A survey in New Jersey (Moldawski, 1990) found 87% of psychologists worked in solo practices, and only 10% were members of MCOs. In recent years, the percentage of clinical psychologists working primarily in a private practice setting has remained stable at about 50% (Wicherski, Woerheide, & Kohout, 1996; Phelps et al., 1998; Williams, Wicherski, & Kohout, 1998). Phelps et al. (1998) also found that 76% of the work done by clinical psychologists continues to be devoted to psychotherapy and assessment, suggesting that there has been little diversification of activities. In contrast, data suggest there has been an increase in the percentage of neuropsychologists in private practice. In 1988, 21% of neuropsychologists were employed primarily in private practice, although an additional 46% maintained a private practice in addition to other employment (Putnam, 1989). An increase in neuropsychology private practice was seen in 1992, with 35% of practitioners working primarily in private practice and an additional 32% doing some private practice in addition to other employment. A recent survey by Sweet, Moberg, and Suchy (2000) found a steady increase in private practice neuropsychologists from 1989 to 1999. For ABPP boarded neuropsychologists, the increase was from 25% of those surveyed to 34%, and for APA Division 40 member non-boarded neuropsychologists, the increase was from 39% to 58%. It is my belief that there continues to be a need for independent practitioners, and this will continue into the foreseeable future.

Stout (1997) estimated that fees for psychological services were reduced from 10% to 35% by managed care. However, this does not appear to have translated into reduced income for neuropsychologists in general. Surveys indicate that the median annual income for neuropsychologists was $59,500 in 1988 (*M* = $71,078) and this increased to $76,022 (*M* = $95,955) in 1992 (Putnam, 1989; Putnam & Anderson, 1994). The median increased at an annual rate of 7%. However, income for clinical psychologists has not increased in recent years (Wicherski et al., 1996; Williams et al., 1998). The median salary for clinical psychologists was $56,000 in both 1995 and 1997. In the more recent survey 58% of clinical psychologists noted a reduction in income as a result of managed care, and this reduction averaged 15%. Earlier data from New Jersey indicated that 25% of psychologists experienced a reduction in income from 1991 to 1992 (Shapiro, 1995). Phelps et al. (1998) found that 65% of independent practice clinical psychologists reported reduced income due to managed care. More experienced (and therefore probably higher paid) practitioners were particularly hard hit. Information regarding the financial impact of managed health care on neuropsychologists is limited.

Changes in the doctor–patient relationship

Frank and Lave (1992) point out that the relationships among the various parties involved in paying for, delivering, and benefiting from health care have changed, and they describe these changes from the perspective of *agency*. This term, from economics, refers to relationships in which one party acts on behalf of another party, and these relationships are often governed by contractual relationships. In health care, providers are hired by patients to provide direct treatment, and also to advise and help manage health problems. The provider assumes a broad advocacy role for the patient. Managed care alters this relationship; UR procedures oversee the activities of treating providers and may determine that his or her treatment and recommendations are not necessary or cost-efficient. The MCO may also guide referrals and dictate level of care. Through these activities, the MCO acts as an agent for the patient, sometimes in conflict with the treatment provider. The agency relationships become increasingly complex and the advocacy component of the provider–patient relationship may be diminished. In managed care, the MCO, through the case manager, takes on an increasing role in deciding what care is necessary and what referrals should be made. The specialty provider assumes the role of a technician or craftsman, applying specialized skills to the patient's care, but beyond this having a limited role in advising or directing the patient.

These changes in relationships can present significant professional issues for psychologists. Phelps et al. (1998) noted that 49% of clinical psychologists felt that working in MCOs resulted in ethical dilemmas. Prominent among these is a loss of patient confidentiality resulting from UR (APAPD, 1994a; Cullen, 1997). Phelps et al. also found psychologists were concerned about being supervised or managed by nonpsychologists (29%) and similarly, the APAPD study found that many psychologists felt that UR personnel were making decisions without an adequate understanding of psychological services.

MCO contracts

When a provider negotiates to be on an MCO panel, the typical approach by the MCO is to propose a reduced fee for services, and in return the MCO's members will be referred only to panel members. This sounds like an arrangement that would increase referrals, although the provider to member ratio is typically not specified and the provider must rely on the good will of the MCO in this regard. Some MCOs actually charge a fee for the privilege of being on a panel or an 'administrative fee' for each referral that is received. What isn't mentioned is that judicious use of specialists is a major aspect of cost savings and accordingly, MCOs take steps to prevent referrals to specialists.

The manner in which neuropsychological services are accessed varies across insurance companies. These services may be accessed through either medical or mental health portions of the plans, and some have provisions for accessing neuropsychology through either mechanism. When a neuropsychologist receives a referral from a mental health 'carve out' program, some restrictions in addition to those incumbent to medical referrals may apply. An initial patient screening may need to be done and cost effectiveness of both evaluation and treatment may come under particularly strong scrutiny. Also, benefits (reimbursement rates, co-pays) may be different from those that would apply to a medical referral.

In the same sense that MCOs emphasize access to their member base to providers, they frequently tell members that access to care will not be restricted. However, this does not necessarily mean that members will receive the specific care that they want, or even the care that their PCP recommends. Specifically related to neuropsychological assessment, MCO manager informed this author that psychological testing was not a benefit. At another company, a manager stated that although psychological testing was a benefit, it was *almost never* approved.

Personal Perspective

As managed health care gained a foothold in the 1980s, the reaction among my colleagues was uniformly negative, although none were quite as intense as Shore (1995), who compared MCO practices with the regimes of Mussolini, Hitler, Lenin, and Stalin. Nevertheless, the new health care system posed definite threats to professional autonomy, the doctor-patient relationship, and the provider's income.

In my community, health care practitioners exhibited a number of different responses to these changes. Some moved rather smoothly into managed health care, and it seemed that many of these individuals had previously cultivated close relationships with insurance carriers and seemed to understand the benefits of these alliances. Others fought vigorously, challenging every denial of service, every case management effort. Many of these individuals were subsequently excluded from consideration for panels. Some scoffed at offers to join panels, and began experiencing financial consequences when panels closed. Still others felt managed health care couldn't succeed, and even today some colleagues express the belief that we will somehow return to a fee-for-service system. Those practitioners who found themselves not included on provider panels had relatively few options. These included development of 'cash and carry' practices; emphasizing other areas of practice (e.g., forensic work); leaving independent practice to work for a clinic, hospital, or university; or contemplating a mid-life career change. There are colleagues who have employed each of these solutions.

In a basic sense, health care is the business of helping people. It is a big business, with a lot of money at stake, but at its core is the promotion of the welfare of our citizenry, on a patient-by-patient basis. One cannot fault society for wanting to contain health costs, or government for responding to these concerns via legislation (after all, that's how government solves problems). One cannot blame employers for wanting to keep employee benefits packages affordable when these companies have to make a profit in an ever more competitive global marketplace. One cannot blame insurers for wanting to make a profit any more than one would blame providers for earning their livings in the health care industry. Yes, health care is the business of helping people, and those of us who emphasize the 'helping' part need to balance out those who focus on the 'business' piece.

The competitive forces that have become active in the U.S. health care delivery system may ultimately result in a viable and reasonable means for delivering quality health care at affordable prices to the largest number of citizens possible. Competition is a common way for our society to resolve issues; it is the cornerstone of the adversarial process in our courts, the basis for debates that guide decisions in congress, and the foundation of our economy. Yet by its nature, competition is not an intrinsically gentle or fair process; it begets winners — and losers. For this system to work, it is important that all sides be represented, and that no party gain an excessive advantage (Feldman,

1992a). Those who have a major interest in health care include businesses, insurance companies, consumers, providers, and government. Of these parties, it appears insurance companies have an advantage at present and that this advantage comes from their dominance in some markets and favorable legislation, notably ERISA. As the health insurance industry consolidates and each company gains additional financial and market clout, this advantage will increase. Providers appear to be at a disadvantage because of supply and demand issues along with unfavorable legislation, notably antitrust statutes. Thus, at least in my community, MCOs have been able to drive hard bargains with individual providers, especially in well-represented specialties. Yet our city has the most profitable hospital in the state, and in part this may be because our city has only two hospital corporations, affording them a favorable negotiating position. Typically, when one side in a dispute becomes too powerful, we look to the government for regulation. Sometimes this happens via legislation. Alternatively, the strong tradition of case law in the U.S. illustrates the importance of litigation as a means of resolving conflicts and clarifying issues. As market forces, legislation, politics, regulation, legal challenges, and various professional standards continue to influence our health care system, a number of different solutions will be considered (Bingaman, Frank, & Billy, 1993; Daschle, Cohen, & Rice, 1993; Durenberger & Foote, 1993; Kerry & Hofschire, 1993) and through the ongoing processes of debate and compromise, guide the shape that it will take in the future.

The impact of dual contracts

As noted at the beginning of this chapter, managed health care is marked by dual contractual relationships. As with indemnity plans, the insurance company has a contract with the insured. But a unique feature of MCOs is that it also has a contract with the provider. It is remarkable that, with this simple step, insurers created a dramatic alteration in health care delivery. The MCO has a well-defined, contractual relationship with both parties in the treatment setting, the patient and the provider. These dual contractual relationships allow the MCO to have a far greater presence in the consulting room.

In indemnity plans, the contract between the insurance company and the insured spelled out the obligations the insurance company has to the insured. In contrast, managed care contracts define a number of obligations for both insured members and providers. In indemnity plans, insured parties are typically free to seek treatment with any provider from any specialty they chose. In managed care, members must obtain treatment from a panel of providers, and usually initial treatment must be with a PCP, typically a family practice or internal medicine physician. The PCP makes referrals to specialists as necessary. Specialists are often not empowered to refer to other specialists; rather they must make a recommendation to the PCP, who can then follow through with subsequent referrals.

The dual contractual relationships of MCOs also underlie their position in making treatment-related decisions. In indemnity plans, the insurer is typically required to pay usual and customary fees for reasonable treatment. If reimbursement for a particular service is disputed, it is difficult for the insurer to prevail. An insurance company case manager is at a distinct disadvantage disputing a claim with a fully licensed, trained, and experienced provider who has direct contact with the patient and responsibility for the patient's care. However, MCO contracts usually require providers and patients to submit to UR, which is performed by staff that have varying degrees of clinical expertise. UR decisions must be accepted, with the understanding that appeals processes are available. Thus, there are clear mechanisms in managed care for reimbursement to be denied on clinical grounds.

Of equal importance, MCO reimbursement may also be denied on *administrative* grounds, and in this domain the case manager clearly has the upper hand. For example, certain services may need to be preauthorized; no preauthorization, no reimbursement. A member may be required to obtain a referral from the PCP to see a specialist; no referral, no reimbursement. An emergency department physician may be required to notify the MCO within 24 hours of a patient's being seen; no notification, no reimbursement. This last example is particularly interesting because the 24-hour notification rule seems arbitrary and not medically indicated or necessary. Many more examples come to mind, but the upshot is that the more rules there are, the more control the MCO has, the more ways that members and providers can err in following the rules, and the more reasons that reimbursement might be withheld. The really elegant part is that this can be done without ever addressing whether the treatment was reasonable or necessary.

By contracting with providers, MCOs can essentially hire and fire panel members at will. As a private company, an MCO can contract with anyone it wants to, without the competitive process that typically regulates government contracting. If a new provider is needed for a panel, the company's contract manager may select a person by an informal process, such as checking with the medical director, administrative colleagues, or other providers. Thus, a provider's reputation may be a very important aspect of being invited onto a panel. Providers may also be removed from a panel without cause, simply by having their contracts terminated. However, there usually is a reason for contract termination and this may include complaints from patients, failure to comply with MCO requirements, or unusually high levels of service utilization (e.g., consistently using up all of the patient's psychotherapy benefits in a short period of time). Although an insurance company should have the ability to work with whomever it chooses, the provider contracting process may become overly one-sided and arbitrary, and some states are taking steps to remedy this.

What can Neuropsychology Do?

If psychology is in a vulnerable position because "corporate America does not understand the nature of psychological services" (Cummings, 1988, p. 427) then neuropsychology is surely in a precarious situation. It seems crucial for the field of neuropsychology to step up and meet the challenge of managed care squarely. Individual practitioners confronting insurance case managers on a case-by-case basis is inherently inefficient and there are many issues that are much better addressed on an organizational level via such mechanisms as policies and standards. There are two fronts on which the health care delivery system can be engaged at present.

The first of these areas has to do with neuropsychology as a science. Neuropsychology needs to demonstrate its relevance to patient care. What do we, as a science, know? What do we add to the understanding of the patient? What is our unique contribution to the patient's care? What helpful recommendations can be made based on neuropsychological assessment? Ultimately, how does neuropsychological assessment improve the patient's treatment (Hayes, Nelson, & Jarrett, 1987; Stout, 1997)? Literally thousands of neuropsychological studies have been done and at least partial answers are available for most of these questions. Efforts are under way to compile this information and summarize it in a useful form (Reynolds, 1999). These efforts need to be regarded seriously by our profession, and the focus should be on what we know, what we contribute. Substantial philosophical differences were noted between the psychological training and medical school classes in this author's training. Psychology classes emphasized picking studies apart, finding methodological flaws, and reaching conclusions with great hesitancy. Certainly this is prudent when dealing with subject matter so complex as human behavior. This attitude seems to infuse the profession and is reflected in scholarly writings. However, it can be frustrating to read a psychological review paper that, after covering dozens of research studies and perhaps all of the extant studies in a given area, reaches the conclusion that we essentially don't know anything because of the various flaws in each of the studies. In contrast, lectures in medical school were liberally peppered with remarks such as "this is our current thinking on the subject," "this is a first approximation of the process," or "here is a useful guideline." While we should not abandon scientific rigor, some attention should be given to practical utility. Picture the situation of a patient coming to an emergency room with his hand severed, and the physician saying, "You know, there is quite a bit of controversy about how to treat that type of injury."

In the future, neuropsychology should emphasize research that has practical utility. Much needs to be done in demonstrating that neuropsychology provides unique information to case formulation, and ecological validity research will contribute to this. For example, neuropsychological research has begun to address driving ability and could contribute importantly to such decisions as release from the hospital, return to work, or need for supervision. Yet only limited ecological validity research exists to date (Sbordone & Long, 1996), and the frequency of these studies does not appear to be increasing. There is a tremendous need to develop and validate treatments for brain-impaired individuals, yet such studies rarely appear in neuropsychological journals. It is disappointing that neuropsychology, the profession that deals with 'brain–behavior relationships', is often relegated to a peripheral role in brain injury rehabilitation programs and there are some rehabilitation programs that do not even have a neuropsychologist on staff. It is clear that our field has the ability to respond to challenges such as these. For example, recent criticism of the ability of neuropsychologists to detect malingering was met with an explosion of relevant studies, and now the ability to detect malingering is actually a strength of forensic neuropsychological assessment.

The second issue has to do with neuropsychology as a profession. One often hears our professional organizations described as guilds. The definition of 'guild' is, in part, "an organization formed for mutual aid or protection, to set standards, and to protect the interests of its members." By this definition, none of our professional organizations comes close to being a guild, unfortunately. If neuropsychology is to be a part of future health care, then the profession must develop a mechanism for having a unified voice with the insurance industry and government policy makers. Sadly, at present our profession is fragmented; we have three major professional organizations, two major professional boards, and the ever-present split between academia and practice. While disagreement can lead to healthy dynamic tensions (Feldman, 1992b), there is also a time to come together. To not recognize this is to fiddle while Rome burns.

Although this makes for good rhetoric, the reality is that it is not easy for neuropsychologists to come together. Some recent examples highlight this. The definition of 'neuropsychologist' has been an ongoing controversy. The issue of having two professional boards (American Board of Clinical Neuropsychology, American Board of Professional Neuropsychology) is a source of ongoing dissension, and one that is periodically debated, often with much rancor, on Internet discussion groups. There are critics of both ABCN and ABPN, and those who criticize the concept of even having board certification. As another example, the Houston conference was an effort to establish some basic guidelines for education in neuropsychology (Hannay, Bieliauskas, Crosson, Hammeke, Hamsher, & Koffler, 1998). This too was met with suspicion and criticism, even from those who chose not to attend. Some colleagues may recall that a few years ago the late Oscar Parsons asked whether there was any interest in a cooperative effort to nationally norm a core neuropsychological battery. The reaction was so negative that it is doubtful that anyone will ever do that again! One of the criticisms was that if a basic 'core' battery was suggested, then this would be the only battery that insurance carriers will pay for. Undaunted by the current lack of standardization in neuropsychological assessment, insurance carriers are happy to make decisions about which tests they will reimburse and which they won't (Reynolds, 1999). How naïve science can be in the light of practical economics!

A recent personal example illustrates this point. I recently submitted a request to an insurer for preauthorization to assess a patient for ADHD. The battery included the WISC-III, WRAT-3, and a variety of neuropsychological measures. I was informed that formal evaluation for ADHD was not covered unless it was comorbid with another disorder, and most of the tests were not approved. I would be allowed an hour to administer a Stroop and Trail Making. Suggesting such an inadequate battery is inconsistent with the notions of quality improvement espoused by many insurers at present, and fuels criticism of this system of health care delivery. But it also underscores how poorly understood neuropsychology is by insurance case managers (and in this case, the decision was made by a psychologist), and how blind application of reimbursement policy without an understanding of neuropsychology can lead to inappropriate decisions. It also points out a shortcoming of the diversity of approaches employed by neuropsychologists along with a lack of minimum standards of assessment.

What can Neuropsychologists Do?

It seems that surviving in private practice requires a combination of clinical skill, business sense, and good fortune. In the past, a surfeit in one area could make up for deficits in the other two to some extent. The competitive environment that now accompanies managed health care has made it harder to flourish on one's strengths and easier to perish because of one's weaknesses. One could reasonably add to the controversy surrounding the modern relevance of the Boulder scientist-practitioner training model by suggesting it be replaced with a scientist-practitioner-business person model. Practitioners whose training did not include business practices may need to take remedial action, and the book by Yenney and APAPD (1994) can be helpful. Alternatively, the practitioner may want to hire a business consultant and APAPD (1994b) provides some useful, common sense guidelines for selecting this type of service.

There are a number of specific steps the neuropsychologist can take to maintain an independent practice in the present managed care environment. Basically, these relate to dealing with the MCO effectively, maintaining a flow of patients, reducing costs, and working more efficiently.

Contracting with MCOs

The first decision faced by the practitioner in dealing with a particular MCO is whether to join, and APAPD (1996) provided some helpful guidelines that assist the practitioner in making this decision. To determine if an MCO is an appropriate business partner, the practitioner should explore the following issues: staffing patterns (are they consistent with quality care?), annual staff turnover (over 15% may cause concern), membership (number of organizations, number of members, and growth), staff to member ratios, reimbursement rates (including how they are set, allowances for inflation, and recent changes), panel member satisfaction, appeals processes, and accreditation (NCQA or JCAHO). The practitioner might want to interview a few panel members regarding their experiences, and might also want to obtain financial documents from the MCO to assess the company's financial health. Final assessment of the MCO should be based on the information obtained along with how helpful the MCO is in this process.

In practice, on only the rare occasion may it be necessary to turn down an offer to join an MCO, and there are often indirect advantages to joining even less desirable MCOs. One reason is that the insurance industry is presently in flux, with many mergers and acquisitions, and along with these business deals there is often a merger of the companies' panels. Thus, being a panel member for a smaller, less desirable company can lead to being on the panel of a larger company, even when the larger company had previously denied one's application. Another potential benefit is that being on several MCO panels may 'look good' when one applies for membership on additional MCO panels.

It is important to carefully review MCO contracts before signing them, as their terms vary considerably. These contracts typically obligate providers to take reasonable steps such as maintaining a prescribed level of malpractice insurance, keeping their license current, and practicing in a reasonable fashion (e.g., within ethical guidelines). However, MCO provider contracts may include additional, sometimes controversial clauses. Some, such as 'gag' clauses that prevented providers from discussing certain treatment alternatives with patients or criticizing the MCO, have received wide publicity (Stout, 1997). No-cause termination clauses are common, and contracts may also include no-compete covenants (Higuchi & Coscia, 1995). Contractual clauses may be objectionable but still legal, making it difficult for the neuropsychologist to contest them after the contract is signed. The neuropsychologist may find discussion and negotiation with the MCO prior to signing the contract beneficial. Alternatively, bringing the matter to the attention of the local psychological association may be fruitful. Local and national organizations have had some success in getting MCOs to alter contract language (Higuchi & Coscia, 1995).

The increased paperwork required by MCOs starts at the very beginning, with the application for panel inclusion. MCO applications can be lengthy and require a substantial amount of time and effort to complete. Unfortunately, each MCO has its own application forms and so each application has to be approached independently. The application may also require additional documents, such as a copy of the applicant's professional license, proof of insurance, and letters of recommendation. Some MCOs charge an application fee as well. Maintaining membership on a panel typically requires that renewed license and insurance information be sent in periodically.

In some cases, the provider will need to make a formal proposal for inclusion on a MCO panel. These proposals should be carefully crafted to be precise yet informative and thus can entail a significant time investment. The practitioner should give careful thought as to whether it is worthwhile to undertake this endeavor. APAPD (1994c) suggests that the following areas should be covered in a proposal: a brief introduction, needs assessment, practice products and services, and evaluation procedures. Those with board certification should mention this credential, because it is an element of the structural aspect of QA, discussed earlier. In fact, some MCO applications include questions about board certification (i.e. "Are you board certified? If not, when will you be taking the board examination?"). Of course, once a proposal is developed it can serve as a template for proposals to other MCOs.

In the event that the application process is unsuccessful and the neuropsychologist is excluded from the panel, there is typically little available recourse (APAPD, 1994d). The neuropsychologist may want to get a written explanation for the denial to help with reapplication. If the MCO covers out of network providers, then the neuropsychologist may be able to accept referrals of the MCO's members under this provision. If the state has an 'any willing provider' statute or freedom of choice legislation, the neuropsychologist may have some recourse under these regulations. If the MCO is ERISA exempt, then most state laws won't be applicable.

Another potential problem is being removed from the panel, and typically the provider contract allows this to be done without cause (APAPD, 1993b). If this happens, the neuropsychologist should review the provider contract to determine whether the termination is legal and appropriate. If it is, then the MCO provider relations office can be contacted to determine what means for appeal or reconsideration are available. If a favorable response is obtained, confirm this in writing and then proceed with whatever steps the provider relations office suggested. In the appeal process, the neuropsychologist should emphasize his or her unique qualifications, the beneficial impact of his or her services on patient care, and positive aspects of the working relationship with the MCO. If the response from the provider relations office is not favorable, then the neuropsychologist may consider contacting the local psychological association and then proceeding with an official complaint to the MCO, copied to appropriate state regulatory agencies.

MCO payment methods and billing issues

Neuropsychologists who are used to being paid at an hourly rate may be unfamiliar with some of the reimbursement models used by MCOs (Stout, 1997). In HMOs, of course, the neuropsychologist is either an employee or a partner in the business and pay is generally on a salary basis. Payment may also be on a capitated basis, with the neuropsychologist receiving a set fee (usually per month) per enrolled member. The neuropsychologist agrees to provide whatever services are necessary for this fixed amount. This is a common payment method for IPAs. Network models, such as PPOs and EPOs, tend to pay on a per-service basis. Payment may be per hour, per evaluation, or per test. When contracting with an MCO, it is important to determine what reimbursement method is used and to then convert it into familiar terms (e.g., estimating how many referrals might be made in a capitated model, how long each test or battery will take, and then estimating the number of hours that will be required) to determine if the reimbursement rate is acceptable.

Billing requires a great deal of expertise and collection demands persistence. Frequently, MCOs emphasize prompt or 'hassle-free' payment but this is rarely stipulated in the contract and there is no provision for penalties should this promise not be kept. In fact, MCOs have introduced one new billing problem; variable rates and co-pays that from plan to plan. As a personal example, one MCO I work with has five different co-pay amounts depending on which specific plan the patient is under, and within a given plan different co-pays apply to different diagnoses. Failure to collect co-pays may be grounds for removal from the MCO panel and, in the case of Medicare, can constitute fraud.

Reimbursement is contingent on having all of the necessary patient information (often including a preauthorization number), and using the proper diagnostic and procedure codes. Claims forms must be filled out completely and carefully. Different companies may use different diagnostic codes (e.g., DSM or ICD) or different revisions of CPT codes. Computerization of billing is nearly essential, particularly given the increasing trend toward electronic billing, which is now required in 7 states (Frank & VandenBos, 1994). Billing should be done regularly, at least weekly or biweekly (APAPD, 1995).

Payments should be carefully reviewed for errors. In my experience they are relatively frequent and nearly always in the insurance company's favor. When claims are denied or underpaid, review them for clerical errors or misinterpretations. Return the claim for reprocessing, with a brief explanation of any problems that were found. A standardized letter asking for reconsideration can be helpful. Recurring errors may reflect a problem in the claims processing system and a discussion with the MCO can often clear these up (Peck, this volume).

Maintaining referrals

There are four elements to maintaining referrals. First, it is important to maintain the flow of referrals. In private practice it has always been important to network, to educate potential referral sources about the services neuropsychologists provide, and to do marketing as needed (Cummings, 1988; Maloney, Fixsen, & Phillips, 1985). Within the managed health care system, these activities continue to be appropriate and necessary. Targeting individuals for marketing or networking can be fairly easy. It is important that the insurance company has some understanding of neuropsychology and the services that can be provided by neuropsychologists. Medical directors or supervisors at the insurance carrier would be the most appropriate individuals to contact because they direct decision making and, in some situations, have the ability to affect policy. Networking with providers should be guided by the referral mechanisms of the company. Some insurers require that the PCP, typically an internist or family physician, make referrals. Some companies require a specialist, typically in psychiatry or neurology, to make the referral. More stringent is the requirement that both the specialist and the PCP agree on the referral. The providers who are capable of making the referral for neuropsychological services would be the obvious choice for networking/ marketing efforts.

Second, when a referral is initiated, the neuropsychologist can take proactive steps to facilitate the referral process. Many insurers now require a referral request form be completed. Some of these forms are short and easily completed. However, because these referral forms aren't standardized across insurers and because some of them are quite lengthy and detailed, completing them can be time consuming. Many require detailed information about the patient's status, the reason for referral, information on how the evaluation will positively impact care, what prior testing has been done and whether this was reviewed, and a list of proposed tests. Some require a full five-axis DSM-IV diagnosis, which seems unusual because neuropsychological testing is often done *to establish* the diagnosis.

Often the referral source is not sufficiently versed in neuropsychology to complete these forms accurately, and it also seems that the process of having to complete these forms can serve as a deterrent to making a referral. To facilitate referrals, the neuropsychologist may offer to either assist in completing the forms or to take on the responsibility entirely. In completing these forms, it is advisable to keep information simple and understandable. Remember that case managers are often not entirely clear what neuropsychology is, and they can be uncertain as to whether neuropsychological assessment is a mental health or medical benefit, an important distinction for many insurance carriers because of mental health carve-outs. An example might be helpful. As part of a diagnostic work-up, a neurologist refers a patient who is having seizure-like episodes and it is unclear whether these are epilepsy or pseudoseizures (e.g., psychogenic). The question is whether this patient has a psychological or neurological disorder. In completing the referral request, the justification for evaluation could be "to differentiate organic versus psychological factors contributing to apparent seizures." In some cases, this may cause the wheels at the insurance company to come to a resounding stop. The problem is, should this evaluation be covered by mental health or by medical benefits? This problem has happened more than once in my practice. A better justification would be "to determine if this individual is suffering the effects of brain damage." This would clearly fall under medical benefits and does not raise unnecessary controversy. Of course, this justification is proffered with the understanding that as part of this determination, psychological issues would need to be explored.

The third means of maintaining referrals is to take appropriate action when referrals are blocked. Whereas occasional difficulties with referrals occurred in the past, these problems are much more frequent now. In the past it wasn't much of a burden to write a letter or make a telephone call once in a while to clarify the reasons for a referral. However, problems happen so often now that it would be an administrative hardship. Some companies make it extremely difficult to argue one's position, and may require hours of phone calls to various representatives throughout the insurance company, with no real progress towards resolving the matter.

Because denials are more frequent and often more difficult to resolve, the practitioner may find it impossible to intercede effectively in all cases where a referral is blocked. It is important to allot this type of administrative time effectively. When a neuropsychologist begins working with an MCO, it is important to know the specific policies and procedures used by the company in making referrals, and this information is often (but not always) contained in a provider manual. Working within these guidelines, the first few denials by the MCO may be treated as 'test cases', to determine which steps are most effective in getting the denial retracted. As the neuropsychologist gains experience with various MCOs, efficiency can be increased by interceding with those insurance companies or case managers who seem most responsive, or by using methods that have worked the best. In other words, find a systematic way to work with the system.

Alternatively, the neuropsychologist can simply inform the patient that the service has been denied and consult the patient on how to proceed. Some patients may decide to contest the decision, and there are several options for this, ranging from informal remedies to litigation. An initial, informal, step for the patient would be to discuss the matter with the referring provider. Some MCOs have established mechanisms for appealing their decisions, although the effectiveness of these procedures is often in doubt. A helpful alternative is for the patient to discuss the matter with the human resource manager at his or her place of employment. The employer pays a great deal of money for employee health insurance benefits and often takes a keen interest when employees run into difficulty with the insurance carrier. Some patients may decide they want the evaluation and pay out of pocket. An extreme approach would be for the patient to contact the state insurance commission or an attorney. Regardless of what steps are taken, attrition in referrals should be planned for as it is unavoidable.

The fourth part of maintaining referrals is fostering a positive relationship with the MCO. An initial step is to read the provider contract and manual carefully — they are not all the same! Each company has different procedures and smooth functioning within that company requires that the provider and office staff are familiar with these. It is important to work within the guidelines of these contracts.

Maintaining personal contact with case managers is also useful. Concerns regarding referral patterns, expenses, or clinical practices can be discussed openly and resolved. As a personal example, I recently received several referrals of somewhat questionable appropriateness from one MCO. I initiated a meeting between with the MCO case manager and the referral source, at which point we were able to discuss concerns and clarify the circumstances under which these referrals would be made. During the meeting, the case manager indicated she had also become concerned about these referrals and she appreciated having the matter resolved in a positive, proactive fashion.

Summary

Managed health care has revolutionized the health care delivery system within which clinical neuropsychologists work. With it comes a new vocabulary, changes in the doctor-patient relationship, restrictions in practice, and external oversight of decisions that have traditionally been exclusively under the purview of the practitioner. To a large extent, managed health care has not been a positive experience for practitioners. Although it is easy to cast aspersions on things that we don't like, it is more productive to attempt to understand them and try to cope with them. Reviewing the history of managed health care provides a basis for understanding the forces governing this movement, and also the perspective that managed health care is not an evil entity descending on us but rather a concerted effort to solve a pressing social dilemma. There has been a great deal of give-and-take on all sides over the years and only recently has the health care practitioner been subjected to this process. Our health care problem isn't solved by a long shot. Health care costs continue to escalate. Companies facing an increasingly competitive business environment find it hard to afford health care benefits for their employees. Patients have fewer choices and higher out-of-pocket expenses. Health care providers face increased paperwork and reduced reimbursements. Many MCOs struggle to maintain profitability even with stringent cost-containment strategies. The government continues to have input via legislation and oversight. There is an ongoing dynamic dialog among these parties and the health care system will continue to change. To survive, the profession of neuropsychology must continue to promote it's relevance to patient welfare. The individual practitioner must adapt better business practices. We all must be flexible and willing to compromise.

References

Altman, L., & Price, W. (1993). Alcan Aluminum: development of a mental health carve out. In W. Goldman & S. Feldman (Eds.), *Managed mental health care* (pp. 55–65). San Francisco: Josey-Bass Publishers.

American Academy of Neurology (1996). Assessment: neuropsychological testing of adults. Considerations for neurologists. Report of the Therapeutics and Technology Assessment Subcommittee of the American Academy of Neurology. *Neurology*, *47*, 592–599.

American Board of Quality Assurance & Utilization Review Physicians (1997). *A practical guide to legal issues in utilization and risk management*. Gaithersburg, MD: Aspen Publishers.

American Psychiatric Association (1988). *The coverage catalogue*. Washington, DC: APA Press.

American Psychiatric Association (1994). *Diagnostic and statistical manual of mental disorders* (4th ed.). Washington, DC: American Psychiatric Association.

American Psychological Association Practice Directorate (1993a). *Practice pointer: What to look for in your state utilization review law*. Washington, DC: American Psychological Association.

American Psychological Association Practice Directorate (1993b). *Practice pointer: How to handle 'no cause' terminations from managed care panels.* Washington, DC: American Psychological Association.

American Psychological Association Practice Directorate (1994a). *APA member focus groups on the health care environment: a summary report.* Washington, DC: American Psychological Association.

American Psychological Association Practice Directorate (1994b). *Practice pointer: using business consultants to your advantage.* Washington, DC: American Psychological Association.

American Psychological Association Practice Directorate (1994c). *Practice pointer: What to include in a managed care proposal.* Washington, DC: American Psychological Association.

American Psychological Association Practice Directorate (1994d). *Practice pointer: How to handle exclusion from an MCO panel.* Washington, DC: American Psychological Association.

American Psychological Association Practice Directorate (1995). *Practice pointer: evaluating your insurance claims procedures.* Washington, DC: American Psychological Association.

American Psychological Association Practice Directorate (1996). *Practice pointer: criteria for reviewing an organized delivery system.* Washington, DC: American Psychological Association.

Appelbaum, P.S. (1993). Legal liability and managed care. *American Psychologist, 48*, 251-257.

Avnet, H. (1962). *Psychiatric insurance.* New York: Group Health Insurance.

Bennett, M.J. (1992). Managed mental health in health maintenance organizations. In S. Feldman (Ed.), *Managed mental health services*, (pp. 61–82). Springfield, IL: Charles C. Thomas.

Berlant, J.L. (1992). Quality assurance in managed mental health. In S. Feldman (Ed.), *Managed mental health services* (pp. 201–221). Springfield, IL: Charles C. Thomas.

Bickman, L., Guthrie, P. R., Foster, E. M., Lambert, E. W., Summerfelt, W. T., Breda, C. S., & Heflinger, C. A. (1995). *Evaluating managed mental health services: The Fort Bragg experiment.* New York: Plenum.

Bingaman, J., Frank, R.G., & Billy, C.L. (1993). Combining a global health budget with a market-driven delivery system. *American Psychologist, 48*, 270–276.

Binner, P.R. (1986). DRGs and the administration of mental health services. *American Psychologist, 41*, 64–69.

Congressional Budget Office (1993). *Trends in health care spending: an update.* Washington, DC: Congressional Budget Office.

Cullen, E.A. (1997). 'Dr. David' tames one managed care goliath. *Practitioner Focus, 10(2)*, 1, 14.

Cummings, N.A. (1988). The dismantling of our health system. *American Psychologist, 41*, 426–431.

Cunningham, R., & Cunningham, R.M. (1997). *The Blues: A history of the Blue Cross and Blue Shield system.* DeKalb, IL: Northern Illinois University Press.

Dangerfield, D., & Betit, R.L. (1993). Managed mental health care in the public sector. In W. Goldman & S. Feldman (Eds.), *Managed mental health care* (pp. 67–80). San Francisco: Josey-Bass Publishers.

Daschle, T.A., Cohen, R.J., & Rice, C.L. (1993). Health-care reform: single-payer models. *American Psychologist, 48*, 265–269.

DeLeon, P.H., Uyeda, M.K., & Welch, B.L. (1985). Psychology and HMOs: new partnership or new adversary? *American Psychologist, 40*, 1122–1124.

Donabedian, A. (1980). *Explorations in quality assessment and monitoring. Volume 1: The definition of quality and approaches to its assessment.* Ann Arbor, MI: Health Administration Press.

Drum, D.J. (1995). Changes in the mental health service delivery and finance systems and resulting implications for the national register. *Register Report*, *20*(3), 4, 5, 8–10.

Durenberger, D. & Foote, S.B. (1993). Beyond incrementalism: designing an infrastructure for reform. *American Psychologist*, *48*, 277–282.

Feldman, S. (Ed.). (1992a). *Managed mental health services*. Springfield, IL: Charles C. Thomas.

Feldman, S. (1992b). Managed mental health services: ideas and issues. In S. Feldman (Ed.), *Managed mental health services* (pp. 3–26). Springfield, IL: Charles C. Thomas.

Frank, R.G., & Lave, J.R. (1992). Economics of managed mental health. In S. Feldman (Ed.), *Managed mental health services* (pp. 83–99). Springfield, IL: Charles C. Thomas.

Frank R.G., & VandenBos, G.R. (1994). Health care reform: the 1993-1994 evolution. *American Psychologist*, *49*, 851–854.

Gabel, J., DiCarlo, S., Fink, S., & deLissovoy, G. (1989). Employer-sponsored health insurance in America. *Health Affairs*, 8, 116–128.

Goran, M.J. (1992). Managed mental health and group health insurance. In S. Feldman (Ed.), *Managed mental health services*, (pp. 27–43). Springfield, IL: Charles C. Thomas.

Hager, M. (1983). $290 billion a year — and growing! *Consumers Digest*, *25*(4), 10–12, 50–51.

Hall, M.A., & Ellman, I.M. (1990). *Health care law and ethics*. St. Paul, MN: West Publishing.

Hannay, H.J., Bieliauskas, L., Crosson, B.A., Hammeke, T.A., Hamsher, K.deS., & Koffler, S. (1998). Proceedings of the Houston conference on specialty education and training in clinical neuropsychology. *Archives of Clinical Neuropsychology*, *13*, 157–249.

Hayes, S.C., Nelson, R.O., & Jarrett, R.B. (1987). The treatment utility of assessment: a functional approach to evaluating assessment quality. *American Psychologist*, *42*, 963–974.

Higuchi, S., & Coscia, J. (1995). Provider contracting issues are central to legal agenda. *Practitioner Focus*, *8*, 1–4.

Hughey, V. (1997). *24-hour health care coverage and workers' compensation*. Carson City, NV: Nevada Legislative Counsel Bureau.

Institute of Medicine (1989). *Controlling cost and changing patient care*. Washington, DC: NAS Press.

Kerry, B., & Hofschire, P.J. (1993). Hidden problems in current health-care financing and potential changes. *American Psychologist*, *48*, 261–264.

Kiesler, C.A. (1992). U.S. mental health policy: doomed to fail. *American Psychologist*, *47*, 1077–1082.

Kiesler, C.A., & Morton, T.L. (1988). Psychology and public policy in the "health care revolution". *American Psychologist*, *43*, 993–1003.

Kiesler, C.A., & Sibulkin, A. (1987). *Mental hospitalization: myths and facts about a national crisis*. Newbury Park, CA: Sage.

Kiesler, C.A., & Simpkins, C. (1991). The de facto national system of psychiatric inpatient care: piecing together the national puzzle. *American Psychologist*, *46*, 579–584.

Knapp, S., & Bowers, T. (1996). A survey of Pennsylvania psychologists on managed care and other issues. *Psychotherapy in Private Practice*, *15*, 33–43.

Kunnes, R. (1992). Managed mental health: the insurer's perspective. In S. Feldman (Ed.), *Managed mental health services* (pp. 101–125). Springfield, IL: Charles C. Thomas.

Letsch, S.W. (1993). National health care spending in 1991. *Health Affairs*, *12*(1), 94–110.

Maloney, D.M., Fixsen, D.L., & Phillips, E.L. (1985). Marketing your produce: the psychologist as communicator. *American Psychologist*, *40*, 961–962.

Manning et al. (1984). A controlled trial of the effect of a prepaid group practice on use of services. *New England Journal of Medicine*, 1505–1510.

Martinson, J.N. (1988). Are HMOs slamming the door on psych treatment? *Hospitals*, *62*, 50–56.

Mechanic, D. (1987). Correcting misconceptions in mental health policy: strategies for improved care of the seriously mentally ill. *The Millbank Quarterly*, *65*, 203–230.

Merlis, M. (1993, January 22). *Medicaid: an overview*. (Congressional Research Service report for Congress).

Moldawski, S. (1990). Is solo practice really dead? *American Psychologist*, *45*, 544–546.

Pallak, M.S., Cummings, N.A., Dorken, H., & Henke, C.J. (1993). Managed mental health, Medicaid, and medical cost offset. In W. Goldman & S. Feldman (Eds.), *Managed mental health care* (pp. 27–40). San Francisco: Josey-Bass Publishers.

Passkey for health insurance licensing, (5th ed.) (1993). Chicago: Dearborn-R & R Newkirk.

Pearson, J. (1992). Managed mental health: the buyer's perspective. In S. Feldman (Ed.), *Managed mental health services*, (pp. 127–142). Springfield, IL: Charles C. Thomas.

Pedulla, D.M., & Rocke, S. (1999). Demystifying ERISA: understanding the basics of a complex law. *Practitioner Focus*, *12*(1), 3, 18.

Phelps, R., Eisman, E.J., & Kohout, J. (1998). Psychological practice and managed care: Results of the CAPP practitioner survey. *Professional Psychology: Research and Practice*, *29*, 31–36.

Physician Payment Review Commission (1994). *Annual report to Congress 1994*. Washington, DC: Psysician Payment Review Commission.

Puente, A.E. (1994). Billing recommendations and CPT codes for neuropsychological assessment. *Bulletin of the National Academy of Neuropsychology*, *11*, 14–15.

Putnam, S.H. (1989). The TCN salary survey: A salary survey of neuropsychologists. *The Clinical Neuropsychologist*, *3*, 97–115.

Putnam, S.H., & Anderson, C. (1994). The second *TCN* salary survey: A survey of neuropsychologists part I. *The Clinical Neuropsychologist*, *8*, 3–37.

Reynolds, C.R. (1999). President's message: on mangled care and other matters. *Newsletter 40*, *17*, 1–9.

Rocke, S. (1999). Psychology deals with ERISA's impact in court. *Practitioner Focus*, *12*(1), 3, 15.

Sbordone, R.J., & Long, C. (Eds.). (1996). *Ecological validity of neuropsychological testing*. Delray Beach, FL: GR Press/St. Lucie Press.

Schieber, G.J., & Poullier, J.P. (1991). International health spending: issues and trends. *Health Affairs*, *10*, 106–116.

Shapiro, A.E. (1995). Managing managed care. *Psychotherapy in Private Practice*, *14*, 57–66.

Shapiro, A.E., & Wiggins, J.G. (1994). A PsyD degree for every practitioner. *American Psychologist*, *49*, 207–210.

Shore, K. (1995). Managed care: the subjugation of a profession. *Psychotherapy in Private Practice*, *14*, 67–75.

Stevens, R. (1989). *In sickness and in wealth: American hospitals in the twentieth century*. New York: Basic Books.

Stout, C.E. (1997). *Psychological assessment in managed care*. New York: John Wiley & Sons.

Sweet, J.J., Moberg, P.J., & Suchy, Y. (2000). Ten-year follow-up of clinical neuropsychologists: part I. Practices and beliefs. *The Clinical Neuropsychologist, 14*, 18–37.

Sweet, J.J., Westergaard, C.K., & Moberg, P.J. (1995). Managed care experiences of clinical neuropsychologists. *The Clinical Neuropsychologist, 9*, 214–218.

Tanney, F. (1989). Comment on Zimet's mental health care revolution. *American Psychologist, 44*, 1334–1335.

VandenBos, G.S. (1993). U.S. mental health policy: proactive evolution in the midst of health care reform. *American Psychologist, 48*, 283–290.

Vein, C.A., & Cullen, E.A. (1996). APA influences evolution of NCQA accreditation standards. *Practitioner Focus, 9*(3), 1.

Virginia lawsuit propels legal initiative to curb MCO abuses (1999). *Practitioner Update, 7(1)*, 1, 4.

Wicherski, M., Woerheide, K., & Kohout, J. (1996). *Salaries in psychology 1995.* Washington, DC: American Psychological Association.

Williams, S., Wicherski, M., & Kohout, J. (1998). *Salaries in psychology 1997: report of the 1997 APA salary survey.* Washington, DC: American Psychological Association.

Yenney, S. L., & American Psychological Association Practice Directorate (1994). *Business strategies for a caring profession: a practitioner's guidebook.* Washington, DC: American Psychological Association.

Chapter 6

NEUROPSYCHOLOGY RESEARCH IN A PRIVATE PRACTICE SETTING

M. Frank Greiffenstein

Introduction

Neuropsychology has its share of myths, one of the more enduring of which is that private practice neuropsychologists (PPN) are unable to conduct peer-reviewed research (Dodrill, 1997). This belief has some historical foundation in the long-standing antagonism between pure scientists and pure clinicians. Graduate schools used the Boulder Model of training as a template for producing a seamless combination of the practitioner and scientist roles (Raimy, 1950). Sadly, the Boulder Model is an ideal that has had little influence on professional behavior (Davison, 1998; Wegener, Hagglund, & Elliott, 1998). Contemporary surveys still show strongly positive attitudes toward this concept of paired roles, and many psychologists identify themselves as examples of such a model. Yet, this ideal is not concretely actualized as most clinical psychologists still do not engage in or publish research.

Another myth is that neuropsychologists are more research oriented than their generalist clinical counterparts are. My tabulation of original research articles in The Clinical Neuropsychologist (TCN) 1990–2000 shows low representation by first authors with solo or incorporated group practices. The modal number of publications per year was one, and the maximum was four (in 1995). This lack of research production is even more striking when one considers the growth of private practice. Putnam and Anderson (1994) found that 35% of neuropsychologists were in solo or group practices while Sweet, Moberg and Westergaard (1996) found 47% of Division 40 members to be private practitioners. Most recently, 58% of APA Division 40 members reported employment in private practice (Sweet, Moberg & Suchy, 2000; see also Chapter 3). Clearly, the growth in private practice neuropsychology has not been matched by growth in publications. If anything, PPN are increasingly *uninvolved* in research endeavors.

Several factors may be inhibiting the research involvement of practicing clinicians. First, there is the large discrepancy between training and employment settings. Abrahamson & Pearlman (1993), commenting on the general field of clinical psychology, note the lack of postgraduate employment opportunities that support internalization of the dual role. In 1988, only 23% of neuropsychologists worked in a medical school setting where such an ideal is most likely to be realized (Putnam & DeLuca, 1990). By 1994, only 14% worked in a medical school setting (Putnam & Anderson, 1994). Sweet et al. (2000) pointedly discussed this development in their survey of ABPP and Division 40 members. PPN may feel special pressure to produce income and market their services, leaving little opportunity for research.

The second inhibiting factor is attitudinal. PPN may have antagonistic attitudes toward research-oriented neuropsychology. To paraphrase Meehl (1954), research neuropsychologists may be perceived by PPN as "atomistic, dead, pedantic, rigid, sterile and blind" while PPN view themselves as "global, deep, genuine, meaningful, sensitive, real, living, concrete." This antagonism is only worsened by contemporary professional trends. Schools of professional psychology, Master's level counseling programs, neuropsychology certification workshops and remote-campus credentialing programs are producing neuropsychology practitioners with limited knowledge of scientific issues. The third inhibiting factor is conceptual: Science and practice may never be unified because of differences in paradigms (Strickler, 1997). Researchers and PPN may not share similar concepts, orientation to problems, vocabularies, methodologies or even the same social backgrounds. If there is no agreement on what constitutes scientific evidence, if there is no consensus on crucial vs. trivial findings, then there is little hope for rapprochement. A good example of this is the controversy between PPN who insist that subjective complaints have validity as indicators of closed head injury and the research consensus that such complaints are common and nonspecific. Indeed, the chief weakness of PPN is isolation from a shared community of research vocabulary and ideals. This may be why certain diagnostic myths persist between PPN and academics.

The purpose of this chapter is to offer neuropsychology practitioners guidelines for making research an important part of practice. This chapter first describes the circumstances enabling research, and then provides a systematic outline for conducting research. Sections include defining the population of interest, hypothesis generation, database construction, methodological considerations, data analysis, common logical pitfalls, writing and submission. The final section presents a real world example of the author's archival research that illustrates the steps in concrete fashion. Peer reviewed, high quality, practical research is possible from the private practice setting.

Research Enabling Factors

A number of developments have made private practice research possible. The first enabling factor is the personal computer (PC) revolution. The importance of the PC cannot be overstated. The PC has freed the neuropsychologist from dependence on university based mainframe computers and software. Complex data analyses that used to take up large memory space on mainframes can now be run on inexpensive computers in the office or at home. The clinician no longer needs to be physically present at or formally affiliated with a university to run data analyses.

The second research enabling development for PPN is the large increase in journals devoted to neuropsychology. In the earliest phase of professional neuropsychology, academic neuropsychologists had the best chance of getting papers published in journals such as *Neuropsychologia* and *Cortex*. The focus of these journals was predominately of theoretical interest. Only the *Journal of Consulting and Clinical Psychology* and a few medical journals offered the occasional neuropsychology paper dealing with everyday diagnostic issues. Currently, more than a dozen journals are devoted just to neuropsychology (Sweet et al., 2000). Many other medical, psychology and scientific journals accept neuropsychology submissions. Further, some of these journals appeal directly to the interests of PPN (e.g., *The Clinical Neuropsychologist*). PPN cannot argue that there are too few outlets for their work.

The third research enabling development for PPN is the commercial availability of inexpensive but powerful database and statistical software. These tools are becoming more 'user friendly.' For example, *SPSS* (Norusis, 1993) has moved from the mainframe to a Windows desktop operating system. Built-in menus and tutors allow clinicians to work out design problems without seeking help from consultants (or that semi-retired statistics professor who no longer remembers your name).

The fourth development is easier access to knowledge and scientific literature. The explosive growth of the Internet, the World Wide Web and local area networks have had effects similar to that of the PC, namely, freeing the clinician from dependence on large institutions (see Chapter 7). Abstracts and reprints are easily obtainable at no or nominal charge. Whole articles can now be stored and downloaded because of inexpensive optical storage systems. There are fewer frustrations in getting a pristine reprint of an article, because software such as Adobe Acrobat® allows perfect copies of reprints to be downloaded off the Internet. PubMed™ and LoansomeDoc™ are excellent online interactive databases free of charge. PPN who have staff privileges can apprise themselves of special services offered by the hospital library such as a free article clipping.

Another enabling factor is an emerging paradigm shift. Strickler & Trierweiler (1995) offer an interesting synthesis of the scientist-practitioner roles. Their model for clinical practice is termed "The Local Clinical Scientist." The essential idea is that the practitioner functions as a scientist in a local setting.

The Local Clinical Scientist deals with immediate clinical issues in the office with the same rigorous, disciplined and critical thought that characterizes the scientist working in the laboratory. The same skepticism and curiosity of a scientist are applied not only to the local patient group, but also to private practice neuropsychologists' own belief structures (e.g., potential diagnostic myths). The chief limitation of this approach is generalizability, but the hope is that general principles may emerge if there is replication of results among many local scientists.

The final factor is purely inspirational. Medical scientist-practitioners proposed the most enduring first principles of neuropsychology. Broca, Wernicke, Ribot and Goldstein were all practitioners who developed brain–behavior laws based on systematic observation of their own patients. In fact, a major part of the modern neuropsychology's foundation is the traditional clinical-anatomic method — an empirical protocol that required the medical doctor to follow patients from disease onset to the autopsy table. Clinical material is the most powerful heuristic available.

Practical Guidelines for Designing Studies in Private Practice

1. Select the population of interest

As a 'local' scientist, focus on the patients you are most likely to encounter. Estimate the diagnostic base rates in your practice for the past year. Two to three groups may account for most referrals. If for example half of the referral base is litigating late postconcussive patients or dementia patients, then data collection should be focused on these groups. If the primary referral source is psychiatric, examine for base rates of such disorders as mood disorders, schizophrenia, etc. There are many interesting neuropsychological issues with these patients that bear more thorough examination.

2. Hypothesis generation

The first critical cognitive activity of the researcher is generation of research ideas. All remaining steps of the research process will flow readily if one begins with a clearly stated research idea. For example, the database construction phase is much easier to manage once a research idea is concretely formulated. There is no 'cookbook' approach to hypothesis generation. Effective hypothesis generation is the spontaneous end product of a clinician's synthesis of academic, test methodology, and experiential knowledge.

There are, however, some concrete guidelines for generating research ideas. First, state in simple terms the area in which you wish to do research (e.g., "I want to examine executive cognitive skills in borderline personality patients"). Second, develop basic knowledge about what research has been conducted to date. It is very important to develop a good summary of the relevant literature. *Medline* or the APA journal *Neuropsychology Abstracts* are excellent resources. Start the hypothesis generation process by reading one or two good review articles. Next, collect key articles relevant to the chosen patient population or test instrumentation. This step does not require encyclopedic knowledge of neuropsychology in general nor of any narrow issue in particular. The focus should be on key, crucial articles. Dodrill (1997) rightfully complains about the poor quality and redundant nature of neuropsychological research, a problem that can be resolved only with a good understanding of what has been done. This requires a discriminating and skeptical approach as outlined in the 'local scientist' model. Third, determine your cognitive satisfaction level with the conclusions reached by researchers. The 'key' research approach outlined above does not imply limiting oneself to the best research. Questionable research can be an excellent starting point if such research has been influential in shaping clinical decision-making. For example, are you confident that the Tinker Toy test is a valid measure of executive cognitive skills, or are you annoyed at the myth driven nature of conclusions based on this test? Do you disagree with the findings of Greiffenstein, Baker, & Gola (1994) regarding questionable test taking motivation by late postconcussion patients? In such sentiments, you may have the beginnings of a research topic. Mere dissatisfaction with a published result because it is undesirable for your practice is not sufficient grounds for a new study: The specific conceptual, paradigmatic or methodological issues underlying your concern have to be identified and articulated.

3. Database construction

The next step is the construction of a relational database (RDB; McGee, 1997). Data are continuously and automatically entered into a computerized database in this system. The database developer must first define the variables to be coded. Ideally, effective database construction depends strongly on hypothesis generation, not the other way around. The variables you select for systematic collection will flow naturally and flow best only after you have defined the research issue in concrete, measurable terms. Simply creating a RDB with multiple variables of convenience is a mindless activity, and the clinician rapidly finds himself/herself rapidly overwhelmed with the sheer volume of variables in the absence of an organizing theme. To use the parlance of the Internet, keep the principle of GIGO in mind (Garbage In, Garbage Out).

Realistically however, most busy clinicians are unlikely to have the time to develop a systematic research program organized around a theme. One way of resolving the time limitation issue is to develop a root database. This relational database quantifies cases with a small set of variables. The root database is constructed by entering a small set of identifying information on every client. For example, a root database may contain only the patient's name, age, sex, education, lesion location and disease type. This database can be managed by an office manager, an assistant or by the clinician once a month. Clinicians with better financial resources could also hire a graduate student or clerk to enter data.

When PPN eventually develop research ideas, the 'select cases' feature of the RDB program can be used to identify subgroups of clients relevant to the chosen topic. For example, a clinician that specializes in brain cancer may become interested in the effects of right frontal tumors on visual memory in females. The select cases command calls up cases of high school educated females above age 20 with right frontal lesions. Most database programs (like *SPSS*) have an 'exclude cases' command that deletes cases not meeting the selection criteria. This subset from the root database can be renamed and saved. This constitutes the new study database. The study database is then expanded by adding new variables such as test scores, psychosocial status (employment, marital status, psychiatric status etc.) and medical status variables (e.g., radiation vs. chemotherapy, total *Gy* dosage). A sample root RDB is presented in Table 1.

The study database should be divided into two general areas — independent and dependent variables. Independent refers to the grouping or blocking criterion while dependent refers to the variable of interest. Most of

Table 1. Sample root database

Variable name (Code)	Variable type	Field size	Coding instructions
Name (Name)	String	15	10 letters of last name, 5 letters from first
Age (AGE)	Numeric	3	In years
Schooling (EDUC)	Numeric	2	Years *completed*
Gender (SEX)	Numeric	1	Male = 1, Female = 2
Employment (EMPLOY)	Numeric	1	In workforce = 1, Not in workforce = 2
Disease Category (DX)	Numeric	2	Normal = 1, Trauma = 2, Tumor = 3, Atrophic = 4, Other =5
Lesion Type (LES)	Numeric	1	None = 1, Focal = 2, Multifocal = 3, Diffuse = 4, Other = 5
Lesion Laterality (LESLAT)	Numeric	1	None = 1, Right = 2, Left = 3, Bilateral = 4, Diffuse = 5
Primary diagnosis (PRIMDX)	String	50	Type physician's diagnosis, e.g., Parkinson's with dementia
CT Findings (CTTEXT)	String	50	Type radiologist's summary impressions directly from report

the research PPN perform is likely to be of the quasi-experimental variety, meaning non random assignment to groups. Instead, the groups are naturally predetermined. In a neuropsychology context, disease category is the most common attribute for assignment to groups. A good database should include some element of traditional categories such as lesion laterality (right vs. left), caudality (frontal vs. nonfrontal) and topography (focal vs. diffuse). There are also many other meaningful analytic categories that can serve as independent variables such as EEG findings, age, gender, education, social class, etc. The dependent variables will most likely be test scores, but they can also be social outcome variables, blood-plasma levels of psychotropic medication, or coded behavior observations. Of course, this paragraph refers to categorical distinctions and is only meant as an illustration, not an attempt at exclusion of other forms of analysis. Correlational and regression analyses may be performed on continuous data. The point is that the database should contain some distinction between what is known and what is to be predicted.

4. Research design

Most PPN are likely to work in conditions allowing only nonexperimental research. As defined by Kerlinger (1986), nonexperimental research is systematic inquiry in which the scientist does not have direct control of independent variables because their manifestations have already occurred or because they are inherently not manipulable. Inferences about relations among variables are made, without direct intervention, from concomitant variation of independent and dependent variables. This is also termed quasi-experimental design (Campbell & Stanley, 1963). Like their counterparts at university hospitals, PPN deal with extant groups that select themselves by their neurological attributes: They come to the office with closed head injuries, brain neoplasms, strokes, etc. The PPN cannot create these lesions in randomly assigned patients. The operating assumption underlying the remainder of this chapter is that the practitioner deals predominantly with assessment cases, meaning a research program will take the form of exploring archival data.

There are two essential differences between experimental and nonexperimental designs. Experimental designs allow control over the independent variable and there is greater confidence in assertions about cause–effect relationships ("condition X caused behavior Y"). In nonexperimental research, the conditional logic of "X is responsible for Y" is still possible but less straightforward. However, the nonrandom selection of groups means selection of uncontrolled variables associated with group membership that may confound explanations. For example, it is well known that closed head injury patients are more likely to be young sensation seeking men. A control group of college undergraduates or even social peers may differ in more ways than simply the absence of a closed head injury. Unless very tightly controlled for by selection of a control group with similar premorbid problems, the presence of uncontrolled attributes makes simple causal statements problematic. For example, the causal assertion "mild closed head injury causes impulse control deficits as measured by a conceptual tempo test" is easily disputed if one has two groups differing in more ways than just injury status. The Dikmen, Machamer, Winn, and Temkin (1995) study of closed head injury outcome is an example of successful control of social characteristics that will lead to more defensible causation conclusions.

The manner in which you compare and contrast groups does not have to be complicated. The difficult part is selection of the appropriate control group (or control measure). The comparison group may be as simple as the standardization sample means and standard deviations from a test manual. The ideal control group would be local patients sharing as many relevant psychosocial and medical attributes with the target group as possible. For example, if the interest were in late postconcussion syndrome (patients with persistent functional complaints years after minor head trauma), it would be important to find a similar comparison group. Much depends on the hypothesis. There are literally dozens of research designs from which to choose, but the selection is made easy if you recognize the constraints imposed by the population with whom you work. By and large, the private practice clinician is likely to conduct research on archival data. That is not to say that true experimental research cannot be conducted by PPN. For example, the study of cognitive rehabilitation efficacy requires random double blind assignment to treatment groups.

5. Recognizing common logical pitfalls

The practitioner-researcher also need not be particularly sophisticated about research design, but she should be aware of the most common design pitfalls, technically known as internal and external threats to validity (Campbell & Stanley, 1963). Internal validity refers to uncontrolled factors that compete with the independent variable as the best explanation for results. Another term for this is a confounding variable. Internal threats to validity are dealt with by proper selection of control cases and/or control tasks. In neuropsychology, a common example of threat to internal validity is the co-existence of nonspecific and specific deficits in cerebral dysfunction (Parsons & Prigatano, 1978). For example, a study in which there is one brain-damaged group compared to a normal control group, one cannot be sure that a significant difference on a test score is due to the general decrements in adaptive behavior or due to the specific brain disease localization.

External threats to validity are factors limiting generalization of results to other populations (i.e., the representativeness of your sample). Experimental findings may only be valid for a local sample but may not be valid for any other group with similar characteristics. Self-selection (or case selection) is the chief form that this threat takes. Of course, self-selection is present in any nonexperimental design, but problematic self-selection occurs when a researcher selects cases based on an attribute illogically extraneous to the research problem. A fictional example is the researcher who studies the health outcomes of golfing. The researcher selects cases from an urgent care facility next to a large golf course and finds that 80% of golfers die after being struck by lightning. The golfers select themselves into the study by the attribute of treatment at an emergency room. The researcher concludes that golf is the most dangerous sport in the world. This example may seem absurd, but similar faulty generalizations based on a case selection design can be found in the literature. For example, Leininger, Kreutzer, and Hill (1991) examined the MMPI profiles of "unrecovered" late postconcussion patients and concluded that personality changes from minor head trauma were more dramatic than changes resulting from severe closed head injury. Dikmen, Reitan, Temkin, & Machamer (1992) later cured this fallacy by demonstrating the different result obtained by giving the MMPI to unselected consecutive head injury admissions from first point of care. It can be difficult to control this kind of threat to validity, because this threat can stem from a particular geographical location, unique referral base, point-of care station, institutional idiosyncrasies, and so forth. That is not to say that case selection is an invalid research design. Studying a patient subgroup, especially a poor outcome group, can be important (e.g., identification of risk factors for poor therapy response). The design becomes problematic only if illogical or overly expansive generalizations are made. The best way to deal with threats to external validity is to discuss the limits to generalization in the discussion section of the paper.

Criterion contamination is a particularly common pitfall. Criterion contamination occurs when the independent and dependent variables are hopelessly intertwined, resulting in guaranteed rejection of the null hypothesis. In other words, the independent and dependent variables are nearly identical in content. In extreme cases, the dependent variable is the same one used to form the groups. An example of criterion contamination is the study of anosmia by Varney (1988). He selected cases in which patients with minor head injuries claimed unusually long disability (the grouping variable) following minor head trauma. Employment was his dependent variable, and he found nearly 100% unemployment in his postconcussion patients with alleged anosmia. Varney concluded that subtle frontal lobe damage associated with anosmia causes major psychosocial problems. Note that the criterion of 'long term disability' contaminated the dependent variable of 'employment' because employability is a major facet of disability. The author chose the Varney study as an example only because he is familiar with the anosmia research. Greiffenstein and Baker (2002) formed anosmic and nonanosmic groups based on criteria independent of the dependent variables. They found no differences in employment rate at long term follow-up, nor did they find executive cognitive deficits particularly associated with anosmia.

6. Data analysis

There are many statistical software packages available for purchase. Most of the research that a busy clinician will conduct will require only the most rudimentary statistical operations. There is no need to get an expensive package of statistical software that includes every known statistical procedure.

SPSS for example offers dozens of expensive add-ons, in addition to the core program. Unless your practice is evolving into a contractual research organization, it is best to simply get a package that includes the basic parametric, nonparametric and correlational tools.

Analyze your results as completely as possible. Organize the statistical output into tables and graphs before you even write a word of your results section. A bare minimum of two types of tables or graphs is mandatory for peer-reviewed research. The first is a table of statistics that summarizes group characteristics. Compare means of the group's identification data to see how closely they are matched as this is often important. Any significant differences in your preselected groups need to be addressed (e.g., how do pre-existing differences affect your conclusions, do they weaken the conclusions or actually make them stronger?). The second mandatory table (or graph) is one that summarizes relations between the independent and dependent variables, or one that summarizes correlations. The most rudimentary form is a table summarizing differences on neuropsychological test scores (the dependent variables) between a brain defective group and a medical control group (the independent variable).

7. Paper preparation and submission

Dodrill (1997) provides concrete steps for this final phase of the research endeavor. It is difficult to improve on his advice. Select a target journal for the paper before even starting the manuscript. It is essential to have some understanding of the 'sociology' behind a journal's editorial style (i.e., 'know your audience'). You would probably not send an article on syntactic processing by aphasic patients to *Psychological Assessment*, but you might send it to *Neuropsychologia*. Similarly, an article on the *MMPI* profiles of traumatically brain-injured patients has a good chance at *Psychological Assessment*, but little chance at *Neuropsychologia*. The underlying scheme is that *Psychological Assessment* is concerned with practical assessment issues, while *Neuropsychologia* is devoted to theoretical issues. Other caveats include making sure to include references to recent publications in the same journal on the same topic. Make sure the article has similar length and style to other articles.

Dictate a rough draft according to a simple outline as advised by Ralph Reitan (cited in Dodrill, 1997): Background and literature review, Methods, Results and Discussion. This can be finished in one day. Next, further subdivide the report into sections that are demanded by the target journal. This can be APA style or Index Medicus style, depending on what journal you choose. A useful practice is to keep a file of photocopied 'Instructions for Authors' from all the major journals. Most journals currently maintain websites that contain instructions to authors. This way there is rapid access to stylistics information, making it much easier to change manuscript formats if you are rejected at one journal.

The task of evolving a rough draft into a final formal draft has been made much easier with the commercial availability of linkable word processing and bibliography programs. EndNote© for example is one of a number of a bibliography databases that stores reference material according to just about any stylistic guideline (Niles & Associates, Inc., 1997). More importantly, EndNote© can be dynamically linked with WordPerfect® or Microsoft® Word. Practically, this means you can upload stored references into your manuscript without the drudgery of manually entering and ordering references in text. This is especially helpful if you are writing for a medical journal in which the reference list is constructed based on text order rather than alphabetically. Revise your draft with the principle 'crisp and clear' in mind at all times. Levy & Ransdell (1995) point out that revision "takes less total time than other subprocesses, but it disproportionately determines writing success."

8. Research example

The following is a description of a research study recently conducted in my private practice. The process exemplifies the steps outlined in the previous sections.

The first step was hypothesis generation. A frequently encountered diagnosis in the author's clinic in the past decade was closed head injury and postconcussion syndrome. Part of this clinical work has been devoted to independent medical examinations on head injury claimants seeking compensation. Based on referral patterns, it was decided the general research topic would be in the controversial area of late postconcussion syndrome (PCS). The author examined the neuropsychology literature to get a sense of what studies had been conducted and whether there was a consensus regarding the neuropsychological basis for late PCS. The reviews of Benton (1989), Binder (1986, 1997), Evans (1994), Binder, Rohling, and Larrabee (1997), were helpful for generating possible research themes. The problem of deficit dissimulation appeared to be a major theme in literature about minor head injury disability claimants. The next step was identification of possible weaknesses in this literature: The lack of any large scale epidemiological study of deficit simulation, irreproducible vague criteria for faking, low sample sizes, and treatment of faking as a global trait rather than a task specific response. The study purpose on specific terms was as follows: Examine the frequency of three types of deficit dissimulation in large consecutive series of late postconcussion patients. In addition, what is the relationship between deficit simulation and initial head injury severity in late PCS? This question was derived from the Miller (1972) study. Miller concluded that there was an inverse relationship between injury severity and faking, but his criteria for faking seemed impressionistic and arbitrary.

The second step was database construction. The root database was searched and cases called up in which the history of presenting complaints was one of trauma (see Table 1). This subgroup of claimants was renamed as a new study database (see Table 2). New independent variables were created to categorize trauma severity. Head injury type was coded into three levels of severity and Glasgow Coma Scale (GCS) scores. The dependent variables

Table 2. Example of new variables added to root database for the late PCS study.

Variable (code)	Type	Field size	Coding instructions
Medico-Legal Status (LS)	Numeric	1	Clinical, no compensation = 1, First party suit = 2, Third party suit = 3, Both first + third = 4
Trauma Severity (TS)	Numeric	1	Whiplash = 1, Trauma without LOC = 2, Trauma < 24 h PTA = 3, Trauma 24–48 hPTA = 4, Trauma 49 — 1 week PTA = 5, Trauma > 1 week PTA = 6, Trauma with DAI = 7
Glasgow Coma Scale	Numeric	2	Code 3–15 from ER records
Rey Word List (RWL)	Numeric	2	# of words correctly recognized
MMPI-F T-score (MMPIF)	Numeric	3	*F*-scale *T*-score
Grooved Pegboard, dominant hand (PEGDOM)	Numeric	3	Time to completion in seconds
Grooved Pegboard, nondominant hand, (PEGNDOM)	Numeric	3	Time to completion in seconds

were scores on the Halstead grip strength, the *Infrequency* scale of the *MMPI*, and the Rey Word Recognition List.

The third step was research design. The sampling technique was a consecutive series of patients with late PCS. The reference group consisted of patients with severe closed head injuries with periods of psychosocial disability matching that of the late PCS group. There were two operational definitions of deficit simulation, each reflective of a different level of clinician confidence. Definite simulation was performance worse than one standard deviation below the performance mean of the severe CHI group. Probable deficit simulation was defined as performance below the mean of the severe closed head injury group. The research design also addressed weaknesses in the literature by considering three different forms of simulation: memory, psychiatric and motor defect simulation.

The fourth step was data analysis, a simple frequency count of valid and invalid performances as a function of task type and confidence level. This resulted in a table of probabilities of valid and invalid performances. These simple descriptive statistics were adequate for determining the probability of

Table 3. Percentage of late PCS claimants producing invalid and valid performances.

	Definite criteria	Probable criteria
Any one sign	62.6%	92%
No sign (valid performance)	37.4%	8%
Any two signs	19.72%	29%
All three signs	15.1%	22.2%
Memory sign only	13.1%	19.2%
Motor sign only	9.2%	13.6%
Psychiatric only	5.4%	8.0%

deficit simulation. Table 3 summarizes the findings showing the percentage of late PCS claimants who evidenced at least one, any two, or all three forms of deficit simulation.

To answer the question about any lawful relationship between deficit simulation tendency and original injury severity, three separate ANOVAs were conducted. The independent variable was severity of the injury within the late PCS group. The four levels were neck strain (the mildest) benign head trauma without altered consciousness, head trauma with PTA up to 24 hours, and moderate closed head injury (PTA up to 72 hours). The dependent variables were the scores on the three neuropsychological measures. We found a significant negative linear relationship between initial injury severity and deficit simulation: Late PCS patients with just neck strain (a.k.a. whiplash) performed poorest, a majority of minor concussive claimants performed invalidly, while late PCS patients with an initial moderate closed head injury produced the most valid scores. Clearly, there was a greater likelihood of improbably poor scores in compensation seeking late PCS claimants with the least objective injury (see Figure 1).

The fifth step was paper preparation. The authors concluded that at least one form of deficit simulation was present in the majority of late PCS patients. Another conclusion was that psychotic symptom manufacture was the least common form of deficit simulation. The practical implication was that the *F*-scale of the *MMPI-2* was insufficient to draw conclusions about simulation on neuropsychological or motor tasks. Consideration was given to external validity threats. The authors conclusions were relevant only to patients with unusually poor outcomes from seemingly minor trauma, especially those patients who were receiving or seeking compensation. It has been estimated that poor outcome in minor head injury represents anywhere from 6 to 12% of all mild head injury and whiplash cases. Thus, the authors cautioned it was

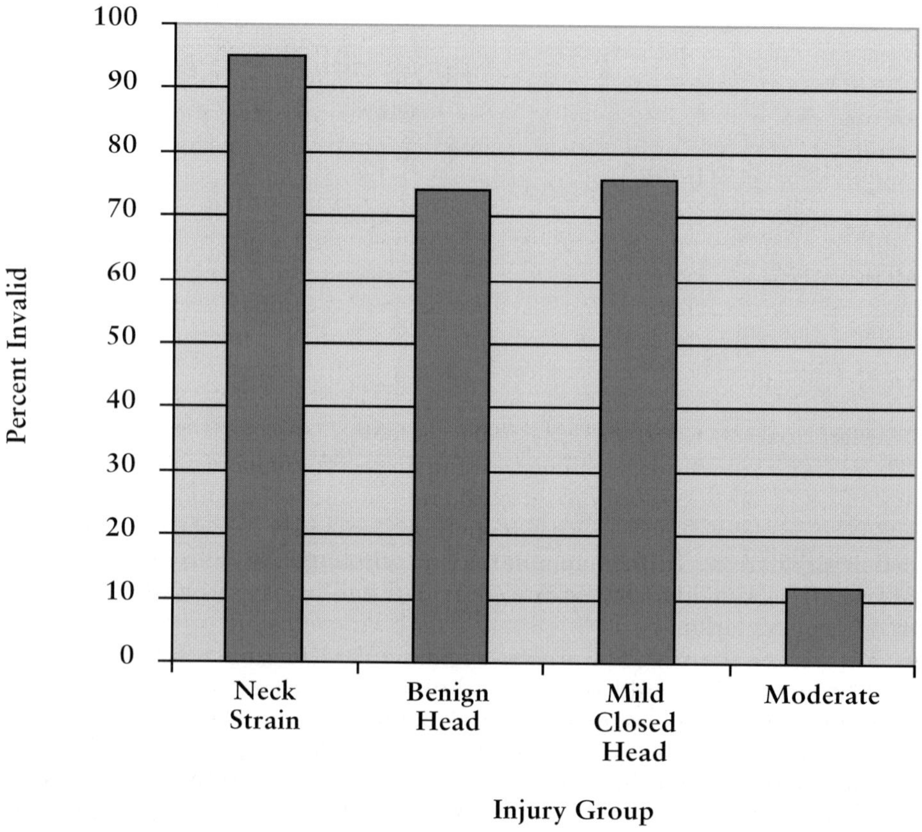

Figure 1. Percentage of compensation seeking claimants showing at least one invalid score as a function of injury severity.

inappropriate to apply our conclusions to any head injured person within the first year of injury. Another caution is that the presence of deficit simulation does not rule out some real form of psychopathology or even neuropathology being present, and that the issues of cerebral dysfunction and deficit simulation should be treated separately on their own merits rather than treated as mutually exclusive concepts.

8. Future directions

Paul Meehl (1978) wrote a scathing critique of clinical psychology research. He argued that clinical psychology lacked the cumulative character of other sciences. The developed sciences integrate theories and established insights into the general body of knowledge, while theories that have been disproved are destroyed, deserving at best a footnote. In clinical psychology, theories are rarely rejected, they simply 'fade away' from lack of conviction, only to be replaced by new fad theory. Interest is rarely maintained to the point that a theory is soundly rejected or accepted. The lessons learned from the negative data are rarely incorporated into the general body of knowledge. Meehl softened his critique by noting that measurement and conceptual difficulties not present in other disciplines plague the social sciences.

The following are a group of research trends that could represent areas of interest for the nascent private practitioner-researcher. These trends, not intended to be either definitive or exhaustive, might provide PPN interested in research with a starting point for a clinical research program.

First, consider focusing on a core set of neuropsychological measures. One of the problems in neuropsychology is the proliferation of test instruments. In some cases, dozens of different tests are used for the same diagnostic issue, e.g., episodic recall measures. Pick up any neuropsychology journal, and you will find research that introduces more memory, executive-cognitive or malingering measures (Ross & Adams, 1999). Neuropsychology needs to organize and summarize the accuracy of core instrumentation. In effect, it may be better for PPN to conduct research with the WAIS-III on 20 different diagnostic groups than to publish research on 20 different IQ tests with the same diagnostic group. Clinical research could certainly compare multiple instruments in the same study, but this requires exceptionally large samples to meet subject-to-variable ratio requirements. Books such as *A Compendium of Neuropsychological Tests* (Spreen & Strauss, 1991) exemplify an approach of concentrating on 'best of breed' measures. That is not to say that the creative PPN should never develop new measures. The point is that such creation should be stimulated by an identifiable diagnostic need. For example, one area where there is a lack of good instrumentation is organic personality changes. Self-report formats (such as the *MMPI-2*) are of limited value with a population whose insight into deficits may be disturbed. Observer rating scales, which cover dimensions of personality commonly encountered in organic populations (such as social disinhibition, apathy, indifference, and depression), would be valuable. PPN are in an excellent position to develop newer measures of personality as PPN observe concrete manifestations of personality disorder everyday. These observations can serve as the basis for writing test items.

Second, treatment efficacy studies are rare but important. Many neuropsychologists offer treatment services to the brain injured, but neuropsychology has failed to conduct the volume of treatment efficacy research necessary to validate our treatment efforts. Managed care organizations and hospitals are demanding greater degrees of justification for treatment from psychologists in general and neuropsychologists in particular. Private practice neuropsychologists who treat the brain injured are in a unique position to conduct this kind of research.

Third, there is a need for more studies of response bias and protocol validity. Neuropsychology lags behind psychopathology assessment in its failure to develop accepted and standardized measures of testing taking validity. The *MMPI* has contained validity scales since inception, and newer measure of personality and psychopathology incorporate validity scales as a matter of course. There has been increasing research into malingering and motivational measures in this decade, but validity measures have not been incorporated into any of the standard batteries such as the Halstead–Reitan or Luria–Nebraska batteries. More research is needed that demonstrates how motivation affects diagnostic error rates. For clinicians that are anxious that administration of neuropsychology validity measures implies mistrust, it is important to bear in mind that deception is common in all forms of psychopathology, not just in litigated head injury cases. Financial incentive is not the only reason for producing invalid results. Quantifying the presence of response bias should be endemic, not alien, to neuropsychology.

Summary

The growing percent of neuropsychologists in private practice is not matched by a proportional increase in journal publications. In the author's opinion, neuropsychology need not display a division between practitioners and researchers. Only PPN can identify the local clinical problems that need to be addressed with measurement tools. Advances in computer miniaturization, the availability of powerful databases, journal proliferation and easy access to scientific literature have provided private practitioners with the means of conducting quality research. The research process can be broken down into concrete steps, although hypothesis generation does require adequate knowledge, training and experiential bases. Creation of a simple database kept on all clients, selection of traditional dependent variables, avoidance of the more common methodological pitfalls and selection of test instrumentation in common usage creates many opportunities for successfully publishing quality research.

References

Abrahamson, D., & Pearlman, L. (1993). The need for scientist-practitioner employment settings. *American Psychologist*, 48, 59–60.

Benton, A.L. (1989). Historical notes on the postconcussion syndrome. In H. Levin, H. Eisenberg, & A. Benton (Eds.), *Mild head injury* (pp. 1–5). New York: Oxford University Press.

Binder, L.M. (1986). Persisting symptoms after mild closed head injury: a review of the postconcussive syndrome. *Journal of Clinical and Experimental Neuropsychology*, 8, 323–346.

Binder, L.M. (1997). A review of mild head trauma. Part II: clinical implications. *Journal of Clinical and Experimental Neuropsychology*, 19(3), 432–457.

Binder, L.M., Rohling, M.L., & Larrabee, G.J. (1997). A review of mild head trauma. Part I: meta-analytic review of neuropsychological studies. *Journal of Clinical and Experimental Neuropsychology*, 2, 421–431.

Campbell, D.T., & Stanley, J.C. (1963). *Experimental and quasi-experimental designs for research*. Boston, MA: Houghton Mifflin Co.
Davison, G. (1998). Being bolder with the Boulder Model: the challenge of education and training in empirically supported treatments. *Journal of Consulting and Clinical Psychology*, 66, 163–167.
Dikmen, S., Reitan, R., Temkin, N., & Machamer, J. (1992). Minor and severe head injury emotional sequelae. *Brain Injury*, 6, 477–478.
Dikmen, S.S., Machamer, J.E., Winn, H.R., & Temkin, N.R. (1995). Neuropsychological outcome at 1-year post head injury. *Neuropsychology*, 8, 80–90.
Dodrill, C. (1997). Myths of neuropsychology. *The Clinical Neuropsychologist*, 11, 1–17.
Evans, R. (1994). The postconcussion syndrome: 130 years of controversy. *Seminars in Neurology*, 14, 32–39.
Greiffenstein, M.F., Baker, W.J., & Gola, T. (1994). Validation of malingered amnesia measures in a large clinical sample. *Psychological Assessment*, 6, 218–224.
Greiffenstein, M.F. & Baker, W.J. (2002). Anosmia and remote outcome in closed head injury. *Journal of Clinical and Experimental Neuropsychology, 24*, 705–709.
Kerlinger, F. (1986). *Foundations of behavioral research,* 3rd ed. New York: Holt, Rinehart and Winston.
Leininger, B., Kreutzer, J., & Hill, M. (1991). Comparison of minor and severe head injury emotional sequelae using the MMPI. *Brain Injury*, 5, 199–205.
Levy, C.M., & Ransdell, S. (1995). Is writing as difficult as it seems? *Memory and Cognition*, 23, 767–779.
McGee, M. (1997). Databases for psychiatrists. *Harvard Review of Psychiatry*, 4, 139–145.
Meehl, P. (1954). *Clinical versus actuarial prediction: A theoretical analysis and a review of the evidence*. Minneapolis: University of Minnesota Press.
Meehl, P. E. (1978). Theoretical risks and tabular asterisks: Sir Karl, Sir Ronald, and the slow progress of soft psychology. *Journal of Consulting and Clinical Psychology*, 46, 806–834.
Miller, H. (1972). Simulation and malingering after injuries to the brain and spinal cord. *The Lancet*, 580–585.
Niles and Associates, Inc. (1997). *EndNote Plus 2.3*. Berkeley, CA.
Norusis, S. (1993). *SPSS for Windows* Release 6.0. Chicago, IL.
Parsons, O. A., & Prigatano, G. P. (1978). Methodological considerations in clinical neuropsychological research. *Journal of Clinical and Consulting Psychology*, 46, 608–619.
Putnam, S., & DeLuca, J. (1990). The TCN professional practice survey. *The Clinical Neuropsychologist*, 4, 199–244.
Putnam, S. & Anderson, C. (1994). The Second TCN salary survey: A survey of neuropsychologists Part I. *The Clinical Neuropsychologist*, 8, 3–38.
Raimy, V. (1950). *Training in clinical psychology*. New York: Prentice-Hall.
Ross, S., & Adams, K.M. (1999). One more test of malingering? *The Clinical Neuropsychologist*, 13, 112–116.
Spreen, O., & Strauss, E. (1991). *A compendium of neuropsychological tests*. New York, NY: Oxford University Press.
Strickler, G. (1997). Are science and practice commensurable? *American Psychologist*, 52, 442–448.
Strickler, G., & Trierweiler, S. (1995). The local clinical scientist: A bridge between science and practice. *American Psychologist*, 50, 995–1002.
Sweet, J., Moberg, P., & Suchy, Y. (2000). Ten-year follow-up study of clinical neuropsychologists: Part I. Practices and beliefs. *The Clinical Neuropsychologist*, 14, 18–37.

Sweet, J., Moberg, P., & Westergaard, C. (1996). Five-year follow-up survey of practices and beliefs of clinical neuropsychologists. *The clinical Neuropsychologist*, 10, 202–221.

Varney, N. (1988). Prognostic significance of anosmia with closed head injury. *Journal of Clinical and Experimental Neuropsycholgy*, 10, 250–254.

Wegener, S., Hagglund, K., & Elliott, T. (1998). On psychological identity and training: Boulder is better for rehabilitation psychology. *Rehabilitation Psychology*, 43, 17–20.

Chapter 7

< E-PRACTICE >: INTERNET RESOURCES FOR THE PRACTICING NEUROPSYCHOLOGIST

H. Risser

> "*The Net's out there waiting for you, and all you have to do is ask.*"
> Neil Randall, *The Soul of the Internet* (1997)

Ask. Most do every day. It is the 21st century, after all. The electronics information age has been here for a while, predating the 1969 birth of the prototypical Internet. Vannevar Bush might well view the recent turn of the century as the unfolding of the electronics *knowledge* age — a time of the direct application of information, something he speculated upon back in 1945. Bush considered then-contemporary thinking about neural associations, intellectual functioning, and memory processing to muse about what he called a 'memex' machine: a way to mechanize the mental pathways of our flights of thinking and the effortless associations that our brains execute with their abilities to integrate and retrieve information. Bush's machine was a fanciful piece of desk furniture. It had embedded cartridges of information made accessible on visual platens, linkages between information made at the discretion of the user, direct photographic capture of written notes, a keyboard, a special lever to navigate around different information sources, and special buttons to support working within an information source. Were he to have left it at that, his thoughts — while having predictive value — might be viewed today as something closer to a Jules Verne anticipation of an Apollo mission to the moon. Bush's lasting prescience, however, appeared at the end of his paper when he peeked into our electronic present: "Must we always transform to mechanical movements in order to proceed from one electrical phenomenon to another? It is a suggestive thought, but it hardly warrants prediction without losing touch with reality and immediateness (p. 108)."

Daily, and without fear of losing reality's touch, today's Internet characterizes computer-mediated electronic communication. It is getting larger, easier to access, more reticulated, and reaches into and out of more lives. Its scope includes the profound and the mundane, the real and the imagined. The Internet far from ideal, though. Risks and irritants exist. Content on the Internet over the past couple of years sometimes seems secondary to commercialization, with once-useful sites becoming paid-subscription-based or peppered with attention-seeking advertisements. Viruses threatening one's hardware and software and "spam mail" cluttering e-mail accounts can challenge the patience and interest of any user. Regular, experienced users of the Net sometimes forget that the learning curve may be less forgiving to newcomers, many not see its value given the time needed to be invested to attain a level of online comfort, and others may find that the risks and irritants simply outweigh any benefits.

Internet novices who are neuropsychologists, though, may be a little easier to entice than other professionals. For decades, the computer had been used metaphorically to understand how the nervous system functions. The first thing to be mindful of when it comes to the Internet — specifically its World Wide Web component — is that the nervous system is itself a useful analogy for appreciating the Internet's structure and function. If any user group can appreciate the irony of this, we are it: to understand the Net, know the brain! Bush appreciated this sixty years ago. More recently, Tim Berners-Lee — the person responsible for creating the Web — credited a conversation with his father about how the brain functions, when he was a high-school student, as the spark that stayed with him: a system that could be based upon connecting previously unconnected material in a manner that was individualized and wholly flexible (Berners-Lee, 1999).

At the turn of the century, health-care professionals accessed the Web at a pace less than that of the general community of users (e.g., HON, 2000), though this gap has been closing (Anonymous, 1999). Neuropsychology's web presence would appear to be lagging a bit behind, relative to psychology, medicine, and health care. Whether this reflects a hesitancy to embrace a digital presence or a cautionary desire to first determine what would be appropriate for online content could be argued. I won't. Reports of physician non-engagement with online environments also find more practical reasons, such as unresolved malpractice- and reimbursement-based issues (Landro, 2002a), time limitations during the work day (HON, 2000), or the so-called 'keyboard barrier' facing professional groups with many members who can't even type, let alone navigate around a computer interface using a mouse (Drezner, 2000). Still, it is paradoxical that our profession does not seem to be nearer to the forefront of embracing an information technology that so closely matches the object of our professional attention.

This chapter presents a vantage point onto what resources are available now to aid neuropsychologists as *consumers* of online knowledge and as *creators* of this applied information for colleagues, patients, and the global community. I am of the opinion that the best use of cyberspace requires the individual to gain a basic knowledge about the Internet itself, in addition to being able to access and provide profession-specific neuropsychological content, so both will be looked at in the chapter. Busis (Busis, 1999; Busis & Honig, 1999) offered a perspective for neurologists, which would also be of interest for neuropsychologists to examine. Emphasis here will be on content that is freely accessible, rather than material with restricted access due to fee-based subscriptions or other membership requirements.

Openly accessible information is, of course, just as available to other professional populations, to patients and their families, to advocates, and to the larger consuming public (Gawande & Bates, 2000a, b, c). Recent survey results from the Pew Foundation (Horrigan & Rainie, 2002) estimate a 36 percent increase between March 2000 and March 2001 in the number of Americans who have used the Internet to track down healthcare-related information, to 64 million from 47 million individuals. An earlier Pew Foundation report (Fox & Rainie, 2000) examined the online activities of these so-called "health seekers" and noted the favorable impact that information obtained online played in medical decision-making for themselves or when obtaining information for loved ones, as well as noting concerns by consumers about tracking down accurate, legitimate information. What is it that your next patient will bring with her into your office? You might be surprised. Useful information will exist alongside the invalid and wacky. Will she bring in a downloaded reprint from this week's issue of the *British Medical Journal*, a hardcopy of the Mini-Mental Status Examination she completed the night before during dinner with the family, or the self-important discussion-forum ranting about miracle cures from someone without any known credentials? Whether one will access it routinely or not, it is beneficial for a practicing neuropsychologist to know something of the Internet's environment and of its potential impact on daily professional life.

The Internet: Think Synaptically

If your notebook, desktop, or hand-held computer is connected to the Internet, it and you are as much a part of the physical and conceptual "Net" as any thing or any one else. From the point of view of the Internet, you are — in essence — a neuron. Your own private axon pokes information out onto the system, such as sending an e-mail message, requesting a document, etc. You capture and receive information from your own dendritic field, which is as simple or complex as your desire and experience allow.

The Internet ('Net' is used synonymously) is a mega-network of many interactive computer networks that are, in turn, comprised of millions of individual users. What makes the Net work are underlying processing protocols that allow communication between any individual links in the mega-network, regardless of the idiosyncratic characteristics of that link. These protocols are called the TCP/IP protocol suite, with TCP referring to 'Transmission Control Protocol' and IP standing for 'Internet Protocol' (e.g., Loshin, 1999). These protocols work by first breaking down all information into small pieces, then bundling these elements into a series of packets. These packets are labeled and handled individually by routers, which help connect networks. Routers electronically peruse each packet to read the destination address, calculate the best route in either a predestined or a dynamic manner at that point in time, and transmit the packet onward and closer to its final destination. Once received there, packets are opened and the pieces of information are reconstructed into their original and meaningful form. Gralla (1999) offers useful graphical renditions of this process and Loshin (1999) provides a basic level of understanding about the workings of these protocols. Online, the websites for LivingInternet.com and the Internet Society provide overviews to the TCP/IP technologies; Table 1 provides the addresses (i.e., the URLs) for these two sites and for a number of other cyberspace websites (some will not be discussed in the text).

The Internet is comprised of different components. These parts include the World Wide Web (WWW; 'the Web'); e-mail; and virtual community modalities: asynchronous discussion forums, synchronous chat rooms, newsgroups, and the so-called MUDs and MOOs. This chapter will discuss only certain facets of virtual communities; MUDs, MOOs, and newsgroups will not be presented. Virtual-reality (VR) applications also fall outside of the chapter, though the interested reader should be aware that VR has begun to generate neuropsychological interest (e.g., Coiera, 1996a; Bloom, 1997; Buckwalter & Rizzo, 1997; Rizzo & Buckwalter, 1997). Finally, the chapter will not discuss considerations about online counseling and psychotherapy services in clinical psychology (e.g.,Nichelson, 1997; Stamm, 1998; APA, 2000; Childress, 2000) and specific telemedical applications (e.g., remote administration of medical tests [Shafqat, Kvedar, Guanci, Chang, & Schwamm, 1999] and surgical interventions).

The WWW

The Web and the Net are not synonymous with one another, though the terms are often used interchangeably. From this point onward, reference will be made predominantly to the Web. A primary online resource about the Web is the WWW Consortium or 'The W3C' (see Table 1). One needs to know the outlines of only three things to grasp the underlying structure of the Web: its mechanics (i.e., HTTP), its language (i.e., HTML), and its synaptic-like operators (i.e., URLs).

HTTP stands for 'Hypertext Transfer Protocol,' which provides the mechanism for the many different platforms that exist on the Web to request and receive information from one another in the relatively seamless fashion

Table 1. **Cyberspace websites.**

Website name and URL	Comment
LivingInternet.com http://livinginternet.com/	History, technical introduction, and current news about the Internet and its components
Internet Society http://www.isoc.org/	Resources about the Internet
W3C: World Wide Web Consortium http://www.w3.org/	Resources about the WWW
Internet.com http://www.internet.com	Internet-related news and features
"Netiquette" by Virginia Shea http://www.albion.com/netiquette/book/0963702513FC.html	Full-text primer for becoming a good online communicator
"The Virtual Community" by Howard Rheingold http://www.rheingold.com/vc/book/	Full-text book about online life
"The Psychology of Cyberspace" by John Suler http://www.rider.edu/users/suler/psycyber/psycyber.html	Psychological examination of online life
CERT Coordination Center http://www.cert.org/	Information about viruses, security threats and incidents, and security methods.
"Web Style Guide" by Patrick Lynch and Sarah Horton http://info.med.yale.edu/caim/manual/	Full-text contents book about website design and application considerations
"Web Teaching Guide" by Sarah Horton http://www.webteachingguide.com/	Adjunctive website and discussion forum
Copyright & Fair Use http://fairuse.stanford.edu/	Primary resources and links to applications
Journal of Electronic Publishing http://www.press.umich.edu/jep/	Quarterly publication examining online publishing issues
Scholarly Electronic Publishing Bibliography http://info.lib.uh.edu/sepb/sepb.html	Resource about electronic publishing
An Atlas of Cyberspaces http://www.cybergeography.org/atlas/atlas.html	Graphical representations of the digital world

Table 1. Continues

Table 1. Continued.

Website name and URL	Comment
Electronic Privacy Information Center http://www.epic.org/	General coverage, but includes specific information about digital health-record confidentiality issues
Resource Center for Cyberculture Studies http://www.com.washington.edu/rccs	Resource about the psychosocial facets of cyberspace
The Berkman Center for Internet & Society http://cyber.law.harvard.edu/	Resource about legal and psychosocial facets of cyberspace
Pew Internet & American Life Project http://www.pewinternet.org/	Ongoing research programs examining the psychosocial impact of the Internet
The International Academy of Digital Arts and Sciences http://www.iadas.net	The group that presents the yearly "Webby" awards. Allows an exploration of creative, technical, and professional trends
MIT Media Lab http://www.media.mit.edu	Applications of digital technology in everyday life
First Monday http://www.firstmonday.dk/index.html	Monthly Internet journal

of the TCP/IP protocol suite. The hypertext protocol defines how Web documents are formatted and displayed (Loshin, 1999), while remaining invisible to the typical Web user but for the 'http://...' that one will keystroke to open up a webpage. The W3C provides a detailed HTTP description (W3C HTTP Working Group, 1998).

HTML stands for 'Hypertext Markup Language.' HTML is the most-common language that is communicated via HTTP. The language is comprised of a series of tags that are added to text to format that text in a manner that can be transmitted and displayed online (Eddy, 1998a). For example, to boldface Bill Gates, one simply keystrokes: <b>Bill Gates</b>. Benignly invisible to a site's visitor, website creators produce HTML tagging with the same fluency as they write in their native language. However, HTML can also remain out of sight to the amateur website creator who uses any of the many contemporary web-authoring software packages. Using these packages in place of learning HTML from the bare bones outward, one may lose the nuances and subtleties that one can use to create professional work products, but one can find a relatively quick and simple manner of creating adequate work products. These programs often convert a creator's instructions into underlying HTML using interfaces and menus that the user works from in order to create the background HTML formatting. HTML has many relatives, including DHTML and XML (Eddy, 1998b) and other tagging systems that can be integrated into regular HTML work products, such as JavaScript (Negrino & Smith, 1999) and CGI (Castro, 1999). At a multimedia level, Macromedia's Flash has been changing the look and sound of contemporary websites (Curtis, 2000).

Learning HTML helps an individual develop a Web presence. One of the documents most frequently accessed by people curious about HTML is a brief document called "A Beginner's Guide to HTML," available at <http://www.ncsa.uiuc.edu/General/Internet/WWW/HTMLPrimerAll.html>. All the foundation tags for creating a basic web page can be found there. A full description of HTML's current version can be found at the W3C site (e.g., HTML, Version 4.01: <http://www.w3.org/TR/REC-html40/cover.html>). Details about using HTML and related languages can be found in a library of how-to manuals and reference guides (e.g., Eddy, 1998a).

Finally, URL stands for "Universal Resource Locator," the now-ubiquitous access-providing address for any web page. URLs are known to every Web user as the way to get from here to there. They are of the general form of <http://www.anyname.com/anypage.html>.

E-mail

Electronic-mail messaging programs and one's e-mail address(es) are a different facet of the Internet and one with its own underlying protocols that interface with TCP/IP. E-mail is a unique form of communication, neither letter- and memo-writing nor conversational speech. Its ability to automatically 'frame' a response (i.e., include the original message bordered by, e.g., '>' s) is a distinctive feature of the medium. Horrigan and Rainie (2002) report that e-mail use in the general American public continues to increase regularly and that, once individuals begin, they typically remain e-mail communicators and conform to certain trends. These trends include (a) the 'wow!' factor of early usage gives way to e-mail becoming a more routine part of life on the job and at home, (b) the frequency of e-mailing specific individuals is reduced but content becomes more serious and more significant in terms of daily-living decisions, and (c) home use drives continued use, but home use begins to include more work-related correspondence.

Most e-mail messages are not encrypted and, therefore, they are not much different from dropping picture postcards into a mailbox — it is possible that anyone could read what is written in one from there to its destination. E-mail messages are broken down and reconstructed as they are sent from your computer to the message recipient in the same manner as described earlier for online content. En route to their destination, messages make stops at a number of nodes (at any one of which, there is the opportunity — but hardly the incentive — for a systems operator to read content) and the message may reside on your service-provider's servers (networking hardware) for long periods after you and your recipient have read, filed, and deleted the message from your respective personal computers. Specter (1999) offered a personal account of his search to find his service-provider's repository of e-mails.

Guides exist as to what is proper style for composing e-mail messages. Virginia Shea's popular *Netiquette* book is perhaps the best-known resource about online manners; it includes a number of sections about e-mail messaging (available online; see Table 1). Style includes those seemingly trivial emoticons (e.g., ' :-)' — the sideways 'smiley' face) that may appear inappropriate, until the first time that one is confronted with needing to modify a verbal statement in a message, but is stymied by not finding the correct way to phrase the statement. Generally acceptable markings and abbreviations also exist, such as putting an asterisk before and after a word to give it emphasis.

In the absence of much guidance, many practitioners now find themselves receiving e-mailed messages from patients, potential referrals, referral sources, and colleagues — all blended in with personal messages, advertisements, etc. It behooves the electronic communicator to learn a bit about the process. It also is useful to examine options that are available in most e-mail programs, but that only a minority of users will use; these include 'bozo filters' (to send messages from known so-called 'clowns' directly — and unopened — into the trash bin or to simply block the receipt of anything from their address) and priority filtering (to create taxonomies and to better organize incoming messages).

For most individuals, there is little need to have over a dozen e-mail addresses, but there are good reasons to have more than just one. A practicing neuropsychologist may wish to have separate e-mail addresses for non-professional communications, for at-work interactions at one's primary employment location, for secondary or ancillary work-related locations, and one or several more public accounts that may be used for handling postings from listservs or interacting with the general public.

There is a growing literature in health care (and in other venues, such as in the legal profession) examining the values and risks of e-mail-based professional communications and what might be done to increase the former and decrease the later. Spielberg (1998) offered an historical overview that is of value to outline the context of using electronic messages in clinical practice. As to actual experiences, Borowitz and Wyatt (1998) provided a statistical analysis of their own practice's e-mail consultation service and D'Alessandro and colleagues (2000) provided information about 300-plus unsolicited messages sent to an author of an online textbook about pediatric radiology.

Guidelines for the clinical use of e-mail were initially suggested by the American Medical Informatics Association (AMIA; Kane & Sands, 1998; Table 2), though each profession will need to consider the specifics of their domains, as they seek to establish recommendations and guidelines (and the same is true for legislative entities). The AMIA guidelines are very useful to examine, if only for instructive purposes. They offer both communication-friendly and medicolegal parameters that are helpful when considering these

Table 2. Websites/pages about clinical e-mail guidelines and issues.

Website/page name and URL	Comment
AMIA Guidelines http://www.amia.org/pubs/other/email_guidelines.html	Kane and Sands (1998)
AMA Guidelines http://www.ama-assn.org/ama/pub/category/2386.html	Initial guidelines
Medem's eRisk Guidelines http://www.medem.com/corporate/corporate_erisk.cfm	Produced by the Medem company in collaboration with a group of medical societies.
American Academy of Family Physicians Primer http://www.aafp.org/quality/email/index.html	An exploration of e-mail applications in medicine
Electronic Patient Centered Communication Resource Center http://www.e-pcc.org	A collection of information by Sands
"E-Encounters" http://www.chcf.org/topics/view.cfm?itemID=12863	A November 2001 report from the California Healthcare Foundation

issues (and can be useful simply in promoting better professional-to-professional electronic interaction, in the absence of resolving any professional-client issues). Other versions of guidelines include an initial set from the AMA, the "eRisk Guidelines" offered in 2000 and 2001 by the Medem corporation in collaboration with a group of medical professional societies, and a primer on the topic provided by the American Academy of Family Physicians (all accessible online; see Table 2).

One mapping point in contemporary discussion on this topic relates to the context in which the practitioner receives an e-mailed message from a patient. That is, whether the message is an unsolicited one from an individual whom the practitioner has had no prior interactions with or whether the message is from (or related to) a known patient, for whom the practitioner has had the opportunity to interact with in person (Eysenbach & Diepgen, 1998; Eysenbach, 2000). D'Alessandro and colleagues presented a sobering account of the extent of personal information that can be sent in an unsolicited manner to health-care professionals who have a Web presence: the author of an online textbook on pediatric radiology available at the University of Iowa's *Virtual Hospital* received a number of messages, though less than five per cent of these messages dealt with radiology per se. E-mails included requests for disease overviews, for diagnoses, and for resolving treatment options, covering a very broad range of content across numerous pediatric specialties.

Given the not-quite-this and not-quite-that aspect of e-mail mentioned earlier (regardless of whom it is at the other end of the message), every sender and recipient needs to be sensitive as to how the content of one's message may be influenced by the online context. Abstractness and humor are easily misinterpreted in cyberspace. Attempts to be concrete by adding additional or redundant information to a message may be misunderstood by the reader as being spoken down to. A sender who views e-mail messages as a way of chatting will probably not be overly concerned with spelling and grammar but, if the message is sent to someone expecting to read the equivalent of a memorandum, both will find the experience a difficult one.

Users of e-mail find themselves in the frustrating situation of having to deal with two devilish aspects of electronic communications: 'spam mail' junk messages and viruses. Risk increases with your use and the extent to which your e-mail address becomes known and used by others (e.g., added to address books and mailing lists). You are at further risk if you need to open e-mailed messages sent to you from people who you do not know; for example, if you distribute your e-mail address on business cards, letterhead, or in public advertising. Self-education and the use of both (a) optional features available in most e-mail messaging programs (e.g., bulk-mail filters, virus checks for received attachments) and (b) antiviral software can minimize the impact of these phenomena and are recommended. An excellent online source of information about viruses and protections against them is available at the CERT Coordination Center website (Table 1). Havoc-producing viruses have garnered national media attention over the past few years, but viral protection should be a daily, regular aspect of online life. Antiviral software is a very important utility to have running on your network-accessed systems; Norton and McAfee are two commercial antiviral companies whose products are easily accessible.

Virtual communities

Figallo (1998) stated, "The Web has provided an environment in which more people than ever before have the space, the tools, and the opportunity to put their personal versions of community into practice [p. 1]." Virtual communities (VCs) are of three types: e-mail based listservs, discussion forums, and chat rooms. The first two are asynchronous, in that the writer and the audience need not 'be there' at the same point in time. In addition to the convenience, this allows for the writer's preparation of messages in the absence of time pressure and for the reader's/respondent's ability to pick and choose where and how to examine material. Listservs may be unmoderated (any member can send a message to the full VC), moderated (members submit messages to the moderator or host or own, who decides in an editorial fashion what to post to the VC and how), or broadcast (VC members receive messages from the moderator or host or owner). Discussion forums (once called 'bulletin boards') may be threaded (i.e., organized by subject and topic heading) or unthreaded, in addition to the types described above. Chat rooms may be text-based or graphic- (avatar-) based, unmoderated or moderated, and usually reflect a thematic subject (even if the theme is an open chat about anything).

Many readers of this chapter will already belong to one or more VCs. If your practice or institution has an intranet-based electronic communications system, then you are a member of one by default. If you contribute to, e.g., an e-mailed-based discussion forum, you are a member of one by choice and have become a "netizen" of the digital world. At the forefront of studying VCs, Howard Rheingold (1993) described himself and fellow netizens as those who "exchange pleasantries and argue, engage in intellectual discourse, conduct commerce, exchange knowledge, share emotional support, make plans, brainstorm, gossip, feud, fall in love, find friends and lose them, play games, flirt, create a little high art and a lot of idle talk [<http://www.rheingold.com/vc/book/intro.html>]."

'Netizenship' has its duties. Every VC has explicit or implicit rules about behavior in that specific community (see, e.g., Shea's primer), and there is a general level of expectation for new members of a community to learn about and conform to those behavioral features, though few would frown upon one or two initial errors by 'newbies' (e.g., Wallace, 1999). Explicit rules are often FAQ-accessible, i.e., available on a page of 'frequently asked questions.' Both Rheingold and Figallo have explored the best ways to build online communities. Guidebooks by A.J. Kim (2000) and Preece (2000) also examine how VCs develop and are sustained. Curiously, few resources examine how VCs might be best closed down when termination becomes necessary, perhaps reflecting the optimism of Internet writers until, say, the rapid demise of 'dot-com' economic bullishness in early 2001.

Neuropsychologists may become VC hosts and leaders. Online resources about the responsibilities of hosting include Rheingold's *The art of hosting good conversations online* (available at <http://www.rheingold.com/texts/artonlinehost.html>) and Collins and Berge's "The Moderator's Homepage" (available at <http://www.emoderators.com/moderators.shtml>).

Examining the experiences of those who have explored VCs is one way to peek at life in cyberspace at its most fanciful and its scariest. The interested reader is directed to any of a number of accounts of virtual life: Dibbell's (1999) *My Tiny Life*, Wallace's (1999) *The Psychology of the Internet*, Turkel's (1995) *Life on the Screen*, Seabrook's (1997) *Deeper: My Two Year Odyssey in Cyberspace*, and Cherny's (1999) *Conversation and Community*. The contents of Rheingold's book and of psychologist John Suler's *The Psychology of Cyberspace* are both available online (Table 1). Online psychosocial interactions deal not only with human members, but sometimes with 'embodied conversational agents,' artificial communicants designed to interact with human participants and provide a full range of facial and behavioral mannerisms designed to supplement their verbal statements (Cassell et al., 2000).

One of the first and most successful VCs in medicine was the listserv-based "ProMED-mail" community. Begun in August 1994, ProMED provided a global community of professionals and interested civilians a venue at which to report and communicate about outbreaks of newly emerging and reemerging infectious diseases in the absence of geopolitical restraints. As many outbreaks occur within political borders that are not amenable to free and quick exchange of information, ProMED rapidly assumed an important back-channel route to get information to and from experts and others. Its June 2000 population of 20,000 members resided in more than 160 countries.

In neuropsychology, David Loring's *NPSYCH* listserv, hosted on Medical College of Georgia webspace at <http://neurolist.mcg.edu>, is the VC with probably the largest number of neuropsychologists as active participants. *NPSYCH* started in 1994 and for the first year predominantly served as a tool for a group of neuropsychologists drawn together by an interest in epilepsy research. With just a couple of minor public announcements, such as a sign posted at an International Neuropsychological Society meeting and a mention in the National Academy of Neuropsychology newsletter, the following years saw continued 'word-of-mouth' membership growth (Loring; personal communication, September 1999). A subsequent change in software (to Lyris) allowed members the ability to search the growing database of posts on a wide range of neuropsychological topics, permitting the community to develop a shared and documented history.

Loring's successful VC had grown to 1081 members from 18 countries as of November 2000 (Loring, *NPSYCH* posting, 3 November 2000). Members are screened prior to acceptance for having some credential related to neuropsychology, either as a professional or as a graduate student. Screening is a common practice for VCs that wish to retain some sense of self-definition. Many communities also maintain rules that provide for the expulsion of members who breach acceptable practices. The NPSYCH community receives upwards of several-dozen posted messages on a daily basis. Like most listservs, the majority of members are so-called 'lurkers' in that they are not necessarily inclined to post messages on a regular basis, but enjoy or find informative enough of the material that is posted to remain members. Conversely, a small number of members post an abundance of the messages there and often one finds the polarizing effect of discussions that are turned to arguments between supporters at the extreme ends of the topic spectrum — a phenomenon common to many VCs (e.g., Wallace, 1999). The Medical College of Georgia's related listserv VC for neurologists — *NEURO* — began at about the same time and had 584 members, residing in at least 51 countries, as of October 1998 (Rivner, 1999). Rivner reported that roughly half the members did not post any messages and that about a third of membership had posted 10 or fewer messages. Thirteen individuals were responsible for at least a hundred messages apiece and one member posted over a thousand messages.

Additional professional-content listservs exist in the neuropsychological community, including one with an emphasis on issues in developmental neuropsychology and another limited in its membership to board-certified individuals.

It would be naïve in the year 2002 to assume that patients referred to you or under your care do not know that they can obtain information over the Web, as well as interact with others (patients, professionals, advocates, charlatans) in VCs. When done well, participation in online supportive VCs can be a useful activity for patients, as well as their families, friends, and loved ones. Possible benefits — in addition to support — can include obtaining knowledge to (a) become a better consumer, (b) monitor and regulate the quality of services provided, and (c) aid in the self-management of illness and disease (Gawande & Bates, 2000c).

Davison, Pennebaker, and Dickerson (2000) noted the particular value of these online communities for those disorders that might carry a stigmatizing or embarrassing impact. A number of VCs exist for various brain diseases. These groups are usually populated by caregivers and family members, as well as by patients; some have professional participation, while others do not. Harvard's Neurology Department of Massachusetts General Hospital has a fairly diverse grouping of discussion forums, text-based chat rooms, and avatar-based chat rooms on general and specific topics in neurology geared to generate discussion between patients, caregivers, and professionals (Hoch, Norris, Lester, & Marcus, 1998; Lester, Norris, & Hoch, 1998). An additional VC example can be found at the Family Caregiver Alliance <http://www.caregiver.org>. Patients or their family members have established VCs dedicated to discussing a particular disease or deficit syndrome; this has been especially the case for caregivers of elderly individuals and those with dementing disorders (e.g., Shellenbarger, 2002).

'Growing' communities of consumers who will return to a website has also become a common part of Web-based e-commerce business plans (e.g., Figallo, 1998); as true in healthcare sites as anywhere else on the Web. For example, patient- and caregiver-oriented discussion forums and chat rooms became common at commercial sites such as PlanetRx.com, once a large online pharmacy e-commerce website, and drKoop.com. The demise of dot.com companies such as PlanetRx.com have added an untoward dimension to this experience: what happens to a community that has been nurtured into development once the website interface has been shuttered? As mentioned earlier, this is an issue in need of fuller exploration.

Content on the Web

'Content' is the information that is actually present at a website once you access it. This section of the chapter will explore accessing, evaluating, and providing content. The homepage of a website, like a book cover, will provide some information about what to expect at the site and will link to all additional sections of the site. Sites commonly have a 'Site Map' (the equivalent of a Table of Contents) and many will provide an internal search engine. Content will range from headlines and reports from the news media, abstracts of papers, the full-text of reports, FAQs, fact sheets, overviews, detailed background papers, and archived material. Content also includes the collection of hyperlinked references to other websites, which may be annotated or simply presented in list or category form. It is increasingly common for websites to include streams of audio, visual, and multimedia (audio-visual) information as part of their content (Novak & Markiewicz, 1998).

From the Web's onset, concern has been expressed about how to assure that valid information from reliable sources could be distinguishable from the undesirable alternatives (Coiera, 1996b; Silberg, Lundberg, & Musacchio, 1997; Hubbs, Rindfleisch, Godin, & Melmon, 1998; P. Kim, Eng, Deerong, & Maxfield, 1999). How to agree upon these assurances, how to implement them, and how to educate the consuming public to recognize the value of this information relative to other online offerings remains major challenges. The Health on the Net Foundation and the Internet Healthcare Coalition are two representative organizations promoting accurate and understandable medical information for public consumption. However, there are also more mundane content issues. Website creators need to assure, for example, that they can present content in a manner which makes sense, does not get lost amid bright colors or clutter, and allows visitors to navigate easily within the webpages of the site and to be able to access other websites via active hyperlinks.

Accessing content

There are different approaches to obtaining content online. One can use a search engine, go to a known site recommended by a colleague or reported in the media, use e-mail to contact others either on a one-to-one or on a community basis to request specific sites to visit, or rely upon simple trial and error. One might view each online session as a proverbial tabula rasa or might stay well within the tight confines of several tried-and-true venues. There is a growing research literature on effective Web-based information-searching strategies (e.g., Choo, Detlor, & Turnbull, 2000; Lawrence & Giles, 1998).

The prototypical behavior on the Web is 'surfing.' Although the term has been turned into a generic for all Web behavior, it actually applies only to one form of accessing content. To surf means to engage the Web by using hyperlinks to travel from site to site, without necessarily having a single destination in mind. Surfing might be delimited by staying within a certain topic or may be free-style, which means that where you end up and how you get there is more a reflection of what you found along the way, rather than following any predetermined plan, which reflects the behavior of direct content access.

Navigational aids are present on the Web and search engines are the most common. Search engines are distinctly different in how they work and the results they produce. A professional using the Web should understand search engines and the factors that distinguish them. One way to do this is by experimentation, ideally using at least a half-dozen different engines (see Table 3 for some examples). Although they are often dismissed as 'vanity searches' and account for a surprisingly large number of searches, I believe that the

Table 3. Search engines and guides.

Website name and URL	Comment
Yahoo! http://www.yahoo.com	Most popular website search engine, employing a large taxonomic system
AltaVista http://www.altavista.com	Webpage search engine
Google http://www.google.com	Critically acclaimed meta-search engine, consistently becoming more popular
Northern Light http://www.northernlight.com/	Mega-search engine. Includes a special section for searching online news-media sources
The Scout Report http://scout.cs.wisc.edu/report/sr/current	Weekly online newsletter evaluating and recommending selected websites
Britannica.com http://www.britannica.com	Online internet guide, containing website reviews
Search Engine Watch http://www.searchenginewatch.com/	Resource about online information searching
ONLINE magazine http://www.onlinemag.net	Monthly columns by Greg Notess: "Internet Search Engine Update" and "On the Net"
Research Buzz by Tara Calishain http://www.researchbuzz.com	Weekly newsletter, current news, and articles about search engines and data management

best way to examine a search engine is to keystroke in your own name and see what happens. You know your own paper trail better than anyone else's and this should permit you to gain some immediate feedback as to what each search engine produces. Yahoo! and AltaVista, for example, have very different work products and both (though popular favorites) can be surprisingly limited in their effectiveness relative to the meta-search engines, such as Google. Yahoo!'s 'What's New' page provides a categorized look at new additions on a daily basis, which can help the regular Web user keep track of what's being added to their database.

At the other end of the spectrum, specialized search engines are those that are specific to certain topical domains (e.g., King, 2000). Several advantages of these so-called niche engines include time savings and theme-limited search results, with some sites providing a vetting of database entries by a staff or an advisory board of professionals and results that include annotated commentary. Medical World Search (once, but no longer, a free service) e.g., limited its database to full-text content from credible health-care sites. Annotated guides with reviews of websites, such as is available at Britannica.com and in the weekly Internet Scout Report online newsletter, provide another source of assistance when searching the Web.

There are other ways to learn about the best uses of search engines. Danny Sullivan's Search Engine Watch offers educational content about how to best use them, with features designed for both novices and experienced users. Additional online resources to keep up to date on search-engine news are Tara Calishain's Research Buzz website and Greg Notess's column in ONLINE magazine (e.g., Notess, 1999).

Evaluating content

Assessing the reliability and validity of health-care content that can be obtained on the Web is one of the most daunting tasks facing professional groups in any health-care domain (as well as those in other professions). One of the earlier attempts, still in practice and having a general degree of acceptance, was the HON Code of Conduct provided by the Health on the Net Foundation <http://www.hon.ch/HONcode/Conduct.html>. This code has a number of principles related to the nature of information to be found at a website, the confidentiality of information about visitors to the website, clear identification of any funding sources, and overt distinction between editorial and any advertising content.

There are a growing number of attempts to offer objective analyses of this task (e.g., Jadad & Gagliardi, 1998; Kim et al., 1999). The American Psychological Association's (1997) initial attempt placed emphasis on whether material was peer-reviewed and printed in acceptable psychology journals prior to being posted online. The American Medical Association (AMA) published guidelines in 2000 (Winker et al., 2000).

Providing content

Any reader of this chapter can develop a Web presence. Though HTML is part of the technical side of web development, it is only one facet of Web designing needed to create this Web presence. The other two are graphic design and content per se. Lynch and Horton's (1999) *Web Style Guide* (also available online; see Table 1) is an excellent resource for a professional seeking to develop a Web presence in his or her work-related activities. Nielsen (1999) offered a detailed examination of website designs that help or hinder the presentation of content. Galitz (1997) provided a comprehensive overview to designing user interfaces that can serve as a useful resource for would-be website developers. Additionally, brief how-to overviews appear frequently in professional journals (e.g., Peters & Sikorski, 1998). Content, of course, will flow from the knowledge base and expertise of the putative website creator and any other contributors to that site.

Many of the issues faced by a website developer are the same as any author or publisher, but with a digital twist. Intellectual property and copyright issues (see. e.g., Stanford University's *Copyright & Fair Use* website; Table 1) are specific realms that come to mind. Other issues of a more editorial nature are unique to electronic life, such as the naming of URL links to specific pages. Unfortunately, these links often lack in longevity, as websites change and are moved from server to server over time. Linking to other content may also provide problems in this regard. The easiest way to lose returning visits to one's website is to not routinely check the status of the hyperlinks there to assure that they still point to active webpages elsewhere.

Neuropsychology-relevant Content

Every neuropsychologist can tailor his or her Web experience to fit their own cognitive strengths and weaknesses, their own tastes and needs. However, I would encourage anyone to be as open and as flexible as possible, especially when beginning one's first forays into cyberspace.

Perhaps the most basic approach for those who need structure with the task and the one with (perhaps) the broadest appeal would be to create a foundation of 'anchor' websites — sites that have a basis in being offered by established entities that possess comfortable levels of face validity in real life (see Table 4 for examples). The National Institutes of Health website is a useful place to start. Perhaps most importantly, this is the site where the National Library of Medicine's webpages are embedded and, via them, direct access to millions of medical abstracts in the PubMed database. Searchable access to over 10 million abstracts in a constantly updated database is not a bad way to begin to size up the potential utility of the Web. Even so, there are reports that — even when physicians know of the existence of this resource and accept its value — actual use of it is not always as high as might be predicted (e.g., Chimoskey & Norris, 1999). In addition to clinically and academically useful information, the NIH website offers databases, news releases, archived publications, grant information, and an abundance of patient-directed educational material.

Major academic health care centers and professional organizations/ societies are also potential 'anchor' websites (Table 4). Several notable ones include Harvard's Department of Neurology at the Massachusetts General Hospital, *OncoLink* from the Department of Oncology at the University of Pennsylvania, and the University of Iowa's *Virtual Hospital*. The American Psychological Association, the Canadian Psychological Association, the American Academy of Neurology, and the American Psychiatric Association each have large and content-laden websites. In the late 1990s, an interesting cyber-presence that served as a model about how to have a broad reach within a profession, to other professionals, and to the public was found in the neurosurgical community: the elaborate *Neurosurgery://On-call* website. In

Table 4. Medical/psychological 'anchor' websites.

Website name and URL	Comment
National Institutes of Health http://www.nih.gov/	Comprehensive coverage, including access to each individual institute
PubMed http://www4.ncbi.nlm.nih.gov/entrez/query.fcgi	Part of the NIH website, these pages allow access to millions of medical abstracts
Gateway to Neurology at Massachusetts General Hospital http://neuro-www.mgh.harvard.edu/	Comprehensive resource for information about the diagnosis and treatment of neurological disorders, as well as host site for a number of patient and caregiver virtual communities
OncoLink, from the University of Pennsylvania http://www.oncolink.upenn.edu/	Comprehensive resource for cancer diagnosis and treatment education, information, and news
Virtual Hospital, from the University of Iowa http://www.vh.org	Comprehensive resource
American Psychological Association http://www.apa.org	APA Web presence, includes the full-text context of "The APA Monitor"
Canadian Psychological Association/ Société canadienne de psychologie http://www.cpa.ca/	CPA/SCP Web presence
American Academy of Neurology http://www.aan.com/	AAN Web presence
American Psychiatric Association http://www.psych.org/	APA Web presence
Neurosurgery://On-call http://www.neurosurgery.org/	Example of diverse coverage offered by a medical specialty
National Academy of Neuropsychology http://www.nanonline.org/	Neuropsychology professional society
International Neuropsychological Society http://www.osu.edu/ins/	Neuropsychology professional society
Division 40, Clinical Neuropsychology, American Psychological Association http://www.div40.org/	Neuropsychology professional society

Table 4. Continues

Table 4. Continued.

Website name and URL	Comment
The American Board of Clinical Neuropsychology http://www.theabcn.org	Neuropsychology specialty board
The American Academy of Clinical Neuropsychology http://www.theaacn.org	Neuropsychology organization
Pediatrics http://www.pediatrics.org/	Free full-text access to most of this monthly journal's contents
electronic BMJ: British Medical Journal http://www.bmj.org/	Free full-text access to this weekly journal's contents
Journals of the American Medical Association http://pubs.ama-assn.org/	Access to some content of the AMA's medical journals, including JAMA and Archives of Neurology
Medscape http://www.medscape.com	Comprehensive medical information
Health on the Net Foundation http://www.hon.ch/	Organization promoting informational standards for online medical information
Internet Healthcare Coalition http://www.ihealthcoalition.org/	Organization promoting informational standards for online medical information
Journal of Medical Internet Research http://www.jmir.org/index.htm	Quarterly journal

addition to peer-reviewed journal-type material and other types of traditional content, the site included searchable listings of professionals, news, subspecialty information, and a curious *Cyber Museum*.

In neuropsychology, there has been an interesting difference between the websites for two of our organizations: the National Academy of Neuropsychology (NAN) and the International Neuropsychological Society (INS). By the later years of the 1990s, visitors to the NAN website found a relatively diverse selection of resources, whilst those accessing the INS site found only a limited amount of content, most of it directed at administrative matters related to the Society per se (e.g., membership information). Though each society certainly has its reasons for presenting themselves as they prefer, the NAN site has been decidedly the more web-savvy of the two in terms of content presentation.

At the next level up in building a foundation of one's own 'anchor' sites, but with a good amount of ebb and flow, are peer-reviewed academic journals. Against a backdrop of dramatic increases in online presence — with many subscription-based opportunities to access full content — the availability of free-access content that extends beyond tables of content and abstracts is usually in a state of flux. The journals *British Medical Journal* and *Pediatrics* can be commended for the length of time that they have offered free access to most (if not all) content. A good example of flux can be found in the experience of visitors to the AMA website in the 1990s. Prior to late 1999, content was of limited availability and then, in the autumn of 1999, the AMA reported that *JAMA* and all the AMA specialty journals would have their full contents freely accessible to all at the AMA website, which remained the case until May 2000, when the decision was made to restrict full-text contents to paid subscribers. Other journals (e.g., *Neurology*) have publishers that promote trial periods of full access to contents for several months prior to becoming subscription based. Newer electronic journals (i.e., e-journals), and other journals with a distinctively Web-based perspective, are also available in full-content form on the Web. Issues in the electronic publishing of academic information are explored online in the Journal of Electronic Publishing and a recommended resource is the Scholarly Electronic Publishing Bibliography (see Table 1).

Specific sites that are 'homegrown' by individuals, academic departments, and research or clinical projects can be another source of 'anchor' content, though this requires a greater demand on the user to assess the validity of any site's content and content provider(s) (Table 5). John Lester (1998), the webmaster for the Massachusetts General Hospital's neurology website, provided a brief, informative online paper about the historical value of homegrown websites.

The best known 'homegrown' neuropsychology website is Jeffrey Browndyke's own *Neuropsychology Central*, which is a compilation of multiple links to other online material and includes a discussion forum. My own website, *A Cup of Neuropsychology?* provides my own content, links to current issues of journals, links to interesting full-text content at other sites, and annotated links to other sites.

Several commendable 'homegrown' websites with a broader medical or psychological scope include Neil Busis's *Neurosciences on the Internet*, which offers a very broad and routinely updated listing of links to relevant online material; Alan Gandy's *Pediatric Database [PEDBASE] Homepage*, which offers information about children's diseases; Stephen Barrett's *Quackwatch*, which offers information about fraudulent and dubious medical products and claims; Daniel Sands's *Electronic Patient Centered Communication Resource Center*, which offers information about physician-patient electronic communications; Sandra Steingart's *School Psychology Resources Online*; and Ruediger Oehlmann's *Cognitive and Psychological Sciences on the Internet.* Good examples of research-program-driven websites are David Snowden's *The Nun*

Table 5. Homegrown and specific-purpose websites.

Website name and URL	Comment
Neuropsychology Central http://www.neuropsychologycentral.com/	Jeffrey Browndyke
A Cup of Neuropsychology? http://www.divinestra.com/np.html	Anthony Risser
Neurosciences on the Internet http://www.neuroguide.com/	Neil Busis
Pediatric Database (PEDBASE) http://www.icondata.com/health/pedbase/	Alan Gandy
Quackwatch http://www.quackwatch.com	Stephen Barrett
School Psychology Resources Online http://www.bcpl.net/~sandyste/school_psych.html	Sandra Steingart
Cognitive and Psychological Sciences on the Internet http://www-psych.stanford.edu/cogsci/	Ruediger Oehlmann
The Nun Study http://www.mc.uky.edu/nunnet/	Example of a research-program website (David Snowden)
Traumatic Brain Injury Model Systems http://www.tbindc.org/	Example of a research-program website
Ottawa Health Decision Centre http://www.ohri.ca/programs/clinical_epidemiology/OHDEC/default.asp	Example of a research-program website
Think-and-Link http://www.think-and-link.org/	Example of a research-program website
The Brain Attack Coalition http://www.stroke-site.org/	Example of a selective-topic clinical-medical website (Coalition of organizations concerned with the rapid diagnosis and treatment of acute stroke)
Alzheimer's Research Forum http://www.alzforum.org	Alzheimer disease
The Whole Brain Atlas http://www.med.harvard.edu/AANLIB/home.html	Comprehensive atlas
The Center for Health Design http://www.healthdesign.org/	Architectural design in health care

Table 5. Continues

Table 5. Continued.

Website name and URL	Comment
Bazelon Center for Mental Health Law http://www.bazelon.org/	Legal issues in mental disorders
National Aphasia Association http://www.aphasia.org/	Communication resources for patents and their families and friends
Digital Anatomist Project http://www9.biostr.washington.edu/da.html	Interactive central nervous system atlas
GeneTests-GeneClinics http://www.geneclinics.com/	Genetic disorders
BioMedNet http://www.bmn.com/	Information for biological and medical researcher

Study, the Traumatic Brain Injury Model Systems (TBIMS) site, the Ottawa Health Decision Centre's site, and the *Think-and-Link* program of exploring e-mail applications for persons with acquired neuropsychological disorders. The *Brain Attack Coalition* and *Alzheimer's Research Forum* offer good examples of a selective-topic clinical-medical website. Other recommended sites are listed in Table 5. Kerns, Mateer, and Brousseau (1998), Kuster (2000) and Smith and Senior (2001) list additional websites.

Mega-sites exist with content that cuts across medical specialties. These sites, which may be for-profit or nonprofit in nature, are usually directed toward users who are general medical practitioners. Medscape is one of the oldest of these sites. It took several years for Medscape to develop its own neurology section, although it had close to twenty other sections and some content of a neuropsychological nature was available in the site's psychiatry section. Mega-sites are an area of investor-targeted financial flux, with some sites closing and others vertically expanding to include the general public (e.g., Medscape joined with CBS to supply content at its consumer-health website), third-party reimbursement organizations, and other professionals. Another mega-site example is Physicians' Online (<http://www.po.com>), which is a physician-only site that offers a diverse set on online tools for its subscription-paying membership.

Finally, there are a number of consumer- and general-public-oriented sites (see Table 6). A review by Lewis (1999) of the research literature in this area reported significant changes in levels of patient knowledge after access to electronic resources, such as the *CHESS* (Computerized Health Enhancement Support System). *NOAH*, *MayoClinic*, *Virtual Hospital*, and *Canadian Health Network* come to mind as notable examples for the provision of

Table 6. Healthcare consumer websites.

Website name and URL	Comment
CHESS: Comprehensive Health Enhancement Support System http://chess.chsra.wisc.edu/Chess/	University of Wisconsin
NOAH: New York Online Access to Health http://www.noah-health.org/	Consortium
MayoClinic.com http://www.mayoclinic.com	Mayo Clinic
Virtual Hospital http://www.vh.org/	University of Iowa
Canadian Health Network/Reseau-canadien-sante http://www.canadian-health-network.ca/	Consortium
InteliHealth http://www.intelihealth.com/	Aetna U.S. Healthcare
Neurologychannel.com http://www.neurologychannel.com/	Part of healthcommunities.com
ObGyn.net http://www.obgyn.net/	Comprehensive peer-reviewed information about women's health issues. Part of MedSpecialty.com
Child & Family Canada/ Enfant & famille Canada http://www.cfc-efc.ca/	Consortium

broad-based content for the public. There are also many venues on the Web for more narrowly based patient education, i.e., websites that provide information for specific diseases and disorders. The number of HIV/AIDS public sites that are available provide suitable examples of this, as do the previously cited OncoLink and Gateway to Neurology websites.

Clinical Issues

As this book predominantly addresses issues in clinical practice, several facets practitioners might want to consider to determine how online resources might work for them in their practice settings will be discussed below.

First, know the level of Net exposure that your patients and their caregivers have. Do they use e-mail? Do they search for information online and, if so, how do they go about doing this? Do they seek out the support of peers in virtual communities? Do they expect 'mouse calls' from you? Several years ago, I began routinely asking about these types of activities during my interviews with patients and their families. It helps me (and may help you) gauge what types of information they may have been exposed to, and it will also help you plan any adjunctive Web-based educational activities or suggest any specific online supportive virtual communities. Consider whether you wish to develop an office-based modality of training patients and their families to use the Net to learn about their problems, to keep up to date on emerging treatment options, or to better communicate with others (including you and your staff). Even if you don't, though, be prepared for well-intentioned and informed clients who have done their cyber homework, as well as for other clients who will come to you with handmade diagnoses and requests for confirmation and treatment, with copies of webpages printed out as if in assurance of their self-assessment (e.g., Ward, 1999).

Second, until you develop a formal strategy to computer-mediated communications, be cautious in your online communications. Think about whether you really want to offer electronic options in dealing with patients and other practitioners. If you don't want to pursue that, consider preparing an effective manner to deal with unsolicited requests for information. D'Alessandro and colleagues (2000) offer a standard e-mail reply message, for which they grant permission for any professional to use and/or modify without restriction. You might want to examine it. Develop a plan of action that outlines how you wish to deal with certain scenarios in patient communications. Examine the impact of confidentiality threats, human error, and time allocation in such communications, relative to other modalities. Maintain vigilance for legislative, litigation, insurance-reimbursement issues that might have an impact on the use of Internet-mediated modalities in the states or provinces where you are licensed to practice. Learn about encryption options, which increase the security of digital communications. Some companies have begun promoting and selling healthcare websites that are password-protected and otherwise secured, though not without critics in the healthcare community who seek to promote maintaining a broader set of security options not particularly limited to a small set of commercial options (Landro, 2002b); learn about the benefits and shortcomings of the options that might be available to you and your practice. Be considerate of your peers in your postings to online professional communities and in direct professional-to-professional messages.

Third, learn something about what is happening in the digitization of medical records and how this interacts with issues of privacy and confidentiality. One place to start is the Electronic Privacy Information Center's medical-records pages, available at <http://www.epic.org/privacy/medical/>. Hodge, Gostin, and Jacobson's (1999) review of legal issues relating to digital health information might also be beneficial to examine.

Fourth, use the Net as a collaborative tool within and between institutions and within and between research and clinical applications in private practices. A primer examining some of these tools (written for teachers) is *Electronic Collaboration: A Practical Guide for Educators* and is available at <http://www.lab.brown.edu/public/ocsc/collaboration.guide/>. Clinician-based research and other activities can be facilitated by many different forms of electronic collaboration, from free chat rooms, listservs, and discussion forums to online options that can be downloaded or obtained for a fee. Institutional use of these collaborative features is increasing, e.g., as part of medical residency recruitment efforts (Buterakos & Taylor, 2000). Another example is the *PATSy* program <http://patsy.cogsci.ed.ac.uk//main.html>, an innovative way of using Web-based interfaces in aphasia-assessment training and research. Consider the degree of confidentiality (or lack thereof) for any such service prior to using it.

Fifth, use the Web as a source of your own continuing education and broadening of your own personal knowledge base. Many medical websites offer formal continuing medical education credits to physicians (e.g., the *Virtual Lecture Hall* <http://www.vlh.com>), and there is some indication that psychologist-oriented sites might become more active in terms of online continuing education. It is common for most major conferences to have their own websites (or be a specific section at larger professional-society websites). Many conferences (albeit often those funded by major sponsors) offer significant degree of online participation, sometimes in real time. Some conference sites offer archival access to multimedia streams from the conference site.

Sixth, consider contributing to the process of using the Web as a way to inform and teach others. Distance-learning options are becoming part of secondary, undergraduate, graduate, and post-graduate programs of study. An excellent starting point is Horton (2000), which includes an adjunctive website (Table 1). Other websites are dedicated to examining and promoting online teaching and learning (e.g., *Educause* <http://www.educause.edu/> and *Asynchronous Learning Networks* <http://www.aln.org/>). Specific discussions of educational issues include Bourne (1998), Wegerif (1998), Carswell et al. (1999), Kettner-Polley (1999), and Brown (2001). For better or worse, accredited programs leading to masters and doctoral degrees in psychology with a primary emphasis on education by distance-learning exist. Topical continuing-education courses were offered briefly on the NAN website. However, it is more common for contemporary online learning to be part of undergraduate education. A number of specific digital-classroom interfaces have been developed to support educations uses, such as WebCT, WebCrossing, Caucus, and Blackboard. Think about whether these educational applications are suitable for clinical neuropsychology and, if so, how they might best be added to more traditional educational venues. Think about the general public and consumer education and perhaps making yourself available to host discussion forums on topics in your areas of expertise.

Seventh, be aware of the durability of the Web, but be wary of the fragility of URLs, hyperlinked content, and individual websites. It is unfortunately the situation that just because you find something today, this does not mean that you (or your clients) will find it in the same place next week. If you maintain a website, keep in mind that the surest way to lose your visitor base is by allowing the slow accretion of dead links to occur. Any user of the Web from, say, 1998 until the current day will have a list of valued websites that have become extinct, either as a result of economic changes or as a result of content providers no longer having the time or interest in maintaining their sites. Websites once offering free services are now bankrupt, have bolstered free services with distracting advertising content, or have made these services paid-subscription based.

In sum, the Internet offers a stunningly combined communication modality and way to access information. It also can be fun, challenging, entertaining, and truly educational, as well as daunting, frustrating, scary, and rife with idiocy. Unless you are truly opposed to it, use it with whatever fluency or limitations that you are comfortable with, but do use it. It's always there.

References

American Psychological Association (2000). Psychology and the Internet (theme issue). *APA Monitor, 31(4).* [http://www.apa.org/monitor/apr00/]

Anonymous (1999). Study shows physician use of internet growing. *Medical Practice Communicator, 6(5)*, 8.

Berners-Lee, T. (1999). *Weaving the web.* San Francisco: Harper San Francisco.

Bloom, R.W. (1997). Psychiatric therapeutic applications of virtual reality technology (VRT): Research prospectus and phenomenological critique. In: K.S. Morgan, H.M. Hoffman, D. Stredney, & S.J. Weghorst (Eds.) *Medicine meets virtual reality: Global healthcare grid* (pp. 11–16). Amsterdam: IOS Press.

Borowitz, S.M. & Wyatt, J.C. (1998). The origin, content, and workload of e-mail consultations. *Journal of the American Medical Association, 280*, 1321–1324.

Bourne, J.R. (1998). Net-learning: Strategies on on-campus and off-campus network-enabled learning. *Journal of Asynchronous Learning Networks, 2(2),* 70–88.

Brown, R.E. (2001). The process of community building in distance-learning classrooms. *Journal of Asynchronous Learning Networks, 5(2),* 18–36.

Buckwalter, J.G. & Rizzo, A.A. (1997). Virtual reality and the neuropsychological assessment of persons with neurologically based cognitive impairments. In: K.S. Morgan, H.M. Hoffman, D. Stredney, & S.J. Weghorst (Eds.) *Medicine meets virtual reality: Global healthcare grid* (pp. 17–21). Amsterdam: IOS Press.

Bush, V. (1945, July). As we may think. *The Atlantic Monthly, 176,* 101-108.

Busis, N.A. (1999). Neurology in the electronic information age. *European Journal of Neurology, 6,* 385–414.

Busis, N.A. & Honig, L.S. (1999). Neurologists and the internet. *Archives of Neurology, 56,* 1335–1337.

Buterakos, J. & Taylor, D.K. (2000). Live chat: Use of the internet as a resident physician recruitment tool. *Journal of the American Medical Association, 283,* 2456.

Carswell, L., Thomas, P., Petre, M., Price, B., & Richards, M. (1999). Understanding the 'electronic' student: Analysis of functional requirements for distributed education. *Journal of Asynchronous Learning Networks, 3(1),* 7–18.

Cassell, J., Sullivan, J., Prevost, S., & Churchill, E. (Eds.) (2000). *Embodied conversational agents.* Cambridge, MA: MIT Press.

Castro, E. (1999). *PERL and CGI for the world wide web.* Berkeley, CA: Peachpit Press.

Cherny, L. (1999). *Conversation and community: Chat in a virtual world.* Stanford, CA: CSLI Publications.
Childress, C.A. (2000). Ethical issues in providing online psychotherapeutic interventions. *Journal of Medical Internet Research, 2(1),* e5.
Chimoskey, S.J. & Norris, T.E. (1999). Use of MEDLINE by rural physicians in Washington state. *Journal of the American Medical Informatics Association, 6,* 332–333.
Choo, C.W., Detlor, B., & Turnbull, D. (2000). Information seeking on the web: An integrated model of browsing and searching. *First Monday, 5(2).* [http://firstmonday.org/issues/issue5_2/choo/index.html]
Coiera, E. (1996a). Virtual reality in rehabilitation. *British Medical Journal, 312,* 4–5.
Coiera, E. (1996b). The internet's challenge to health care provision. *British Medical Journal, 312,* 3–4.
Curtis, H. (2000). *Flash web design.* Indianapolis, IN: New Riders Publishing.
D'Alessandro, D.M., D'Alessandro, M.P., & Colbert, S.I. (2000). A proposed solution for addressing the challenge of patient cries for help through an analysis of unsolicited electronic mail. *Pediatrics, 105,* e74.
Davison, K.P., Pennebaker, J.W., & Dickerson, S.S. (2000). Who talks?: The social psychology of illness support groups. *American Psychologist, 55, 5.*
Dibbell, J. (1999). *My tiny life: Crime and passion in a virtual world.* New York: Henry Holt.
Drezner, J.L. (2000). Understanding adoption of new technologies by physicians (editorial). Medscape General Medicine, 7 February 2000. [http://www.medscape.com/viewarticle/408031]
Eddy, S.E. (1998a). *HTML in plain English,* 2nd ed. New York: MIS:Press.
Eddy, S.E. (1998b). *XML in plain English.* New York: MIS:Press.
Eysenbach, G. (2000). Towards ethical guidelines for dealing with unsolicited patient emails and giving teleadvice in the absence of a pre-existing patient–physician relationship — systematic review and expert survey. *Journal of Medical Internet Research, 2(1),* e1.
Eysenbach, G. & Diepgen, T.L. (1998). Responses to unsolicited patient e-mail requests for medical advice on the World Wide Web. *Journal of the American Medical Association, 280,* 1333–1335.
Figallo, C. (1998). *Hosting web communities.* New York: John Wiley & Sons.
Fox, S. & Rainie, L. (2000). *The online healthcare information: How the Web helps Americans take better care of themselves.* Pew Internet & American Life Project. [http://www.pewinternet.org/reports/toc.asp?Report=26]
Galitz, W.O. (1997). *The essential guide to user interface design.* New York: John Wiley & Sons.
Gawande, A.A. & Bates, D.W. (2000a). The use of information technology in improving medical performance: Part I. Information systems for medical transactions. Medscape General Medicine, 7 February 2000. [http://www.medscape.com/viewarticle/408032]
Gawande, A.A. & Bates, D.W. (2000b). The use of information technology in improving medical performance: Part II. Physician-support tools. Medscape General Medicine, 14 February 2000. [http://www.medscape.com/viewarticle/408033]
Gawande, A.A. & Bates, D.W. (2000c). The use of information technology in improving medical performance: Part III. Patient-support tools. Medscape General Medicine, 22 February 2000. [http://www.medscape.com/viewarticle/408035]
Gralla, P. (1999). *How the internet works: Millennium edition.* Indianapolis: Que.

Helwig, A.L., Lovelle, A., Guse, C.E., & Gottlieb, M.S. (1999). An office-based internet patient education system: A pilot study. *Journal of Family Practice, 48,* 123–127.

Hoch, D.B., Norris, D., Lester, J.E., & Marcus, A.D. (1998). Information exchange in an epilepsy forum on the world wide web. [http://neuro-oas.mgh.harvard.edu/cscw98/seizure_paper.html]

Hodge, J.G., Gostin, L.O., & Jacobson, P.D. (1999). Legal issues concerning electronic health information: Privacy, quality, and liability. *Journal of the American Medical Association, 282*, 1466–1471.

HON (Health on the Net; 2000). Surveys: Evolution of internet use for health purposes. [http://www.hon.ch/Survey/analysis.html]

Horrigan, J.B. & Rainie, L. (2002). *Getting serious online.* Pew Internet & American Life Project. [http://www.pewinternet.org/reports/toc.asp?Report=55].

Horton, S. (2000). *Web teaching guide.* New Haven: Yale University Press.

Hubbs, P.R., Rindfleisch, T.C., Godin, P., & Melmon, K.L. (1998). Medical information on the internet (editorial). *Journal of the American Medical Association, 280,* 1363.

Jadad, A.R. & Gagliardi, A. (1998). Rating health information on the internet: Navigating to knowledge or to Babel? *Journal of the American Medical Association, 279*, 611–614.

Kane, B. & Sands, D.Z. (1998). Guidelines for the clinical use of electronic mail with patients. *Journal of the American Medical Informatics Association, 5,* 104–111.

Kerns, K.A., Mateer, C.A., & Brousseau, S. (1998). Internet resources for neuropsychology. *The Clinical Neuropsychologist, 12,* 217–230.

Kettner-Polley, R.B. (1999). The making of a virtual professor. *ALN Magazine, 3(1).* [http://www.aln.org/alnweb/magazine/Vol3_issue1/Kettner-Polley.htm]

Kim, A.J. (2000). *Community building on the web.* Berkeley, CA: Peachpit Press.

Kim, P., Eng, T.R., Deering, M.J., & Maxfield, A. (1999). Published criteria for evaluating health related web sites: Review. *British Medical Journal, 318,* 647–649.

King, D. (2000, May). Specialized search engines: Alternatives to the big guys. *ONLINE.* [http://www.online.com/onlinemag/OL2000/king5.html]

Kuster, J.M. (2000). Internet resources for stroke and aphasia. *Topics in Stroke Rehabilitation, 7,* 21–31.

Landro, L. (2002a). When it comes to e-mail, the doctor is not in. *Wall Street Journal,* 11 February 2002, R12.

Landro, L. (2002b). New guidelines to make doctor–patient e-mails profitable, less risky. *Wall Street Journal,* 25 January 2002, A13.

Lawrence, S. & Giles, C.L. (1998). Searching the world wide web. *Science, 280,* 98–100.

Lester, J.E. (1998). Websites by providers, patients, and caregivers — A review. [http://neuro-www.mgh.harvard.edu/chapterxx.shtml].

Lester, J.E., Norris, D.M., & Hoch, D.B. (1998). Patient support using the world wide web. A paper presented at the 1998 Association for Computing Machinery Conference on Computer Supported Cooperative Work (Seattle).

Lewis, D. (1999). Computer-based approaches to patient education: A review of the literature. *Journal of the American Medical Informatics Association, 6,* 272–282.

Loshin, P. (1999). *TCP/IP clearly explained,* 3rd ed. San Diego: Morgan Kaufmann.

Lynch, P.J. & Horton, S. (1999). *Web style guide.* New Haven, CT: Yale University Press.

Negrino, T. & Smith, D. (1999). *JavaScript for the world wide web,* 3rd ed. Berkeley, CA: Peachpit Press.

Nichelson, D. (1997). Telehealth poses opportunities and challenges for psychology. [http://www.apa.org/practice/pf/aug97/teleheal.html]
Nielsen, J. (1999). *Designing Web usability : The practice of simplicity.* Indianapolis: I: New Riders Publishing.
Notess, G. (1999). Search engines in the internet age. *ONLINE,* May/June, 20–22.
Novak, J. & Markiewicz, P. (1998). *Guide to producing live webcasts.* New York: John Wiley & Sons.
Peters, R. & Sikorski, R. (1998). Building your own: A physician's guide to creating a web site. *Journal of the American Medical Association, 280,* 1365–1366.
Preece, J. (2000). *Online communities: Designing usability, supporting sociability.* Chicester, England: John Wiley.
Randall, N. (1997). *The soul of the internet: Net gods, netizens and the wiring of the world.* London: International Thompson Computer Press.
Rheingold, H. (1993). *The virtual community: Homesteading on the electronic frontier.* New York: Addison-Wesley.
Rivner, M.H. (1999). Neuro@neurolist.mcg.edu: An e-mail discussion list for neurologists. *Neurology, 52,* 1891–1893.
Rizzo, A.A. & Buckwalter, J.G. (1997). The status of virtual reality for the cognitive rehabilitation of persons with neurological disorders and acquired brain injury. In: K.S. Morgan, H.M. Hoffman, D. Stredney, & S.J. Weghorst (Eds.) *Medicine meets virtual reality: Global healthcare grid* (pp. 22–33). Amsterdam: IOS Press.
Seabrook, J. (1997). *Deeper: My two year odyssey in cyberspace.* New York: Simon & Schuster.
Shafqat, A., Kvedar, J.C., Guanci, M.M., Chang, Y., & Schwamm, L.H. (1999). Role for telemedicine in acute stroke: Feasibility and reliability of remote administration of the NIH Stroke Scale. *Stroke, 30,* 2141–2145.
Shellenbarger, S. (2002). Some Internet sites that can help ease burdens of elder care. *Wall Street Journal,* 27 February 2002, B1.
Silberg, W.M., Lundberg, G.D., & Musacchio, R.A. (1997). Assessing, controlling, and assuring the quality of medical information on the internet: Caveat lector et viewor — let the reader and viewer beware (Editorial). *Journal of the American Medical Association, 277,* 1244–1245.
Smith, M.A. & Senior, C. (2000). The Internet and clinical psychology: A general review of the implications. *Clinical Psychology Review, 21,* 129–136.
Specter, M. (1999). Your mail has vanished. *New Yorker, LXXV(37),* 96–104.
Spielberg, A.R. (1998). On call and online: Sociohistorical, legal, and ethical implications of e-mail for the patient-physician relationship. *Journal of the American Medical Association, 280,* 1353–1359.
Stamm, B.H. (1998). Clinical applications of telehealth in mental health care. *Professional Psychology, 29,* 536–542.
Turkel, S. (1995). *Life on the screen: Identity in the age of the internet.* New York: Simon & Schuster.
W3C HTTP Working Group (1998). Hypertext Transfer Protocol — HTTP/1.1 (18 November 1998). [http://www.w3.org/Protocols/HTTP/1.1/draft-ietf-http-v11-spec-rev-06.txt]
Wallace, P. (1999). *The psychology of the internet.* Cambridge, UK: Cambridge University Press.
Ward, B.O. (1999). "Internet-positive patients" driving you crazy? Find out how to get online and cope. *Internet Medicine, 4,* 1–6.
Wegerif, R. (1998). The social dimension of asynchronous learning networks. *Journal of Asynchronous Learning Networks, 2(1),* 34–49. [http://www.aln.org/alnweb/journal/vol2_issue1/wegerif.htm]

Winker, M.A., Flanagin, A., Chi-Lum, B., White, J., Andrews, K., Kennett, R.L., DeAngelis, C.D., & Musacchio, R.A. (2000). Guidelines for medical and health information sites on the internet: Principles governing AMA web sites. *Journal of the American Medical Association, 283*, 1600–1606.

PART III

A SURVEY OF SETTINGS AND PRACTICES IN CLINICAL NEUROPSYCHOLOGY

Chapter 8

THE INDEPENDENT PRACTICE OF CLINICAL NEUROPSYCHOLOGY: ONE PERSON'S PERSPECTIVE

Robert L. Heilbronner

Wasn't it Mark Twain who said, "reports of my demise have been greatly exaggerated?" Similarly, there are those who have prematurely predicted the imminent demise of the independent practice of clinical neuropsychology (see comments by Puente in Johnstone et al., 1995) or have at least anticipated that it will recede to the background with the advent of managed care. Many of the chapters in this book are written by, and intended for, an audience of independent practitioners. This would appear to represent some evidence that independent practice in clinical neuropsychology is here to stay. In fact, a recent survey (Sweet, Moberg & Suchy, 2000) documented that private practitioners constitute the largest group of neuropsychologists practicing in the United States today. (Note: this chapter was written in late 2001/early 2002. A multitude of changes may have already taken place in the health care marketplace since that time which affect the practice of clinical neuropsychology in general and independent practitioners more specifically.)

What are the keys to starting and maintaining a successful independent practice in clinical neuropsychology? First, you have to define what 'success' means to you. Is it achieving a certain level of income? National or international recognition for your work? Free time to pursue other personal interests? No one has all the answers. There are probably as many different ways to conduct an independent practice in clinical neuropsychology as there are independent practitioners. How you choose to conduct your practice depends upon multiple factors, including the current health care climate, the geographic region in which you practice, your philosophical approach to business, and a myriad of other influences. Most people believe that independent clinical practice affords the practitioner the opportunity to pick and choose the kinds of cases you want to take, how many hours to work, how much money to make, etc. Indeed, it is true that independent practice affords a certain degree of flexibility. But, our time is really not our own (contrary to popular belief). It is necessary to respond to referral sources, and quickly too, because the neuropsychologist across town is just a telephone call away.

There are many axioms and recommendations one could make which might help those who are considering independent practice. But, the two concepts which appear to be most important and which may guide one in their pursuit of independent practice are: *personal values* (which leads to prioritizing things) and *flexibility* (or a willingness to expand one's boundaries). Once you have your personal values in order then everything else falls into place. How many hours a week do you want to work? How much money do you want to make? How much time do you want to spend with your family? These questions are easily answered once you have examined your own personal values. Sure, you can always do another evaluation (even see patients on Saturday or Sunday if you like), but how many of your children's soccer games are you willing to miss? How much time would you like to reserve for your family or friends? These things are stated very candidly as the author had to go through a very thorough process of self-evaluation to determine what is important to him. Once that became known, then the approach to practice and to the business of practice fell into place. Not everyone has to go through such a rigorous process of self-examination. But, at the very least, you need to consider some of these things before you make the decision to leave whatever secure job you may have to venture into the uncertain world of independent practice.

The other important concept to consider is flexibility. In independent practice, you need to be open-minded and go beyond the bounds of the traditional neuropsychology laboratory. How much of your time is devoted exclusively to conducting neuropsychological evaluations? Do you do therapy with patients any longer? Would you be willing to go to a patient's home to conduct an evaluation? How about to a homeless shelter to evaluate someone with dementia? It is certainly appropriate to have a focus or speciality area (e.g., dementia evaluations, forensic consultation, etc.), but in independent practice multiple skill domains are required in order to stay viable in the competitive marketplace. Whereas our colleagues who work in medical settings might have a continuous flow of patients from within the medical center, one cannot simply sit back and wait for patients to come to the office. In the private practice world, one has to do the marketing, seek out referrals, and entertain other 'nontraditional' kinds of neuropsychological and psychological activities.

Educational Background and Credentials

The editors have asked the authors to provide readers with a brief summary of our educational background and some of our credentials and appointments. This is so that the audience at least has some confidence that the chapter author is a credible source. But, credentials do not a person make (even in the legal arena). One's experience is perhaps far more critical than the school they attended, the number of diplomas they have hanging on the wall, etc. Having said that, here is an annotated summary of the author's training and credentials.

Dr. Heilbronner received his Ph.D. in Clinical Psychology in 1986 from The University of Health Sciences/The Chicago Medical School (CMS). The program at CMS was one of the first clinical psychology programs located in a medical school and it certainly was one of the first with a separate tract devoted to clinical neuropsychology. Assessment was a strong suit, while traditional psychoanalytic theory and psychodiagnostics were less emphasized, which is unfortunate because even a neuropsychologist has to have a coherent understanding of Freud!

The author did his clinical internship at The Medical College of Virginia. This was a traditional internship with three rotations on inpatient, outpatient, and consultation/liaison psychiatry units. Following the internship, a one-year postdoctoral residency in clinical neuropsychology was completed at The University of Oklahoma Health Sciences Center. After completing the residency, the author began work as a staff neuropsychologist (and eventually became the Co-Director of the Brain Injury Rehabilitation Program) in the Department of Neuropsychology at HCA-Presbyterian Hospital. The focus of the program was neuropsychological assessment, cognitive retaining, and psychotherapy with the goal of facilitating the psychological, social, and vocational adjustment of chronic brain injured patients and their families. In 1989, the author took a position as Senior Psychologist/ Coordinator of Brain Trauma Neuropsychology Services at The Rehabilitation Institute of Chicago (RIC), a large, free-standing rehabilitation facility. Primary responsibilities included the evaluation and treatment of acute and chronic brain-injured patients, supervision of postdoctoral fellows in medical psychology, consultation to members of the brain injury team, and clinical research. At RIC, the psychologists seem to be regarded by many of the physicians and hospital administrators as merely technicians whose only value was 'psychometrics.' This was very frustrating for someone who had come from an environment where neuropsychology and psychotherapy were the primary emphases of treatment. Apparently, this kind of experience, where neuropsychologists are regarded as 'second class citizens' is not at all uncommon among psychologists and neuropsychologists who work in large medical or rehabilitation centers.

The Referral Base

One of the most common questions colleagues and lay people ask about private practice is: "Where do you get your referrals?" The most frequent response is typically: "I don't know" often followed by "...the telephone just rings." I am the first to admit that I wish I had more of a steady referral base. Perhaps, a neurology practice or psychiatry group who refers to me as their only consulting neuropsychologist. But, after a couple of years of marketing, telephone calls, sending out my vita, going to grand rounds, doing lunches, etc. it appeared that either there was no interest or perhaps these physician groups already had someone else to refer to. It became clear then that the quality of the work product (i.e., the neuropsychological report) would be the best, and most important, marketing tool. After being in Chicago for over ten years, most referrals come from people who are familiar with my work or they have obtained my name from someone who may have worked with me in the past. There is nothing wrong with that. But, developing as many consistent referrals sources as you possibly can is strongly recommended. Use your slow times for marketing or dedicate at least one morning per week towards this activity. It is time well spent. For those considering entering into independent practice, make an initial attempt to meet as many people as possible. Get your name out there, send out announcements, give talks to local groups (especially nurses, case managers), etc. It doesn't hurt to try as many avenues as possible. If a presentation led to just one referral, then that's one more than you otherwise would have had.

The Mechanics of Practice

There are many clinical neuropsychologists who have been in independent practice for a long time and they possess some very keen insights into the mechanics of practice. Chapter 4 by Dr. Peck includes a lot of information devoted to the business aspects of neuropsychology. In it, he provides alot of useful information about ways to deal with insurance carriers, minimize expenses, maximize profits, keep track of overhead, etc. His chapter is a useful resource for clinical neuropsychologists in general, but especially for those in independent practice. But, like this chapter, Dr. Peck's chapter reflects his own particular approach to managing his practice. Develop your practice by taking bits and pieces of information from other practitioners, from your own physicians' or dentists' offices, from previous training sites, etc. Your practice should be an extension of yourself and, as previously stated, it should not be conducted without first examining your own values.

There are a number of different models of independent practice. Some of you may be more interested in a group practice model. Others may want to have a number of junior associates who can help to generate referrals and manage the large volume of work that you (hopefully) have for them. Still, others may desire to be a solo practitioner without any associates at all. The important point is that there is no 'right' or 'wrong' way to conduct an independent practice in clinical neuropsychology. You simply have to choose the model which is most comfortable for you.

Most people think that those who are in independent practice have unbridled flexibility and free time. But, one does not always have complete control over when they see a patient, do a deposition, etc. Indeed, an urgent call may come in from a physician who would like his patient seen before discharge from the hospital the next day. More often than not, things will need to be rearranged so that the patient can be seen, but it often comes at the expense of something else, perhaps a daughter's ballet lesson, dinner with your spouse, etc. It would be nice if things could be scheduled at a comfortable pace. Perhaps, one or two full evaluations a week would allow adequate time to write reports before the next round of patients is seen the following week. But, responding quickly to referral sources and providing a rapid turnaround time is one of the best marketing tactics. Thus, it is recommended that you do whatever you can to schedule a referral ASAP even if you have five or six other reports to complete. That way, the referral source knows that you are responsive to their needs and you can be relied upon in the future. Acceptable turnaround time? For most, a telephone call the next day is appreciated and a written report within a week to ten days is good practice. This may not always be possible to do. Indeed, there are times in which other things (personal and/or professional) take precedence. Don't sweat it, but try not to make it a habit!

The author's professional time is devoted towards multiple activities. Approximately 50% of the time is spent conducting neuropsychological assessments, 15% doing psychotherapy exclusively with medical or neurologically-impaired adults, 25% doing forensic-related work (e.g., record review, testimony), 5% supervising colleagues, and 5% devoted towards teaching and research. These percentages can change at any time. During some periods, the legal referrals may be very busy whereas the psychotherapy referrals may be somewhat slower. On other occasions, an influx of treatment referrals may arise whereas the legal referrals may have quieted down. Being flexible and willing to take on other non-traditional activities goes a long way when the regular referrals are slow. Five years ago, I could not have foreseen that part of the time would be spent sub-contracting to an industrial-organizational psychology group and performing personality evaluations on police, firefighter and correctional officer candidates. But, this has become one of the most consistent and interesting components of the practice and the work is interesting because it requires sound general clinical skills and has very little to do with clinical neuropsychology.

The author is in solo practice and does not belong to a group, share overhead or revenues with anyone else. But, he is also a shareholder and Co-Director of a network of clinical neuropsychologists and rehabilitation psychologists (e.g., The NeuroBehavior and Rehabilitation Network: NBRN). This is a business corporation that was co-founded with five colleagues who previously worked at RIC. The network was formed seven years ago in anticipation of venturing into private practice on our own. At that time, The American Psychological Association (APA) strongly advocated that practitioners consider joining forces in order to minimize some of the challenges brought about by managed care. APA believed that referrals were more likely to go to large networks of providers and not to independent practitioners. The network was formed with the hope of increasing our visibility and attractiveness to managed care corporations. However, after a few years it has become clear that none of us were interested in having to deal with the rigors of managed care (i.e., having to write reports to justify further treatment, accept their low rate of reimbursement, etc). A decision was made to shift the emphasis of the network in other directions like generating referrals from Workers Compensation and Disability Insurance carriers, physicians' groups, etc.

There are many benefits to belonging to, and being a shareholder of, a business corporation like NBRN. Some examples include: stationary with common letterhead that lists multiple office locations (which gives the appearance of a group practice), cross referrals, reductions in the cost of liability insurance, and participation in other group insurance plans (e.g., health, dental, and disability). Suffice it to say, there are six different perspectives on how the network should operate or how it should serve the needs of its members. The author has benefited greatly from associating with each colleague and respects how they have chosen to run their practice. Trust and respect for the individuality of each group member is critical to the success of organizations like NBRN.

The Office Environment

The author shares office space with five clinical psychologists (not the same as the NBRN members) and a psychiatrist. Sharing an office with colleagues can be invaluable: it helps to insulate one from feeling isolated (a common occurrence among colleagues who practice alone). Simply going downstairs for coffee in between patients can provide ample relief during busy days or on days when tucked away typing reports. I distinctly remember earlier in my career when I worked in a medical center as part of a Psychology Department: there was a lot of interaction and always someone I could discuss patients with if I so desired. I miss those times, but also value my alone time. Sharing office space provides the best of both worlds.

Practically speaking, the office of a clinical neuropsychologist does not really require much more than a desk, a testing table with two chairs, a computer, telephone, fax machine and a couple of bookshelves. If one's practice is truly a reflection of his/her personality, then it is also true of the office environment: you can design or outfit your office in whatever way you choose. When cost becomes an issue, it forces a person to consider what is necessary, or of primary importance, for the purposes of conducting clinical neuropsychological activities. Anything beyond that might represent overcompensation for feelings of inadequacy! Indeed, many of our neuropsychology colleagues have some very beautiful office suites; but, the author would not feel particularly comfortable referring patients to some of the people who occupy them.

Membership in Professional Organizations

Stating the obvious, it is important to belong to, and support, as many clinical neuropsychology organizations as one's financial resources will allow. In 2001/2002, there were a number of different organizations, with some representing clinicians and others comprised largely of scientist-academic types. There were also two recognized clinical neuropsychology boards (ABPP-CN and ABPN). A number of 'vanity boards' also existed, where one could simply pay a fee to become a member and be 'board certified' (the reader is referred to Chapter 1 for a more extended discussion on the board issue in clinical neuropsychology). At the time of writing this chapter, the most well established neuropsychology organizations include: The National Academy of Neuropsychology (NAN), The International Neuropsychological Society (INS), Division 40 of The American Psychological Association (APA), and The American Academy of Clinical Neuropsychology (AACN). Perhaps others have emerged by the time this text has been published. It is important to contribute one's time and money to these established organizations, as they are our voice and our representative bodies for promoting clinical neuropsychology services to the public, governmental agencies, and other important entities. Without active representation, clinical neuropsychology and clinical neuropsychologists do not stand much chance of surviving in today's environment of managed care and cost-containment.

Setting of Fees

The author has not personally conducted a formal survey to determine what the relative value of clinical neuropsychology services are. That is something being addressed by others, notably Medicare and the insurance industry. Generally speaking, most neuropsychologists establish their fees based upon what others in the neuropsychological community are charging. There may be differences contingent upon geographic region and some may charge more because they are board certified; others may set their fees based upon some other professional or personal standard. Often, there is no choice; fees may be established by someone in the business office at the medical center we consult to. Even more true, reimbursement of fees is set by someone at the insurance company or managed care organization based upon some unknown formula or factors.

When the author was at RIC, patients were billed according to an established fee schedule: it was based upon 15-minute units. It was never known whether or not the institute was getting reimbursed for these services and often the manager of the Psychology Department was not even privy to whether or not, or at what rate, these services were being reimbursed. The point is that there should be some overt connection between the amount billed and the amount received. In independent practice, you should have an understanding of how much you are being compensated for your time. Is it 100%, 80%, 50% reimbursement? Is neuropsychological testing being reimbursed at a different rate than psychological testing? Does Insurance Company A reimburse more or less than Insurance Company B? Answers to these questions are important to know because you cannot expect to be fiscally viable if you don't know how much you are being compensated for your time/services. It is important to do a cost analysis and find out how much time you are spending versus how much you actually make per service rendered (again, refer to Chapter 4 for a more extended discussion on these issues).

Some practitioners bill according to units of time: per hour, per half-hour, per 15 minutes, etc. Others bill by test: e.g., the WAIS-3 costs $250.00, the WMS-3 $200.00 etc. You should charge according to whatever method feels ego-syntonic for you. If you bill by a particular unit of time (e.g., 15 minutes), the insurance may request that you resubmit the charges according to cost per test. This can be infuriating and time intensive to have to resubmit and consider the cost of each test. It is recommended that, even if you bill by some unit of time, you have at your disposal some idea or formal list of charges for each test if you are ever asked by an insurance company to resubmit your charges according to this particular method. If you are figuring out the cost per test, remember to include the time it takes to administer, score, interpret and write the results. In actuality, it does not really matter what you charge because the insurance company has their 'maximum allowable reimbursement schedule' for your particular service or test. You can bill $1,000.00 an hour if you like, but you may receive only $75.00 if that is all the insurance company allows for that service. If you are an 'out of network' provider you might expect to receive even less (or, in rare cases, more). Becoming aware of these things can determine whether or not you decide to become a 'preferred provider' in some panels.

A note about billing for forensic services. Some practitioners bill at the same rate for clinical and forensic evaluations whereas others may charge more for forensic evaluations. As an example, they may charge $250.00 an hour for testing in a clinical evaluation and then $350.00 an hour for testing in a forensic evaluation, even though they are performing the same service. There is support for both approaches and no one can be faulted for adopting one approach or the other. One should be ready to justify why there is a different and/or more expensive rate for forensic versus clinical evaluations. This will likely come up during the course of deposition or trial testimony and may be used to question your credibility as an expert. There may be some local norms or acceptable practice standard depending upon the geographic region in which you practice. Just remember that the setting of your fees (like everything else in your practice) leaves an impression on others.

Coding/Billing/Collection Practices

This is probably one of the least favorite things to talk about and certainly the least favorite part of the author's practice (except for the collecting part!). Like most of you who read this book, the author became a clinical psychologist because of a desire to help people. It was never anticipated that so much time would have to be spent fighting for financial livelihood or having to convince, cajole, and comply with so many people in the claims departments of insurance companies. Practically speaking, the amount of time I spend on the phone trying to get paid is probably far less than most other colleagues doing similar activities. A conscious choice was made years ago not to enroll in too many managed care panels because time was better spent doing other things besides filling out forms to justify further treatment, obtain pre-authorization, etc. One of the benefits of being in independent practice is not having a boss or supervisor to respond to. But, working as a provider of health care services, means that there are still insurance company employees telling us what to do, placing limitations on our practice, and ultimately our professional and personal livelihoods. Nonetheless, here is two cents about coding, billing, and collection.

The codes the author uses most often (probably 95% of the time) are: 96117 (Neuropsychological Testing); 96115 (Neurobehavioral Status Exam); 96100 (Psychological Testing); 90801 (Diagnostic Interview); 90806 (Psychotherapy: 45–50 minutes); and 90808 (Psychotherapy: 75–80 minutes). Most neuropsychologists use 96117 to cover the interview and testing. Others may bill 90801 to cover the interview time (one hour maximum) and 96117 for the testing component. Some practitioners prefer to use 96115 to cover the time spent interviewing a patient because they can bill more than one hour, although this is usually reimbursed at a lower rate than 90801. As a cautionary note, most insurance companies will not reimburse for 96115 and 96117 because they believe that the Neuropsychological Testing and Neurobehavioral Status Exam both include an assessment of the patient's mental status. They will also not reimburse for 90801 and 96117 because Neuropsychological Testing inherently includes an interview component. Puente (2001) has suggested that, if you use 96117 for the testing aspects of your evaluation, you should use 96115 for the interview, because these relate to neurological conditions. If you are using 96100, then the interview portion should be billed as 90801, which are psychiatric codes.

Medicare is used as an example of how the coding, billing and reimbursement process works...or doesn't work. It has some very specific guidelines for neuropsychology-related activities and most insurance companies follow

Medicare's lead to justify cost-containment. In Illinois, psychologists are not allowed to bill more than eight hours for 96117 in any given year. If someone comes back for a reevaluation within a year, it will not be covered unless the provider is willing to spend a lot of time writing letters or making telephone calls to justify the evaluation. Even if the patient agrees to pay out of pocket, it can only be billed *at the Medicare* rate if you are a Medicare provider. Stated again, a Medicare provider can only accept payment *at the Medicare* rate even when the patient is willing to pay the bill personally.

Medicare has some other very specific billing and coding guidelines. They typically will not reimburse for neuropsychology services that exceed nine hours in any given day. That means, if you see a patient for an evaluation in the morning and then another one in the afternoon, you should not bill for more than nine hours of services rendered. Any amount beyond nine hours will potentially 'raise a red flag' and call attention to the possibility of fraud or abuse. Medicare allows a provider to bill a half unit for every unit of face-to-face contact with a patient. So, if you see a patient for four hours of testing, you could add two hours to cover the cost of record review, test interpretation, and report writing time. If you were to see two patients, each for four hours and then add four hours to the total time for writing two reports, that would add up to 12 hours of services rendered on a given day. Whereas that might not be out of the ordinary for most of us, Medicare will not likely reimburse for that many hours of service on a given day. Remember, this chapter was written at the beginning of the new millennium. Things may be different by the time you read this, although I doubt that it would be more in the favor of neuropsychology by this point in time. I hope that I am wrong!

There are still insurance companies who will reimburse X% of what you bill. For example, if you bill $250.00 an hour for Neuropsychological Testing, they may cover 70% or 80% (if you are lucky) and then the patient is responsible for the co-payment. This model of reimbursement is not as prominent as it once was. A much more common scenario is that the provider will be reimbursed at a 'preferred provider' rate if he/she is a member of the panel of providers. If the patient is on a PPO, they usually only have to pay a modest co-payment fee (e.g., $10.00, $20.00) and the PPO covers the balance up to the amount you agreed upon when you joined their panel. If you are not a preferred provider, you can still get reimbursed by the PPO at an 'out-of-network' rate (which is probably less). It is recommended that you (or the patient) contact the PPO in advance to make sure that the service is pre-authorized. But, even if it is pre-authorized, this does not guarantee payment! If a patient has coverage through an HMO, they have to be referred for the evaluation by their primary care provider. Get a copy of the prescription or referral from that physican and have the patient (or your office manager if you have one) contact the HMO to find out if neuropsychological testing is covered under their plan. But, even a referral from a primary care provider does not guarantee payment!

Overhead

Most business people keep track of every single penny that they spend. Indeed, it makes good business sense to keep track of all expenses right down to the very last paper clip. But, time may not always allow one to stay on top of these things until it is too late. It is strongly recommended that anyone who is entering into independent practice establish a system to track expenses from the very beginning. Some common expenses include: office rent, billing and collection services, technician time, test equipment and test forms, books, journals, conferences (including travel, lodging, registration costs), supplies, telephone, faxes, internet access costs, and 'business lunches.' Do not forget to include the cost of professional liability insurance and health, dental, and disability insurance, as part of your office overhead.

Professional Practice Surveys

One of the most useful resources for the practicing neuropsychologist are the surveys which have been presented in *The Clinical Neuropsychologist* (Putnam & DeLuca, 1990 & 1991; Sweet, Moberg, & Suchy, 2000; Sweet, Moberg, & Westergaard, 1996). For those who are interested, these surveys provide answers to many of the most common questions we ask ourselves and that are asked of us by others. Who are the most common referral sources? Are they the same for independent practitioners as they are for those who work in medical settings? What are the salaries of neuropsychologists practicing in the United States? What are the most commonly used neuropsychological tests? These kinds of surveys contain a lot of important information that can be helpful when you are asked by a hospital administrator to provide a list of usual and customary fees or if an insurance company ever questions why you charge as much as you do for your services. This text also will serve as a useful resource for anyone who wishes to obtain information about the business and practice of clinical neuropsychology in their particular work domain.

A Final Word

There are no great words of wisdom or axioms which will guarantee success in the quest to practice the 'art' of independent practice in clinical neuropsychology. It is hoped that what is contained in this chapter will provide at least a starting point and some direction for those who are considering branching out into independent practice. Talk to as many other colleagues as you can to get a sense of their perspective on things. Remember to examine your own values and weigh out your priorities. Be flexible, expand your skills in ways that you might not have previously thought, and be willing to take on challenges that others might not want to take on. These things will help you to decide whether or not you want to pursue this particular direction for your professional future. Do not be afraid to abandon the ivory tower neuropsychology lab and venture into other nontraditional arenas. You can make your practice what you want and meet your professional and personal needs at the same time. For most of us, that would seem to represent the best of both worlds.

References

Johnstone, B. et al. (1995). Psychology in health care: Future directions. Professional *Psychology: Research and Practice, 26*, 341–365.
Puente, A.E. (2001). Reimbursement for professional neuropsychological services. *The 21st Annual National Academy of Neuropsychology Conference,* San Francisco, CA.
Putnam, S.H. & DeLuca, J.W. (1990). The TCN Professional Practice Survey: Part 1. General practices of neuropsychologists in primary employment and private-Practice settings. *The Clinical Neuropsychologist, 4*, 199–243.
Putnam, S.H. & DeLuca, J.W. (1991). The TCN Professional Practice Survey: Part 2. An analysis of the fees of neuropsychologists by practice demographics. *The Clinical Neuropsychologist, 5*, 103–124.
Sweet, J.J., Moberg, P.J., & Suchy, Y. (2000). Ten-year follow-up survey of clinical neuropsychologists. *The Clinical Neuropsychologist, 4(4)*, 479–495.
Sweet, J.J., Moberg, P.J., & Westergaard, C.K. (1996). Five year follow-up survey of practices and beliefs of clinical neuropsychologists. *The Clinical Neuropsychologist, 10*, 202–221.

Chapter 9

PRIVATE PRACTICE WITH A PHYSICIAN PARTNER

John C. Courtney

I came to practice with my physician colleague, Robert M. Shuman, M.D. in an almost accidental sort of way. I had stopped seeing patients in the local hospitals, preferring to work with them (primarily children between the ages of 4 and 18) in an outpatient context. Furthermore, since the bulk of my referrals were outpatients and they came from pediatricians, neurologists, neurosurgeons or other medical professionals, it was not hard to conceive of completely giving up the hassles of inpatient consultation and the well-known complexities of being paid for those services.

My overlearned associate is a board-certified pediatrician, pediatric neuropathologist, pediatric neurologist, and neuroimaging expert. Before his arrival in our community, we were forced to 'make due' with adult neurologists diagnosing and treating children with neurological anomalies. I point this out mostly because I was practicing in my community for four years before his arrival and I had been uniquely inconvenienced by the unavailability of a pediatric neurological specialist. The local hospital where I practiced has a well-staffed neonatal intensive care unit. Consequently, more and more very sick preemies and neonates were living beyond what would have been previously expected. These children were being referred to me with a broad range of problems. Learning disabilities, academic difficulties, and common neurobehavioral disorders usually associated with childhood are not, as I quickly discovered, an area of interest for most adult neurologists.

To complicate matters further, because there had been no previous pediatric neuropsychologist in our area, I found myself in the unenviable position of suggesting heretofore 'esoteric' pediatric neurobehavioral diagnoses and conditions for the children I had been seeing. Frankly, the medical community was not very familiar with what I did and they were skeptical about the value of neuropsychological evaluation of children. This is not to say that the neuropsychologists in my region were not competent, but there remained a difference between how child specialists viewed injury in the context of child development and how it was seen by those not commonly practicing with children. Dr. Shuman's arrival provided some academic and intellectual relief for me, as he had some general familiarity with neuropsychology and psychometric procedures (his undergraduate degree was in psychology), as well as a strong background in pediatric neuropathology.

Shortly after several of my patients saw Dr. Shuman at his office across town, and after we had spoken on the phone a number of times, I requested the opportunity to spend a few hours with him while he examined patients. It has been my practice to do this as referrals from any particular physician increase, particularly if I am unfamiliar with his or her practice. Moreover, it provides me with some qualitative data to impart to patients and parents about the physicians to whom I commonly refer. Working with them for a couple of days allows me to gain some understanding of how they work with patients, how they talk to them, and how patients experience their interactions with these physicians. I knew that Dr. Shuman was well regarded in his field as his reputation had preceded his arrival. He introduced me to his staff, colleagues, and patients as "Dr. Courtney" and with a reasonably clear explanation of what my area of specialization was. While I appreciate being referred to as "doctor," I am also used to being referred to in various other ways by my medical colleagues; a clear sense of collegiality was apparent from the very start of our interaction.

During the examination of our first patient, Dr. Shuman asked for my opinion several times. He took the time to teach (the parents, patients, and me) about what he found as he went along. His background as a teacher first, and a skilled clinician later, was immediately apparent. What I eventually learned, however, was that he was really more interested in 'how' I thought, than what I knew. In other words, I was getting 'checked out.'

We both passed our respective tests of one another, which is not to say that we agreed about what or how we saw our patients' conditions. This kind of discrepancy in diagnostic 'approach and understanding' has produced a respectable 'tension' between us that is practically productive. Our relationship's tension is productive because it does not stem from a mistrust of the other, but rather from an acknowledgement of the strengths and weaknesses both of us bring to patient care. Moreover, because we are both reasonably strong personalities, with more than our share of 'issues' regarding dominance, we are also able to advocate for our diagnostic and treatment recommendations with one another. Ultimately, mutual respect results from our ability to combine our best ideas and skills for the benefit of patients and their families. It has also produced significant personal growth for both of us and I have grown to like him more and more over the decade we have actively collaborated.

These points are meant to affirm that if you are going to enter into practice with a medical professional, it makes sense to have common areas of professional interest and perspective, a willingness to remain firm regarding areas of personal expertise, and an openness to reflect upon and challenge your own limitations. Physicians, as a group, are generally willing to 'run with the ball' toward whatever goal appears appropriate to them. Neuropsychologists are not immune to this phenomenon. However, it is critical that the neuropsychologists not give up their own professional identity only to become professional testers or psychometricians because their community is unaware of what other kind of box fits them best. Neuropsychology has something of real value to offer in the treatment of patients, and the neuropsychologists professionally assertive attitude regarding their skills will make it easier for the physician you will work with to feel comfortably referring to you.

Training

It is likely that part of medicine's difficulty with knowing what to do with neuropsychologists, and psychology in general, is that there is such a profound diversity in the training of each clinician. This is in relative contrast to the system in medicine where training follows a more reasonably rigid set of guidelines. The Houston Conference, while not accepted by all, is clearly an attempt to provide a more apparently delineated method of acquiring the skills necessary to practice. When I entered graduate school in 1982, I started a masters degree program in psychopharmacology at the University of Oklahoma's Health Science Center. Other than my undergraduate courses in the biological sciences and physiological psychology, my real introduction to neurophysiology occurred via research we were doing on the effects of cocaine and caffeine in rats and primates. This required a fairly rigorous preparation in animal neuroanatomy, as we were also responsible for the surgical implantation of intracranial catheters for direct substance exposure.

When I started my doctoral program in Chicago (the Illinois School of Professional Psychology) in 1984, I was ready for a change. I had developed some health problems related to an increasingly sensitive allergy to rats, making the work uncomfortable. While in the psychopharmacology program, I worked as a assistant director at a Rape Crisis and Battered Woman's Center in Oklahoma City. Having no such known allergy to humans, I found the work with my emotionally and physically injured clients fascinating (as well as emotionally draining). Already interested in psychoanalytic theory, ISPP offered a strong program in this area with advanced training with people like Merton Gill, M.D., Robert Langs, M.D. and others that I thought would be productive. While I later opted to refocus my studies towards neuropsychology, I have never regretted the advanced analytically oriented therapy training I received in school, as I believe that it has served to make me a better clinician in whole.

After two years of externship (Cook County Hospital Criminal Health Services Division and the other at the Illinois State Psychiatric Institute/

Institute for Juvenile Resources), I completed my training with an internship at the University of Notre Dame. The externship at ISPI and IJR focused solely on children and, having multiple options for training there, I opted to pursue the psychotherapeutic and neurodiagnostic rotations for severely impaired children. Subsequently, my internship provided rotations through a psychiatric hospital, mental health center, and the counseling center at Notre Dame. However, when I interviewed there, the training director agreed to allow my rotation in the psychiatric hospital to shift to a local regional medical center and private neuropsychological practice. That part of my experience would be supervised by a board certified neuropsychologist who was both on the staff at the hospital and on the University's faculty. As it turned out, I ended up doing about seventy percent of my internship with some sort of neuropsychological focus. The psychiatric hospital and mental health center had just hired a neuropsychiatrist from the University of Oklahoma. He placed a very high premium on neuropsychological evaluation, saw a preponderance of patients with psychiatric problems related to seizure disorders, and referred all of these to our testing service. Atypical behavior and seizures became an area of interest for me that ultimately became the topic of my dissertation.

Following my internship, I took a postdoctoral position at Kingwood Hospital in Michigan City, Indiana. I was offered the position through the recommendation the hospital's medical director who was a neuropsychiatrist and had also been the psychiatrist on staff at the University of Notre Dame. During those two years (1988 to 1990) I saw a far greater variety of psychiatric and neurological disorders. Because of the acceptance of the neuropsychiatrist in that community by his physician colleagues, many other neurological disorders with behavioral sequelae were referred to the testing service. Additionally, I continued to obtain supervision from a board certified neuropsychologist, as well as a very stark perspective of private/for profit psychiatric facilities.

After practicing roughly 12 years, I opted to complete the board certification in pediatric neuropsychology (ABPdN). While somewhat non-traditional in the age of ABCN/ABPN, this additional step reflected what had become much of my area of focus since graduate school. Simultaneously, I have become very politically active in support of the practice of psychology in whole and have been the president of the Indiana Psychological Association (2000–2001). Perhaps when my obligations with regard to the IPA are complete, I may seek certification through the ABPP(CN) or ABPN.

I must admit that as I passed 40 years of age, the pressure I felt to add letters behind my name diminished considerably. However, requiring a continual willingness to have your (my) work critically reviewed by my peers is important and this model is at the heart of any real board certification process. At its best, this is what makes certification so critical. It is also absolutely essential when working with an academically oriented physician colleague who thrives on peer review.

Understanding the Relationship

Any new relationship requires some adaptation. Sometimes this is easy, sometimes it is not. Knowing what you're getting into in advance is always helpful, but even that knowledge is usually incomplete. With that in mind, I've broken down what I believe to be the major areas of adaptation that are likely to cause difficulty for those entering into practice with a medical colleague. While other issues may arise from time to time, the following appear to present the greatest challenges.

Money

It seems obvious enough that since marriages face frequent conflicts over money, so will business partnerships. It should be understood that the better one could address this issue up front, the better the relationship. In the early phase of practice with my colleague, his office staff did my billing for a flat fee. This initially seemed like a reasonable alternative to setting up my own office for billing services. However, aside from the sheer additional strain on manpower required to transfer my accounts from the previous billing agency, setting up new accounts, and keeping track all of my managed care contract requirements, there remained a disparity between the CPT codes used by neurology and those used in neuropsychology. Frankly, no matter how we talk about classifying and advocating for our services as medical, neuropsychologists continue to face an inordinate amount of ignorance from third party payers as it relates to the meaning and purpose of neuropsychological testing. The neurologist's support staff was simply unprepared for this.

Like many in the field, I established my fees based upon those of my colleagues. I charge an amount equal to or greater than that of my psychiatrist colleagues. This wasn't done on purpose after finding out what psychiatrists charge per hour, but rather as a result of assessing the charges of other neuropsychologist in our region. In contrast, the neurologists charge roughly 25 percent more than we do.

Part of the money problem became apparent when I overheard the office staff trying to explain to insurance carriers and patients' parents what I do and how it is different from what a child neurologist does. In retrospect, it is moderately humorous. My skills were somewhere on a continuum from a really fancy psychometrist to someone whose telepathic skills were just shy of 'The Great Kreskin!' It became apparent that my first obligation was to teach the support staff exactly what I did for a living. They, were the first line of contact for me with the world of referrals . I tried, they glazed over. So I wrote a script, they read it over and over until it sounded natural, and they eventually began to understand the differences.

Ultimately the staff improved admirably. My collections became regular and more efficient, although I felt a bit out of place giving his staff directions about how to handle patients and my finances. After all, while I was paying for the service, they were not actually *my* employees. The separation of revenue sources and the streams of income, as it turns out, has strengths and weaknesses. Paying for the services via a flat rate produced very little incentive for his 'salaried' staff to aggressively attend to my billings and the rate did not change with the efficiency in collections. However, if my over-the-counter and third party collections happened to be very good, my expenses were always capped.

In the end, I opted to manage my own billing because I felt that no one watches my money better than I do. I think this was the correct decision for my practice because having control over how my patients are billed made it easier to be personal and precise about it. Consistent with this plan, I incorporated my practice as a separate entity. That said, to the general public, our practices remained nearly seamless. They confuse our addresses, phone numbers, billing, and they also assume that what ever gets written in his records are magically written in mine as well. So, while my corporation is responsible for those bills generated by the clinicians in my office, if I were going to use a physician's billing service again, I would make the following changes:

1. Graduate the fee paid to the physician's billing agency in a fashion that rewards the billing staff directly for increasing efficiency;
2. Before contracting with any billing agency I would produce two separate explanatory documents: one would cover exactly what CPT codes I use, what third party contracts I have, and what kind of history I've had (positive or negative) in getting reimbursed. This would facilitate the start-up time dramatically. Secondly, I would provide the billing agency with a professional description of my services from the outset so that they could argue effectively for reimbursement.
3. I would request some sort of documentation regarding what and who had been billed, the amount of work completed on collecting accounts over 90 days old, and some sort of information regarding what efforts had been made in working with resistant insurance carriers that were not attending to my charges appropriately.

Confidentiality

Prior to working with a child neurologist, and aside from the interactions I had with pediatricians and family doctors, most of my daily contacts had been with other mental health providers. Mental health providers share a common language and a set of rules or understanding regarding patient confidentiality. This is not so clear with physician practices. Patients' cases get discussed via hallway consults, without the patient or their guardian having given consent. This sort of thing is so regular as to make it the rule rather than the exception. In fact, in Indiana, no such consent is necessary for two health professionals wishing to discuss patient care (IC 16-39-2-6). Despite this, I have generally opted to gather releases of information, if for no other reason than the fact that I'd want to give my permission for someone to talk about me if the tables were turned.

Confidentiality has become an awkward issue on a number of occasions. It appears to be the opinion of many physicians, whether explicit or implicit, that the patient–doctor privilege (I use that term synonymously with confidentiality in this context only, recognizing that we are really talking about confidentiality) should really be termed patient's–doctor's privilege. In short, they seem to believe that doctors should be able to talk to one another freely about any particular patient's care without having to bother with releases. In fact, some states have loosened confidentiality guidelines so as to allow physicians to converse regarding patient care issues without a patient's consent, ours clearly is one of them. Psychologists and psychiatrists are the 'oddballs' in this predicament, clearly demonstrating resistance to the trend and requiring releases before they can discuss a case with another professional. How this changes under HIPAA is yet to be seen, but some State's guidelines for confidentiality will likely have to be strengthened under this 1996 law that is set to be implemented by 2003 (PL 104-191).

I have found myself in the position of possessing information about a patient that likely would have been of some benefit to the neurologist. It is my general approach to try to educate families about the need for openness with their treating physician as it pertains to medically important material. As a psychologist, however, it is also my position (and that of the APA and most State psychology boards) that families and patients have a clear right to confidentiality. I have an obligation to respect and protect that right so long as it does not put someone in imminent jeopardy. Unfortunately, what we see as imminent and what our physician colleagues see as imminent are not always the same. My partner and I have worked very hard to come to a mutual understanding about this issue, yet it remains a complex part of our relationship.

Perception of Psychology and Psychotherapy

You will note that I did not frame this section, "Perception of Neuropsychology and Cognitive Rehabilitation." While there are a few areas of contention between neurology and neuropsychology, there appears to be a general respect for the diagnostic material we bring to the table. The fact that neurologists, neurosurgeons and other medical professionals refer to us so readily is reflective of this.

Psychotherapy is another matter; particularly if the material to be discussed is anything other than from a strictly cognitive/behavioral model. My therapy training in Chicago included a healthy dose of psychoanalytic education, coupled with more than just tangential instruction in Family Systems. While I now identify my own therapeutic model of comfort as 'cognitive,' I do not divorce myself from my original dynamic and systemic training. Simply put, I believe that these models offer real and constructive methods for understanding patient behavior . . . even brain-injured patients, as well as providing models for successful intervention with many of them. Additionally, brain injured patients usually have families, thus enhancing the role for integrating therapeutic models.

My medical partner is not alone in regarding psychodynamic interpretations or action (often seen as inaction) as a mentally self-indulgent exercise on the part of the therapist. I have noted that physicians (my partner included) are more prone to 'cut to the chase,' resulting in new disturbing events, making psychotherapeutic work even more difficult for a therapist working with an impatient medical colleague. Consequently, it is not uncommon for me to help patients and families organize the material presented to them by a physician.

The result of having to help patients or their families through the situation mentioned above is not entirely without benefit. A patient or family feeling 'assaulted' with complex information regarding their condition, coupled with their wanting to make sense of it, can make for very productive therapeutic fodder. It allows me to use the therapy tools I have to work with the patient in a way that my partner cannot. This is the essence of a partnership! If he were able to meet all of the patient's needs, there would be no need for a psychologist in this practice. I'm better at neuropsychology and psychotherapy than he is. He is better at reading EEGs, diagnosing and treating complex neurological conditions, and reading MRIs than I am.

Finally, our practice includes a child psychologist, a psychologist who is completing his second postdoctoral program in psychoanalytic psychotherapy (the first in Object Relations and the second in Jungian Analysis), a Marriage and Family Therapist, a doctoral level school psychologist, and a psychiatrist. We have a grand-rounds like staffing every Wednesday and we include both our Dr. Shuman and the child's physician and/or psychiatrist if they are inclined to attend (and they do from time to time). This venue serves as a remarkably effective place to educate our medical colleagues regarding the training and thought process in psychology, neuropsychology, and mental health in general. It also allows for an ongoing effort to constructively integrate somewhat disparate disciplines for the purpose of assisting the patients we all serve.

Closing thoughts

Having written about the associated pitfalls in working with a physician partner, I am compelled to state that it is very difficult for me to imagine practicing without a child neurologist, or at least a pediatrician, as a partner. The admittedly selfish benefits are hard to enumerate. I am more easily accepted by other medical colleagues, have access to health care (hospital based) information that physicians seem to be privy to well in advance of most other health service professionals, and have had a learning experience that could only be likened to a never ending post-doctoral fellowship. Under the supervision of my partner, I read MRIs, EEGs, evoked potentials, and have learned to do a reasonably thorough basic neurological examination. I have learned, firsthand, about what physicians think when they read our reports. I have heard him complain about other psychologists, about me, and I have heard him compliment us as well.

All things considered, I think this sort of multidisciplinary practice produces benefits that far outweigh the risks. Dr. Shuman tells me that he has adapted as well. He's becoming a bit more sensitive to how he explains complex material to patients; he is increasingly quick to refer for psychotherapeutic help *as well as* neuropsychological testing. He has stopped referring the WAIS Verbal IQ as the left-hemisphere IQ, the Performance IQ as the right hemisphere IQ, and he has gained an appreciation for our role with complex and emotionally challenging families. Our growth, therefore, has been mutual and I believe that our patients genuinely benefit from both our areas of agreement as well as our areas of discord.

Would I recommend this sort of practice to other neuropsychologists? Certainly. However, it is important to consider the personality dynamics of the two parties very carefully before joining forces. The impact of leaving such a practice and continuing to survive in a small community might produce obstacles that could be nearly insurmountable and this should be weighed attentively at the very outset. That said, if the relationship is productive, it is hard to imagine how a private practitioner could hope for better than this.

References

Hannay, H.J., Bieliauskas, L., Crosson, B.A., Hammeke, T.A., Hamsher, K., & Koffler, S. (1998). Proceedings of The Houston Conference on Specialty Education and Training in Clinical Neuropsychology. *Archives of Clinical Neuropsychology*, 13, 157–250.

Indiana Code 16-39-2-6, Chapter 2. Release of Mental Health Records to Patient and Authorized Persons. http://www.in.gov/legislative/ic/code/title16/ar39/ch2.html

Public Law 104-191. Health Insurance Portability and Accountability Act (1996). http://www.hcfa.gov/medicaid/hipaa/content/HIPAASTA.pdf

Chapter 10

ON THE PRACTICE OF FORENSIC NEUROPSYCHOLOGY

David S. Bush

> "It is characteristic of all deep human problems that they are not to be approached without some humor and some bewilderment."
> Freeman Dyson, *Disturbing the Universe* (1979)

Introduction

In an era of widespread litigation, which is often based on claims of brain damage and psychological injury, it comes as no surprise that neuropsychologists have risen to a role of prominence on the medical–legal stage. As a group, neuropsychologists are highly verbal and intelligent. They are often skillful communicators who, having been trained in the scientific method, know how to analyze data to support an argument.

Aside from various personal characteristics that make many neuropsychologists uniquely well suited to perform roles of litigation consultant and expert witness, the contemporary practice of neuropsychology adapts quite well to the vicissitudes of the legal world. With its emphasis on quantification and measurement technology, neuropsychologists purport to offer dispassionate explanations of human behavior while relying on objective tests and value-neutral clinical judgments. Although this characterization of neuropsychology practice represents an exaggeration, it has not lessened our attractiveness in the eyes of the legal profession. If anything our apparent capacity to deliver 'hard' science answers to what are usually 'soft' science questions has increased our value to triers of fact, attorneys and the clients they represent. Perhaps not surprisingly then, a recent survey of professional trends has shown that attorneys are now the top referral source for neuropsychologists in private practice (Sweet, Moberg, & Suchy, 2000).

The notion of a subtle but nonetheless devastating brain injury makes for a compelling basis for a lawsuit. That such an injury may escape detection via conventional neurodiagnostic techniques and cause pervasive disruption of a person's ability to lead a productive and enjoyable life, in the absence of any obvious physical disability, helps account for the success of forensic neuropsychology practice. As the construct of the 'invisible' brain injury has gained popularity, often to an extent that has outpaced the available scientific evidence, the professional floodgates have opened. The forensic neuropsychology scene often resembles an idea bazaar where expert opinions are impervious to data and constrained by imagination only. Regrettably, internecine squabbling over what constitutes appropriate training and credentials in the field has precluded standardization and paved the way for 'experts' of all stripes to venture forth.

The ascendance of managed care has slashed reimbursement rates for clinical services and put doctorate-level practitioners in competition with lesser trained providers who are usually willing to provide seemingly comparable services for substantially lower fees. This dynamic has prompted many generalists to seek alternative modes of practice and pursue re-specialization in neuropsychology, presumably with a view toward forensic practice.

This chapter is about the *practice* of forensic neuropsychology, not forensic neuropsychology. No doubt, there are as many ways to successfully conduct the practice of forensic neuropsychology as there are successful neuropsychologists doing this type of work. My focus is to provide an overview of an established solo neuropsychology practice, which involves a significant component of forensic referrals. At mid-career, I have hopefully gleaned some insights that others will find useful.

Pathway

My path to neuropsychology was indirect and somewhat unanticipated. Having completed a doctorate degree in clinical psychology at Washington University in St. Louis in 1982, I entered the field at a relatively young age and at a time when the clinical job market was not exactly vibrant. In retrospect, my professional prospects were narrowed by my own uncertainty of the direction I wanted my career to take. Although I was not actively pursuing post-doctoral training in neuropsychology, I enthusiastically accepted Dr. Joe Bleiberg's offer of a fellowship at the Rehabilitation Institute of Chicago and was excited by the prospects of continuing my clinical and academic training within the Northwestern University Medical School system.

In Chicago, I was fortunate to receive excellent supervision in methods of neuropsychological assessment, which incorporate an understanding of underlying psychodynamics and interpersonal process. To this day, one of my core values as a clinician is that the practice of neuropsychology should never be divorced from the practice of clinical psychology and an understanding of the phenomenology of a human being experiencing an alteration of their brain functioning. I was also fortunate to be exposed to a broad range of individuals struggling with the social, psychological and neuropsychological consequences of life-altering injuries and illnesses. These patient groups were at varying phases of the recovery process, from acute spinal cord injuries to chronic rehabilitation cases. This exposure helped sensitize me to illness and injury as a psychological process that occurs along a developmental arc. As a post-doctoral fellow, and as a staff psychologist for the three years that followed, my clinical experiences at Northwestern were fortified by the access I had to a range of training opportunities in the behavioral and neurosciences afforded by a major medical school setting.

Toward the end of 1986, I received an offer to join two physicians, both of whom were double-boarded in neurology and psychiatry, in a newly established practice in northern Palm Beach County (Florida). By this time, I decided that the organizational politics of an institutional setting were not for me and felt ready to begin full-time private practice. My major trepidation about moving to Florida was that I would be giving up the diverse patient population of an urban university medical center for a disproportionate number of elderly retirees referred for questions of dementia. Fortunately, I was able to quickly jettison these concerns as it was not long before I was busy providing treatment and assessment services to as broad a patient base as I was seeing in Chicago. Obviously, establishing myself with two enterprising physicians helped me to 'hit the ground running' while simultaneously insulating me from several of the risks and difficulties inherent in starting a practice. Also, there were not many seriously-trained neuropsychologists in southeast Florida in the mid-1980s, and the part of the state I moved to was growing rapidly. My arrangement with the physicians proved successful and in relatively short order our group expanded.

By the time I was first exposed to a forensic case, I was already a fairly busy private practitioner with no substantial knowledge of the unique demands posed by medical–legal work. Not even knowing the difference between a plaintiff and a defendant until well after my deposition had been taken on several occasions was, perhaps, the best evidence of my forensic naivete! My attraction to the work derived from a long-standing but latent ambition to teach, an enjoyment of report writing and an appreciation for the quasi-supervisory function that forensic work can offer (i.e., being forced to examine and articulate the basis of one's thoughts and beliefs about a clinical case).

Following the rise of managed care, and contemporaneous with an unsolicited increase in medical–legal referrals, it became harder to justify the excessively high overhead expenses of operating a neuropsychology practice within a neurology group. In 1997, I left the group practice to establish a solo office in the same community. Today, the practice consists of a psychometrician, a secretary, an office manager, an outside transcriptionist and myself. The physical space is approximately 2000 square feet on two levels in a mixed-use condominium office building close to major exits off of I-95 and the Florida Turnpike. The upper level, which consists of approximately 500 square feet, is used exclusively for storage. The lower level is made up of a waiting area, a business office, two testing rooms, a nook, a bathroom, a conference room, a storage/work area and a private consulting room. Not infrequently, I am asked to conduct neuropsychological evaluations in adjacent counties and other parts of the state. On such occasions, we request that a conference room of a conveniently located hotel be reserved.

Our medical–legal referrals typically involve civil litigation and are generated throughout the state of Florida, but primarily south Florida. On average, approximately two-thirds of this work is referred by defense attorneys and one-third by plaintiff attorneys. Most frequently, these cases involve claims of acquired cognitive impairment due to head trauma and other accidents. A smaller but significant percentage of these referrals involve claims of toxic exposure, medical malpractice, Posttraumatic Stress Disorder, chronic pain and other psychiatric conditions. Often, worker's compensation and disability insurance companies generate medical–legal type referrals. We regularly evaluate individuals referred for questions of different types of competency, including testamentary capacity, which is not surprising given the demographic make-up of south Florida.

Establishing a Referral Base

It is ironic that the Editors have requested a section on marketing because, over the years, I have done very little to actively promote a forensic practice. Admittedly, I became established at a time and place when medical–legal referrals were readily available to those willing and able to do the work. Nevertheless, I continue to believe that the best method of drawing forensic referrals is to achieve the best possible clinical training and adhere to the highest possible scientific and ethical standards of practice. Of course, it helps if one enjoys the unique demands of forensic work; it can be quite stressful and is not for everyone. As in all areas of life, a little self-knowledge is a very good thing.

In retrospect, my entry to forensic practice was facilitated by already having a reasonably steady flow of non-forensic referrals. This enabled me to not feel overly dependent on any single referral source. It is likely that many colleagues, especially those at the beginning of their career, make the mistake of taking on complex forensic cases too soon and without adequate supervision. Such practice places one at risk for aversive professional experiences, which can preclude a more successful expansion of one's professional repertoire later. My personal view is that board certification should constitute a prerequisite for accepting medical–legal referrals without outside consultation.

Given the types of conditions that lead people, especially younger people, to neuropsychologists it is almost inevitable that every active clinical neuropsychologist will be drawn into the medical–legal arena at some point. Each such case poses an opportunity to increase skills and publicly represent one's expertise. Clearly, publications and talks to professional groups will increase the neuropsychologist's visibility and contacts. Affiliations with hospitals, academic departments and medical groups lend credibility within the context of a still emerging profession. Several years ago, I spent a significant amount of time and money on the preparation of an office brochure, which describes my credentials and professional interests. It was an artistic success but, to the best of my knowledge, the production costs were never recovered by increased referrals. Informal checks of how new referral sources have obtained my name have always implicated word of mouth as the premier method of gaining new business.

The extent to which many neuropsychologists ignore the image conveyed by their offices and their apparent lack of awareness of good business practices is surprising. Although many neuropsychologists are highly conscientious about clinical details, they seem much less aware that, in addition to practicing an applied science, they are in a service business. As much as possible, it is important to determine and be attentive to the needs of those we serve. Being available and responsive to referral sources seems obvious, but appears to be regularly overlooked. I have always been willing to discuss new cases with lawyers at no charge. This has consistently been a useful strategy for conveying interest in the work and transmitting preliminary impressions that are often helpful to a lawyer in the process of making decisions about how to proceed with a case. Sometimes this leads to a decision to not go forward with a referral, but the collegial consultation provides an opportunity to strengthen a professional relationship and is, inevitably, good public relations. Conversely, I have always politely declined invitations to socialize with attorneys/clients. Fraught with dangers of unconscious bias and over–identification, inherent in any social exchange, such interactions run the risk of a conflict of interest and, in my opinion, should be avoided for the same reasons that psychologists do not fraternize with patients.

A neuropsychologist's staff holds his professional reputation in their hands. This includes their answering service (or voice mail system), the transcriptionist who prepares their clinical reports and correspondence, their office support staff and, of course, their psychometricians. Carelessness, inefficiency, discourtesy and a lack of professionalism at any level of the practice reflect poorly on the neuropsychologist and will have an adverse marketing effect. Making a follow-up phone call a few days after receiving an initial inquiry or sending a report is almost always appreciated. Being proactive about faxing a curriculum vitae and fee schedule in response to a prospective new case communicates interest and availability. The neuropsychologist's personal appearance and the ambience of an office are factors that influence judgments about professional credibility. In the conference room of our office there are a series of blown-up charts, diagrams (e.g., the bell curve; statistical conversion tables; the Glasgow Coma Scale; a list of non-neurologic factors that can impact neuropsychological test scores; etc) and other teaching aides that can be displayed on a tripod. In response to recurrent questions during depositions and conferences, these 'visuals' have been accumulated over several years. They help reinforce the inevitable parallels between the roles played by the forensic neuropsychologist and university teacher; a comparison that I find to be the best metaphor for understanding the function of a neuropsychologist working in a forensic context.

Many neuropsychologists may misconstrue attention to these 'extra-clinical' details as unnecessary. While it is true that technical excellence does not demand an efficient support staff, a comfortable office or a reliable telephone answering system, these are factors that inevitably impact a professional's desirability in the eyes of the consumer. Limitations in the neuropsychologist's ability to accommodate attorneys and other clients occur often in the course of forensic work. However, good clinical and ethical practice can be compatible with good public relations.

Tasks of Forensic Practice

Within the context of providing forensically-related services, my neuropsychology practice consists of seven principle procedures: 1) conducting evaluations; 2) reviewing records; 3) report writing; 4) conferencing with attorneys; 5) conducting case research (i.e., literature reviews); 6) preparing affidavits; and 7) testifying in depositions, trials and hearings. (Keeping up with the research literature has not been explicitly mentioned, as it is assumed doing so is a priority for all serious neuropsychologists who subscribe to the scientisit-practiontioner model.) I will comment on each of these tasks.

Conducting evaluations

In my practice, one and a half days are scheduled for a neuropsychological evaluation. Evaluation fees are set by procedure, rather than hourly-based, and include the review of a reasonable amount of records (i.e., 1–2 hours). When additional time is needed to review records, the referral source is informed and the time is billed at an hourly rate. Due to the substantial time commitment, pre-payment in full is required by three business days in advance of an evaluation appointment. However, pre-payment is routinely requested by ten days in advance. A referral source is notified if pre-payment has not been received by this time and thereafter as needed. Appointments are not held when pre-payment has not been received or special arrangements made, though this is seldom necessary. In the event of a cancellation with less than seventy-two hours advance notice (weekends excluded) or a no-show, a 50% rescheduling or disruption fee is triggered. One of the major management difficulties of forensic work is the inevitability of unanticipated schedule disruptions and the associated potential for the interruption of reliable income. The best remedy to this dilemma is to insist on pre-payment or, when not possible, to obtain a written agreement of financial responsibility. A meaningful disruption policy is imperative. Office policy should be stated clearly on the medical–legal fee schedule, which can be faxed to a referral source at the time of an initial inquiry and the booking of a new appointment. The fee schedule should include a tax identification number.

I have never accepted a '*letter of protection*' (i.e., an agreement to defer payment pending the availability of monies generated by litigation) or any type of lien for an evaluation or other professional service. Such arrangements appear ethically untenable because they place the neuropsychologist in a position of having a vested interest in the outcome of a lawsuit. Under such circumstances, claims of objectivity trigger incredulity. Whenever a lawyer asks whether I accept 'L.O.P.s,' I always remind them that under Florida law an attorney is permitted to fund the cost of their client's evaluation. Usually, we never hear from them again.

The elements of the evaluation are not substantially different from non-forensic cases. For independent or compulsory examinations, the individual being evaluated should be informed about the neuropsychologist's neutrality toward the outcome of their claim or litigation and the non-confidentiality of the findings. When appropriate, the absence of any direct feedback, advice or treatment should be made explicit. (Interestingly, on numerous occasions I have offered to meet with an independent examinee for feedback, provided their litigation was resolved and both attorneys agreed. I have offered to do this at no charge. To date, I am still waiting for the first person to accept my offer!) The examinee should be told that a written report will be submitted and that the neuropsychologist reserves the right to include any information that emerges during the course of the examination. The examinee can be cautioned to not divulge any information they do not want the lawyers or other participating parties to learn about. (Over the years, a few lawyers and some neuropsychologist colleagues have challenged me about the wisdom of this latter forewarning, but I remain convinced that it facilitates rapport under difficult circumstances and, often, increases a person's willingness to disclose.) Consent to these terms should be obtained verbally and in writing. Occasionally, an examinee refuses to sign a consent form or has been advised by counsel not to sign anything pursuant to the request of an independent examiner. In these instances, the matter is not forced. I merely inform the person about the terms of the examination and document their verbal agreement. In the case of a minor or incompetent patient, it is of course necessary to obtain consent from a legal guardian.

The interview typically lasts approximately two to two and a half hours on average. Following a break, the testing process begins. I utilize a *flexible battery* approach comprised of tests that appear with relatively high rates of frequency across published surveys of contemporary test usage (Guilmette, Faust, Hart, & Arkes, 1990; Butler, Retzlaff, & Vanderploeg, 1991; and

Lees-Haley, Smith, Williams, & Dunn, 1996) with symptom validity measures. During breaks examinees are encouraged to help themselves to coffee, water and soft drinks. (As most neuropsychologists know, observing a person during a break is diagnostically informative. Often, such observations are robust sources of 'extra-test' data that are relevant to referral questions.) A courtesy phone for local calls is always available in the waiting room.

Record reviews

A careful, thorough review of all relevant records is a critically important aspect of good forensic practice. It is an integral component of the important distinction Matarazzo (1990) made between psychological testing and psychological assessment. Psychological testing represents a relatively unidimensional activity, performed by various professions, while psychological assessment is a complex integrative activity, performed by an *artisan*, and yields a *portrait* of an individual. Neuropsychologists are unique in their ability to integrate data, derived from diverse sources, and articulate a cohesive narrative shaped by the results of empirical research. Yet, having had the opportunity to read hundreds of neuropsychological reports, it is apparent that a significant percentage of practitioners are either unimpressed by or unaware of the importance of data contained within records. Nevertheless, like observations made of 'extra-test' behavior, data contained within records are often as relevant, if not occasionally more relevant, than test scores.

In my practice it is not unusual to spend dozens of hours reviewing records in a single case. This can be tedious, labor-intensive work but is almost always revealing of highly significant information relevant to an understanding of the effects of an injury or life-event. So often the neuropsychologist will find documentation in the contemporaneous medical records (e.g., evidence of a mild, uncomplicated head injury) that is discrepant from alleged damages that form the basis of litigation (e.g., disabling amnesia). Carefully reviewing post-accident records can illuminate temporal patterns that either support or contradict self-reported histories and what is known about the expected course of a given injury or condition. Similarly, scrutiny of pre-accident medical, school, vocational and legal records will often demonstrate pre-existing factors that should either increase or decrease a clinician's confidence in a particular diagnostic inference.

In general, attorneys are advised to retain the neuropsychologist to review records in a case prior to making a decision about whether to go forward with an examination. This allows the neuropsychologist to form certain preliminary impressions about a case and convey information that may have a bearing on the lawyer's decision to proceed. We request a retainer fee that amounts to four hours of review time and, when needed, bill at an hourly rate for any additional time. I am in the habit of dictating notes as I conduct the review and marking important pages with adhesive tabs. While dictating notes increases expenses due to transcription costs, it substantially improves my efficiency (one can continue reading while dictating). My handwriting is very poor and I like having typed notes to refer back to in the event that I eventually examine the person and prepare a report. Also, when conferencing with an attorney after the review is completed, I will always offer them a copy of my typed notes, which they have no difficulty reading.

Report writing

Every neuropsychologist has their own particular style of handling reports. To be sure, there is no single right or wrong format. Each neuropsychologist should determine what constitutes important content, along with the particular needs of the user(s) of the report, and present this as clearly and as succinctly as possible. In forensic work the neuropsychologist's report is usually entered into evidence and serves as an outline for subsequent examination and cross-examination. Thus, my preference is to generate a report that is detail-oriented and maximally thorough. By making explicit one's clinical reasoning process, and the data that substantiate the diagnostic inferences and conclusions, the neuropsychologist is in effect generating a schematic that their future testimony can follow. Over the course of reading hundreds of neuropsychological reports and depositions, the pitfalls associated with insufficient or incomplete clinical analysis at the time a report is generated are apparent. When a neuropsychologist produces a report that reflects a failure to consider compelling alternative hypotheses or significant data, their credibility is diminished even when the ultimate conclusions about a case may be correct. My approach to forensic report writing is to always try to ask myself about the data that comprise and corroborate my opinions and statements. In essence this is no different from what all good clinicians try to do when formulating a case, though the requirement for being *data-bound* must be especially stringent in forensic contexts. The benefits of publicly acknowledging those aspects of a case that are not well understood or can not be presently explained should not be underestimated.

My forensic reports are usually fairly lengthy, depending on the amount of records I have reviewed. Following brief sections containing Identifying Information and the Reason for Referral, there is a section subtitled 'Informed Consent' where I mention informing the examinee about the terms (i.e., non-confidentiality) of the examination and obtaining their consent to proceed. It is critically important to list the sources of all records reviewed, as the neuropsychologist will be expected to cite the basis for each and every opinion. The person or agency that provided the records should be stated because it is not unusual to obtain case materials from more multiple sources (such as when test data are received directly from another neuropsychologist). I usually preface my summary of the records by stating that I will limit my comments to data that I consider relevant to a formulation of the person's current neuropsychological status and their probable relationship to the accident or incident in question. In this way the rationale I am relying on for the editorial decisions that follow is clear. My summary of the records proceeds in chronological order beginning with the contemporaneous documentation of the accident or event that occasions the claim. Afterwards, information contained within any pre-accident records is discussed. When the neuropsychologist determines that potentially important records are lacking, this should be documented and it may sometimes be necessary to defer reaching a conclusion until after the additional information is received. I have difficulty reading other people's handwriting. Consequently, is not unusual for me to comment on a given record being illegible. In this way, I am acknowledging having seen the record but not knowing its content.

Following a detailed summary of the records, the next sections of my reports summarize the Interview Information and Behavior Observations. There are statements about behavior observations that I might include in a clinical report, but not a forensic report. Usually, these statements pertain to inferences derived from counter-transference reactions. While clinically relevant, they are typically too speculative within a forensic context and could be easily construed as prejudicial. For example, many years ago I described an individual undergoing an independent examination as 'quietly hostile.' This observation was based on my 'gut' response to the examinee's attitude and was not explicitly anchored by any of his overt statements or behaviors. During cross-examination, his attorney fixated on this detail and, in actuality, did an effective job of creating an impression of bias. After listing the tests administered, I proceed to the Results section. Years ago, I adopted a format for this section that organizes tests according to major cognitive domains (i.e., 'Attention/Concentration/Information-Processing Speed'; 'Learning/Memory'; 'Language/Praxis'; etc.). Within each section, I cite only quantitative data, usually percentiles, and completely avoid any presentation of what each test purports to measure and what the scores may mean. I find such presentations of test findings to be cluttered and almost impossible to read.

In the Conclusions/Recommendations section, the major inferences derived from the relevant records are stated (e.g., "Using standardized criteria, Mr. Jones sustained a mild and medically uncomplicated closed head injury. These criteria are: ..."). Next, the individual's clinical course and their major subjective complaints are summarized. The test results, including any contradictory findings, and the conclusions are described, which hopefully take into account a consideration of all of the available data. After stating the conclusions, recommendations are outlined. This includes the need for any additional information that may be required before opinions can be finalized. Even in cases where the purpose is limited to diagnostic issues, I almost always comment on the implications that I think my conclusions have for the person's ability to work or attend school, their need for future evaluation/treatment and, where applicable, the need for supervision. My experience has been that it is inevitable that a neuropsychologist will be asked to opine about such matters.

On occasion specific research citations are cited to substantiate my conclusions. This usually occurs in cases where other experts have already offered opinions that seem egregious. At the end of a report, I state that my conclusions are based on the currently available data and are offered within a reasonable degree of neuropsychological probability. I also mention that my conclusions may be subject to some degree of revision in the event of information not yet received. The importance of carefully proofreading a forensic report cannot be overemphasized. Any neuropsychologist engaged in forensic work should expect their reports to be scrutinized. In much the same way that supervision did during training, anticipating questions and challenges can help sharpen the neuropsychologist's analysis and increase diagnostic confidence. My bias is that spelling and grammar count! Finally, it is not unusual to be questioned about a case many months, and sometimes years, after an evaluation was conducted. A detailed and carefully crafted report will make testimony more effective and less stressful.

Conferencing with attorneys

Conferences with attorneys usually take place after I have reviewed records. They also occur following an evaluation, but this almost always happens prior to a deposition or trial and after I have submitted my report. Conferences may take place in person or over the phone, though they are always pre-arranged to insure that I have an adequate opportunity to prepare. Often, I will compose an informal outline in advance of a conference to make sure I cover issues that I expect are important to the attorney. Our office requests pre-payment at the time the appointment is scheduled. The fee is based on an hourly rate, which is stated on the fee schedule.

I conceptualize a conference with an attorney as an opportunity to *translate* from the language of neuropsychology to plain English. The purpose is to clarify what I think about a case and intend to say when questioned about my opinions. Again, knowing in advance what one thinks about a case and why guards against any threat of a conference degenerating into a negotiation process where the attorney inappropriately attempts to shape the neuropsychologist's opinions. Sometimes, I am made aware of new information about a case or information not previously available. On such occasions, the neuropsychologist should request that the information be forwarded in its original form, as soon as possible, and maintain a circumspect position about the effect it will have on their conclusions.

Cases that involve serial neuropsychological examinations are almost always especially difficult. For one thing, there is more technical data to analyze and explain. For another, such cases are usually the most contentious and require an attorney to have a very clear understanding of the technical nuances leading to a disagreement between the experts. When faced with such cases, I try to approach the conference as a private tutorial session, which often includes reading assignments provided ahead of time. Those attorneys who are willing to invest the necessary effort and time are, inevitably, the ones that are most satisfying to work with. Taking the time to prepare graphs and summary tables that make trends in the data easier to understand, and can later be used as trial exhibits, is almost always quite helpful.

Conducting case research

One of the best parts of doing forensic work is that, unlike the clinical environment, the neuropsychologist is compensated for utilizing a labor-intensive approach to assessment cases, which is always preferable. Quite often this entails an investigation of specific topics raised by a medical–legal case. Recent examples from my practice include the risk of neuropsychological injury secondary to chiropractic manipulation; psychogenic stuttering following closed head injury; the parameters of ordinary forgetfulness and the neuropsychological effects of coronary artery bypass surgery. Obviously, the internet allows for fast, efficient literature searches that can be conducted from the home or office by individuals, such as myself, who do not have easy access to a university or medical library. For the most part, attorneys seem very appreciative of these efforts; understandably so, as there have been a number of cases where the outcome seemed directly tied to a cogent presentation of relevant research findings.

Time spent conducting case research is billed on an hourly basis at a rate that is stated on the medical–legal fee schedule. Before undertaking a special literature review, I inform the attorney about the purpose of the inquiry, estimate the time involved and obtain authorization to proceed.

Preparing affidavits

An affidavit is a sworn written statement given voluntarily before a qualified witness (our secretary is a notary public). Affidavits are often used in preliminary legal proceedings and, in my practice, I am frequently asked to produce them. In Florida, there is case law that allows for the videotaping of independent examinations, though the majority of board-certified neuropsychologists in our state regularly resist these attempts; a position that is congruent with the official position of the National Academy of Neuropsychology (2000). Over the years, I have submitted numerous affidavits to sensitize the courts as to why I believe that the videotaping of neuropsychological examinations is contraindicated. I have also submitted affidavits on a range of other issues. Some examples of these topics include: a) justifying the need for one and a half days to conduct a neuropsychological examination, b) explaining why it is necessary to review a person's pre-accident psychiatric records, c) stating my reasons for refusing to pre-release the names of tests I intend to use in an examination and d) explaining my reluctance to conduct an examination in the presence of a lawyer or an observing psychologist. Frequently, these affidavits are supplemented by corroborating documents (i.e., research articles, letters from test publishers, etc.) referred to as exhibits.

Testifying in depositions, trials and hearings

There are a number of books aimed at psychologists and other professionals interested in developing their skills as an expert witness (cf., Blau, 1984; Shapiro, 1984; Brodsky, 1991,1999; Klawans, 1991; Tsushima & Anderson, 1996). To be sure, this is a complex topic and one that is well beyond the scope of this chapter. Even though I have been called on regularly to testify for many years, the art of expert testimony is not a topic that interests me and I have not paid any serious attention to the available literature. I am, however, able to share some basic strategies that have seemed to serve me well.

In terms of practical considerations, we always block off two hours for a deposition. The fee schedule reflects a two-hour minimum and, again, pre-payment in full is required by seventy-two hours (weekends excluded) in advance. In my experience it is highly unusual for a deposition involving neuropsychological evidence to last one hour or less. My secretary will keep me apprised of upcoming depositions to insure adequate time for preparation. Prior to a deposition copies of the curriculum vitae should be placed on the conference table. A current account statement should be made available. It is critically important to have immediately accessible all of the case records and any other materials that have been relied on. Years ago, I began keeping a list of all depositions and trial appearances. When such records are kept, they must be furnished upon request according to Florida Civil Rule of Procedure (Rule 1.280) and on the basis of Florida Statute (*Elkins v. Syken*). Due to the unpredictable nature of trials, the scheduling of a courtroom appearance is inevitably much more disruptive to the neuropsychologist's schedule. This is compounded by the associated need for intense, time-consuming preparation and a generally heightened level of anxiety. My experience has been that a retaining lawyer can give much more reliable information about the exact date and time of a courtroom appearance after the trial has begun. At that point, my office will maintain close contact with the attorney's secretary as a way of minimizing schedule disruption. Our fee schedule reflects a five-hour minimum for the scheduling of a courtroom appearance but, much more often than not, a full day is required and pre-payment under the usual terms is requested. Even on those infrequent occasions when I have traveled to the local courthouse, been called at the pre-arranged time and dismissed in relatively short order, I find I am often too exhausted, or otherwise distracted, to see patients that day. For particularly complex cases, I will often block time off in my schedule in advance of a courtroom appearance in order to prepare. Otherwise, most of my preparation takes place in the early morning, evening and on the weekend. While the need for advanced preparation is never insignificant, I find it is largely a function of how recently my deposition was taken. Not surprisingly, cases involving multiple sets of neuropsychological test data almost always require maximal preparation time.

Within the context of being an expert witness, the metaphor of neuropsychologist as teacher is especially apt. From this vantage point, the neuropsychologist's primary role is to articulate what the relevant data are and clearly explain the conclusions they do and do not support. I always try to avoid any sense of attachment to the outcome of a forensic case and prefer to focus my energies on how best to explain to myself and others what I believe to be factual and why. By conceiving of my function as a teacher, not an advocate, I seldom have a problem acknowledging when I do not know the answer to a question or (heaven forbid!) neglected to consider a reasonable alternative. A teacher/expert should, ideally, rise above the adversarial fray and, as much as possible, maintain faithfulness to the data as best as he understands them. Admittedly, these standards are often a kind of platonic ideal and can be quite difficult to adhere to when one is under attack.

Closing Statement

There is an old Zen story about a swordsman who dedicated his life to avenging the assassination of his master. After many years of searching, he finally finds his master's assassin and fights him to the ground. As he unsheathes his sword and tells the assassin to prepare to die, the assassin spits in the swordsman's face whereupon he returns his sword to its sheath, mounts his horse and begins to ride away. The assassin calls out "Why didn't you kill me?" The swordsman responds "Because I was angry." The meaning of this story is that, rightly or wrongly, the desire to avenge a master's assassination is principled, but that acting in anger is undignified. One of the major challenges of practicing forensic neuropsychology is that it often provokes strong affects. When doubts about our work are raised in public, along with attempts to undermine our integrity, we are all narcissistically vulnerable. The most effective experts, however, will maintain their equanimity in the face of attack. Their actions and statements are governed by principle, not impulse. In our field, this means adherence to the values of science and the Ethical Principles of Psychologists and Code of Conduct (APA, 1992), especially as they relate to issues concerning boundaries of competence, the basis for scientific and professional judgments and validity considerations (see also Binder & Thompson, 1995).

Neuropsychologists involved in forensic work face thorny ethical dilemmas and questions about what constitutes appropriate professional action on a more or less regular basis. Business pressures and, occasionally, the harassing behavior of interested parties often compound the complexity of these dilemmas. Being able to discuss these scenarios with trusted, experienced and board certified colleagues is invaluable, though it may become necessary to cite their names on the record. Sometimes, it is also necessary to rely on one's personal attorney to clarify proper courses of action. The neuropsychologist doing forensic work is well advised to have available a 'team' of trustworthy consultants willing to offer advice as needed. This is not a line of work for the faint-hearted. However, it can be quite gratifying for those who enjoy an intellectual challenge and an ongoing opportunity to introspect about the basis of their clinical formulations.

Acknowledgment

The author wishes to express appreciation to Drs. Paul Lees-Haley and Jerry Sweet for their helpful critiques of an earlier draft of this chapter.

References

American Psychological Association. (1992). Ethical principles of psychologists and code of Conduct. *American Psychologist, 47*, 1597-1611.

Binder, L.M. & Thompson, L.L. (1995). The ethics code and neuropsychological assessment Practices. *Archives of Clinical Neuropsychology, 10*, 27–46.

Blau, T. H. (1984). *The psychologist as expert witness.* New York: John Wiley & Sons.

Brodsky, S.L. (1991). *Testifying in court: guidelines and maxims for the expert witness.* Washington D. C.: American Psychological Association.

Brodsky, S.L. (1999). *The expert expert witness: more maxims and guidelines for testifying In court.* Washington D.C.: American Psychological Association.

Butler, M., Retzlaff, P.D., & Vanderploeg, R. (1991). Neuropsychological test usage. *Professional Psychology: Research & Practice, 22*, 510–512.

Dyson, F.J. (1979). *Disturbing the universe.* New York: Harper & Rowe.

Elkins v. Syken, 672 So.2d 517 (Fla.1996).

Fla. Rule of Civil Procedure, Rule 1.280.

Guilmette, T.J., Faust, D., Hart, K., & Arkes, H.R. (1990). A national survey of psychologists who offer neuropsychological services. *Archives of Clinical Neuropsychology, 5*, 373–392.

Klawans, H.L. (1991). *Trials of an expert witness: tales of clinical neurology and the law.* Boston: Little, Brown & Company.

Lees-Haley, P.R., Smith, H.H., Williams, C.W., & Dunn, J.T. (1996). Forensic neuropsychological test usage: an empirical survey. *Archives of Clinical Neuropsychology, 11*, 45–51.

Matarazzo, J.D. (1990). Psychological assessment versus psychological testing, validation from Binet to the school, clinic and courtroom. *American Psychologist, 45*, 999–1017.

National Academy of Neuropsychology (2000). Presence of third party observers during neuropsychological testing, official statement of the national academy of neuropsychology. *Archives of Clinical Neuropsychology, 15*, 379–380.

Shapiro, D.L. (1984). *Psychological evaluation and expert testimony.* New York: Van Nostrand Reinhold Company.

Sweet, J.J., Moberg, P.J., & Suchy, Y. (2000). Ten-year follow-up survey of clinical Neuropsychologists: part II. Private practice and economics. *The Clinical Neuropsychologist, 14*, 479–495.

Tsushima, W. T. & Anderson, R.M. (1996). *Mastering expert testimony, a courtroom handbook for mental health professionals.* Mahwah, New Jersey: Lawrence Erlbaum Associates.

Chapter 11

ADULT PRACTICE IN A UNIVERSITY-AFFILIATED MEDICAL CENTER

Ivan J. Torres and Neil H. Pliskin

Introduction

The practice of Clinical Neuropsychology within a medical school setting shares many of the same challenges encountered in other settings, and many of these issues are echoed throughout this book. Nevertheless, several elements combine to make work in the medical center setting unique for (neuro)psychologists. In some respects, the neuropsychologist is working as an 'outsider' within a setting that inherently runs according to a medical model of training and service delivery (i.e. typically as a member of a psychiatry, neurology, or other medical department). Within such a setting, a tendency can exist for resources and decisions to be preferentially managed by physician colleagues. By virtue of being a part of an academic institution, neuropsychologists in this setting also often function in multiple roles. Along with providing patient care, a successful clinical practice can serve as a foundation for educational training and clinical research programs. Thus, in addition to attending to important concerns directly related to maintaining a practice, the neuropsychologist working within this setting must also be mindful of how decisions shaping practice are likely to influence training and research goals. In some instances practice considerations can be influenced by educational and research agendas.

It is important to acknowledge that among colleagues, other medical professionals, administrators, and departmental hierarchy in a multidisciplinary setting such as a medical school department, there may variably in understanding what neuropsychology has to offer. Moreover, the extent to which neuropsychological programs are supported by these agents can be strongly influenced by the latter's biases and perceptions. For obvious reasons it is especially important for neuropsychology to receive support from within the department in which it resides. To this end, ongoing effort needs to be directed toward educating and conveying information about the breadth of services that can be provided, the scope of patients that can be served, and the extent to which these services can be reimbursed. In today's environment, this latter point poses a particular challenge, and this topic will be addressed in more detail later in the chapter. It is thus important to convey that 1) the neuropsychological services provided will enhance the department's mission of helping patients and they are an important component in the evaluation and treatment of psychiatric, neurological, and medical illness, 2) neuropsychology's contribution to the clinical, teaching, and research programs can enhance the department's recognition within and outside the medical center, and 3) the provision of these services can be fiscally feasible and even advantageous. An informed departmental leadership will also be able to acknowledge the indirect advantages of having a strong clinical program. In addition to generating new sources of patients, establishment of intra and inter-departmental relationships can lead to the development or enhancement of research programs. The potential financial and academic gains (e.g. grants, publications) to the department are readily apparent. Also, many neuropsychologists, by virtue of their advanced research degrees and academic backgrounds, can contribute to and design research programs that many physicians cannot. Additionally, the establishment of an excellent clinical service serves as a core for medical and psychological educational training programs. The direct gains for the department include participation of psychologists in medical training, as well as attracting excellent psychology and other trainees that are drawn to a reputable training program.

Finally, in some respects, neuropsychologists can feel at times as though they are functioning on 'foreign soil' within an academic medical school setting. For instance, the needs of the medical students and medical programs are often given extra weight. This is due, at least in part, to the fact that medical students pay tuition which supports the university, and which serves as a source of revenue for the department. By contrast, psychology programs within an academic medical center setting have to be self-sustaining. Within a medical school environment, a neuropsychologist may also encounter a higher incidence of misconception, negative bias, or limited understanding of what neuropsychology has to offer. However, if these biases are understood as resulting from lack of education about neuropsychological training, roles, and potential contributions, then the neuropsychologist can work to gradually change perceptions through interaction, excellence in education, and superior service provision.

This chapter will provide a description of a neuropsychology clinical practice within a medical school psychiatry department. Although the general description of our neuropsychology service may briefly describe some aspects of the pediatric program, the more specific points pertain exclusively to the adult section. It is hoped that the somewhat detailed coverage of our program will provide the reader with an estimate of the staff and material resources necessary to run a neuropsychology practice in this setting. The chapter will also broadly cover many of the advantages, disadvantages, and specific challenges inherent in practicing within the medical school setting. The issues that are deemed most relevant, including discussion of the establishment, nature, and maintenance of referral relationships, the interplay between clinical and academic/teaching goals, and business/financial considerations will also receive detailed coverage.

About The Authors

The authors are full-time faculty members within the psychiatry department at the University of Chicago who specialize in adult neuropsychological assessment. Dr. Torres is an Assistant Professor of Clinical Psychiatry who has been in the psychiatry department for approximately four years, and who functions as the Associate Director of Adult Neuropsychology and the Director of Practicum Training in Adult Neuropsychology. He received predoctoral training in Neuropsychology at the University of Memphis, within the Neuropsychology track specialty that is part of the clinical psychology program. This was followed by a clinical internship in Neuropsychology at the West Haven VA Medical Center. In addition, he completed a two-year post-doctoral fellowship in Neuropsychology/Neuroimaging in schizophrenia, within the Clinical Research Center (Psychiatry Department) at the University of Iowa. His research interests include the neuropsychology of schizophrenia, neuroimaging of memory disorders, and effects of brain radiation therapy on cognitive function.

Dr. Pliskin is a board-certified clinical neuropsychologist and an Associate Professor of Clinical Psychiatry and Neurology. He has served as Director of Neuropsychology for the past 12 years and also serves as the training director for the clinical psychology internship and fellowship programs within the department. He received his predoctoral training in neuropsychology from the Chicago Medical School, followed by a clinical internship at the National Institute of Mental Health – St. Elizabeth's Hospital and a postdoctoral fellowship in clinical neuropsychology at the University of Oklahoma Health Sciences Center. His research areas include medical neuropsychology, multiple sclerosis, and electrical injury.

The Practice Setting

The authors are part of a larger group of five adult and two pediatric neuropsychologists who have full time faculty appointments in the Department of

Psychiatry and collectively make up the Neuropsychology Service. This service is composed primarily of several independent clinics operating within the outpatient departments in sections of adult and child/adolescent psychiatry. In both child and adult neuropsychology, formal outpatient clinics operate four days per week, although the inpatient neuropsychology consultation service is continuously active and 'on call' during the week. Of the seven faculty, four (two adult, two pediatric) have full-time clinics at the university hospital setting, and three have primary functions at satellite clinics. In addition to individual offices for each faculty member at the university hospital, two full time technicians (one adult, one pediatric) share an office, and there is a neuropsychology computer lab with four IBM computers, which is shared by practicum students and part-time technicians. Neuropsychology trainees at the internship and post-doctoral fellow levels also have individual offices. There are five testing rooms that are available at the university hospital setting, which are shared by four full-time and two part time faculty. Additional lab or research space is scarce and its availability is generally contingent upon grant funding. Specific practice patterns for the authors include formal outpatient clinics as well as shared coverage of inpatient referrals throughout the week.

Referrals/Professional Relationships

Variability in referral source needs

Before considering how referral sources are identified and maintained in the medical school setting, it is important to define the active and potential referral sources within this environment. In this setting, upwards of 80% of referrals are generated directly by internal and community-based physicians in a variety of medical disciplines, including neurology, neurosurgery, general medicine, geriatrics, primary care, and psychiatry. The remainder of referrals arise from a variety of other sources including attorneys, non-physician health care providers, and self-referrals.

Although physicians initiate most referrals, it is important to acknowledge the tremendous diversity of referral questions and patient needs that are encountered in this setting. Significant variability exists in terms of referral source sophistication and their pre-existing knowledge of the potential benefits that can be gained from neuropsychological services. The clinical questions or concerns among referral sources also vary. It is one job of the neuropsychologist to consider these issues carefully in order to maximize his or her effectiveness. In addition, the interactions between the neuropsychologist and referring physician should not be perceived as exclusively a unidirectional flow of information from referral source to consultant or vice versa. In many instances, the interaction can and should take the form of helping to shape the referral question by assisting the referral source with discussing the issues at hand. Situations often require that we implicitly or even explicitly educate referral sources about what it is that we do, and how we can contribute to caring for patients. A further elaboration of this teaching process can include provision of inservices, grand rounds, or other lectures to active or potential referral groups in order to educate them about how their care could be enhanced by neuropsychological services. Similarly, offering lectures and experiential opportunities to other department's residents can be an effective way to market. Several articles on neuropsychological assessment in medical settings can also be useful for this purpose and are liberally distributed in the process of teaching physicians and residents (Auerbach, Cicerone, Levin, & Tranel, 1994; Keefe, 1995; Report of the Therapeutics and Technology Assessment Subcommittee of the American Academy of Neurology, 1996). Experience indicates that following such presentations, referrals to our clinics are increased. Another modality that is used to market services, targeting either potential or diminishing referral sources, involves distribution of pamphlets and letters to groups or individuals. Regardless of the means of communication, the described process requires the clinician not only to be sensitive to the referral source's knowledge, previous training, and expectations, but also to educate and help shape referral questions in a manner that is interpersonally sensitive and does not elicit defensive responses.

The patterns of professional interaction and service delivery can vary based upon several factors, one of which is the extent to which neuropsychology services are integrated into a specialized multidisciplinary treatment team. As an example, in our setting, neuropsychology is an integral part of several established specialty programs treating a targeted group of patients. Examples of these include the Epilepsy Surgery Program, the Center for Comprehensive Care and Research on Memory Disorders (Dementia Clinic), the Electrical Injury Program, the Brain Tumor Program, and the Lupus Clinic. Within these settings, the importance of neuropsychology has been well established and neuropsychology represents an important component of the treatment team. As part of existing treatment protocols, all or nearly all patients that are seen through these clinics are routinely seen for neuropsychological evaluation. Moreover, mechanisms have been established for provision of feedback, reports, and other support. Patient staffings are commonly conducted in multidisciplinary meetings, and in addition to written reports, the neuropsychologist provides feedback to the group within these staffings. While it is not the focus of this chapter to describe in detail the role of the neuropsychologist in each of these individual settings (this is better elaborated in other chapters), functions and roles can vary quite significantly across various programs. For example, whereas the important contribution within the Epilepsy Surgery Program relates primarily to identification of focal brain dysfunction for the purpose of possible treatment through surgical resection, the goals within the dementia setting have more to do with differential diagnosis and assessment of functional status (e.g. ability to live independently). Regardless of the service needs, we consider the establishment of neuropsychological services within a specialized multidisciplinary team as optimal, given the obvious advantages this provides to clinical, training, and research goals.

In addition to providing service as part of a multidisciplinary team, a significant proportion of patients are referred by individual clinicians, and these patients are seen in non-specialized outpatient neuropsychology clinics within our department. Although many of these referrals come from established referral connections with individual physicians, in many instances the referral sources are new and unknown to the neuropsychologist. It is with the latter type of referral that it can be most useful to discuss cases with the referral source prior to the evaluation in order to help shape the referral question. Evaluations conducted in the outpatient clinics are also likely to be the most comprehensive both in terms of testing procedures and written reports. The reason for this is that referral sources often send patients because of vague cognitive or behavioral complaints, and in an effort to understand patients, comprehensive cognitive and personality/emotional assessment must often be integrated with historical information. Within this context, our role is primarily diagnostic, and in order to sift through competing diagnoses, comprehensive evaluations are often necessary for accurate case conceptualization.

In contrast, when the neuropsychologist's role is defined as a member of a larger multidisciplinary treatment team, evaluations tend to be less comprehensive. For example, the need to summarize history in an extensive manner is often unnecessary, as the treatment team typically already knows this information. Rather, the goal is to provide much more succinct reports summarizing neuropsychological findings. Thus, in providing findings pertinent to our defined 'piece of the puzzle,' it is often the case that reports can be more abbreviated and directed. To summarize, depending on both the nature of the referral as well as the setting in which the service is delivered, the role of the neuropsychologist can vary from being a consultant addressing a specific question to playing a central role in directing and providing treatment care.

Educational training programs

A critical function of our neuropsychology program is to serve as a major neuropsychology training site at the graduate (practicum), internship, and post-doctoral levels. In contrast, other programs may choose to focus on one level of training. In an average year, the externship program offers advanced training in neuropsychological assessment and rehabilitation for 8–10 students from local graduate clinical psychology programs, in both child and adult areas. The internship program is an APA approved neuropsychology training program that adheres to Division 40 training guidelines and the Houston Conference recommendations for training in Clinical Neuropsychology (Proceedings of the Houston Conference on Specialty Training in Clinical Neuropsychology, 1998). The program trains two neuropsychology interns in adult and/or pediatric neuropsychology. The post-doctoral fellowship training program also adheres to Houston Conference guidelines for training, and consists of a two-year slot that is renewed on alternating years. At all levels of training, students are involved in clinical and didactic training with the opportunity for research involvement. The faculty are heavily involved in most aspects of training which include formal training seminars in the clinical neurosciences, neuroanatomy, and related specialty topics. The faculty also provide weekly individual and group clinical supervision. In addition, one form of research mentoring involves serving on thesis and dissertation committees for students conducting research in neuropsychology and clinical neuroscience.

Clearly, the breadth of training opportunities that can be offered to students are dependent upon relationships established with referral sources within the medical center. Because our center is heavily involved in training at multiple levels, it is important to provide a breadth of experiences in clinical neuropsychology. Moreover, this is obviously facilitated by having increasing numbers of faculty, as this enhances the likelihood that the various disciplines in need of neuropsychology services can be covered. The establishment and maintenance of professional and collaborative relationships with medical colleagues can also lead to further training opportunities for students in our programs. For example, our students routinely have the opportunity to participate in bedside neurology rounds or brain pathology labs that are based in other departments.

Research considerations

One of the attractive aspects of working within a medical setting is the opportunity to pursue research interests. Participation in research in an academic medical center is facilitated by direct access to clinical populations, the opportunity to collaborate with researchers from similar or distant disciplines, and the ability to capitalize on resources available within a medical academic institution. The provision of clinical services often serves as the core to either establishing research programs directed by the neuropsychologist, or engaging in ‘opportunistic’ collaborations with other investigators. It has been our experience that once medical colleagues understand the utility of neuropsychological contributions, they often become interested in establishing research collaborations. This can often lead to the enviable situation of having options for working with any of a variety of patient populations. For example, the neuropsychologist interested in investigating memory disorders can choose to work with a host of different populations (e.g. dementia, epilepsy, brain tumors, etc.). Finally, as part of a recognized discipline within a multidisciplinary treatment team (e.g. the epilepsy surgery program; dementia program, etc.), the opportunity to participate in individual or center grants can be tremendously enhanced. To summarize, this discussion underscores the importance of establishing successful and reputable core neuropsychological services, as these often serve as the backbone to establishing neuropsychology research programs.

Personnel

Across the full neuropsychology service including all satellite settings, the service staff consists of three full-time bachelor's level neuropsychology technicians, in addition to approximately five ¼ to ½ time graduate level part-time technicians. Additionally, one secretary is shared among all the neuropsychology faculty. The coordination of scheduling is conducted through the psychiatry department's intake office. The staff in this office are responsible for taking telephone requests for referrals, scheduling patients, ordering medical records, and verifying insurance coverage. Similarly, the processing of billing forms is conducted within the departmental billing office (to be covered in more detail later). Finally, legal consultation is available for all members of the medical staff through the medical school office of legal counsel. The aforementioned resources, although generally provided by the department and the medical school, are ultimately bundled into the clinical revenue targets that are calculated for each individual clinician within the department.

Mechanics/Conduct of Practice

General procedures

With little exception, most of the neuropsychological assessments are conducted through a close collaboration between the neuropsychologist and a student or technician. The level of independence afforded to the student depends on the level of training. Nevertheless, all patients are interviewed with the attending neuropsychologist's presence in the patient room, and the technician or trainee conducts the psychometric testing. A typical clinic day involves meeting with students/technicians in the morning to discuss cases for the day, covering issues relevant to the cases, and creating a battery of tests to address the referral question. After patients arrive, a brief interview is conducted to 1) understand the general nature of the patient's presenting complaints, 2) assess the patient's general mental status and identify potential barriers to testing, 3) gather any materials the patient may have brought with them to help facilitate integration of historical material (e.g. medical records, history questionnaires, scans, etc.), and 4) explain the procedures of the day to patients and family members, and answer any preliminary questions they may have. After a morning of testing, the clinic group meets again early in the afternoon to discuss emerging findings and make modifications to the initial battery of tests. Consistent with recent trends, a hypothesis-testing flexible battery approach is employed within our service (Sweet, Moberg, & Westergaard, 1996). The afternoon meeting is followed by a more extensive interview with the patient, and the rest of the afternoon is devoted to completion of testing. Depending on the nature of the referral question or level of impairment, patients are generally evaluated between three and eight hours.

After students have scored their protocols, patient files are checked and double checked by one of the senior technicians. It is also standard practice to schedule patients and families for follow up feedback sessions in order to discuss results of the neuropsychological evaluation.

Responsiveness to referrals

Several major goals of any successful neuropsychology practice include accurate diagnosis, provision of useful recommendations and written reports to referral sources, and completion of these tasks in an efficient, timely manner. Diagnosis often takes the form of differentiating brain dysfunction from psychologically-based disorders, or of identifying specific organic mental disorders. Although diagnostic questions are often, although not always addressed, referrals almost always involve specification of cognitive strengths and weaknesses and their functional implications. While the ability to accurately diagnose and to identify functional strengths and weaknesses is obviously important, this ingredient alone is not sufficient for a successful practice. The most thoughtful, accurate, and comprehensive conceptualization of a case can be of little practical use if findings are not presented clearly to the intended audience. Similarly, a well-communicated report (or verbal feedback) may have little utility if it is delivered too late to impact upon treatment decisions. For this reason, the neuropsychologist in the academic medical center setting must also be sensitive to the specific needs of referral sources, as this is ultimately linked to the needs of patients. As is the case in other settings, responsiveness to referral source needs also leads to subsequent referrals.

In our setting, responsiveness in terms of turnaround time for reports is an ongoing challenge. Several training related factors can serve as barriers to quick and efficient turnaround times. As previously mentioned, all scoring protocols have to be checked and re-checked for accuracy. Additionally, depending on the student's sophistication with report writing, multiple drafts often have to be re-edited before a final report is generated. Despite these necessary sources of delay, the great majority of reports are completed within one to two weeks after the patient is seen in the outpatient clinic.

Inpatient vs. outpatient settings

Although a considerable majority of our service has always been outpatient based, we have regularly provided consultation to inpatient units within the hospital. This is not surprising, given that many of the referring physicians familiar with our services also care for acutely ill hospitalized patients. Inpatient referrals can take on several forms, including evaluation of delirium versus dementia, assessment of functional level to assist with issues such as ability to live independently, and evaluation of acute treatments on cognitive function (e.g. effects of LP, shunt operations, medication changes, ECT, etc.). Inpatient evaluations often differ qualitatively from outpatient evaluations in several respects. First, the discrete referral questions that are posed commonly can be answered with briefer evaluations and reports. Moreover, the process requires the clinician to conduct more bedside and qualitative evaluations where formal psychometric findings are often less appropriate. Finally, the dynamic inpatient environment requires more flexibility on the clinician's part, given the variable access to patients on the medical units. The need to interact with referral sources and to provide timely feedback becomes especially critical in inpatient settings. Given this immediate need for prompt feedback, verbal feedback is often provided on the day of testing, and a final report is completed and placed in the patient's chart within 1–2 days of patient contact.

Business

For many years, academic medical center neuropsychology programs operated without close scrutiny paid to their billing and reimbursement practices. In today's environment of manage care, declining reimbursements, and governmental regulations, the reimbursement for neuropsychological services has been dramatically altered (Sweet, Westergaard, & Moberg, 1995). Now, neuropsychology programs are expected to cover all costs related to expenses including salary, overhead, supplies, and technical support. In the past, many neuropsychologists working within academic settings billed for their services but often times never received detailed financial information related to reimbursement or productivity. This has changed dramatically. Neuropsychologists in academic settings are now required to devote detailed attention to their practices and costs, in a similar way that private practitioners have done for years. Our department establishes a financial target of "amount billed" for each individual provider within the neuropsychology program. This target is built upon the amount of charges that would be required to generate sufficient revenue to cover the provider's costs to the department. The breakdown of the total costs to the department include:

Expenses:
Salary plus Benefits (23% of salary)
Administrative Overhead – includes space, utilities, etc. (22%)
Taxes:
Billing Service Tax (8%)
Dean's Tax (11%)

These expenses and taxes are deducted from the total amount billed, which is then adjusted by the current collection rate (approximately 55%) in order to derive a final revenue target necessary to cover costs. This final dollar amount is then converted to number of hours necessary to generate the revenue and then is converted to a weekly target. As is apparent from the high rate of administrative overhead and the significant 'Dean's Tax,' working within a major medical center clearly does not afford one the control (or access to revenue) that is present in private practice. By contrast, certain expenses are also covered broadly by the academic medical center including liability insurance and CE budget that typically are paid by the private practitioner.

Coding, Billing, and Collection Practices

Within our practice, the billing procedures are conducted in cooperation with the departmental billing office. The neuropsychologist completes the initial diagnostic coding process with little contribution from the billing office. The billing office may monitor that basic coding requirements are met for some carriers like Medicare. Among these guidelines are the assurance that there is an appropriate attending on the bill (which in our institution needs to be an MD physician), and that certain coding modifiers are included with the bill (AH modifier). The billing office on occasion supplies clinicians with other very general coding guidelines established through the department's participation in mental health contracts or carve outs. Finally, the billing office also monitors bills for obvious errors that can occur such as leaving out a diagnosis, failing to specify the name of the provider, failing to fill in the hours billed or billed amounts, etc. The billing office, however, provides no input regarding the diagnostic codes that should be used, which may be different from other institutions. Thus, if specific payers have idiosyncratic rules about particular diagnostic codes that may offer better reimbursement rates, the burden is on the clinician to become familiar with these rules. In order to complicate the situation, these specific rules can vary among different payers. One of the general practice principles we have adopted is to preferentially bill conditions under medical, as opposed to psychiatric codes, whenever possible. This practice is based on the idea that payers frequently reimburse medical services in a less restrictive fashion.

Our billing practices have historically involved billing for units (hours) of CPT code 96117, but based on ongoing developments in our field, some of us have experimented with billing 96115 for a clinical interview, used in conjunction with 96117 for testing. For neuropsychological assessment, our practice has been to bill at a ratio of 1.5 hours for every one hour of testing in order to cover records review, test scoring, and report generation. A dementia evaluation consisting of 3–4 hours of testing, for example, is often billed at 5–6 hours. In contrast, a comprehensive full day evaluation consisting of 7 hours of testing is typically billed at 10 hours.

In terms of payer mix, approximately one third of our work is Medicare based. Within the state of Illinois, neuropsychological assessment is not reimbursed under Medicaid. Thus, the few Medicaid patients that we see essentially represent pro-bono work. The remainder of the patients we see are paid through HMO/PPOs, contracts (State mental health facilities, department of child and family services), private insurance, or self-pay (including medical-legal work). Once bills have been submitted, the billing office is responsible for processing these charges further then sending them on to our billing service to handle collection activities. Across the various payers that have been recognized, we generally achieve reimbursement around 55% of that billed. Obviously, the poor reimbursement rates obtained through Medicare, Medicaid, and many private insurance carriers and HMOs is offset by better rates of reimbursement obtained through medical–legal work, contracts, self-pay, and some private insurance carriers. As a result, and consistent with general trends, neuropsychologists in this setting have to work harder, see more patients, and work longer hours than ever before to maintain the level of revenue they generated more easily in the past (Sweet et al., 1995, 1996).

While provision of inpatient services has historically been an important component of practice in our setting, several emerging external factors have influenced our practice in this arena. Perhaps the most significant of these has been the trend toward declining reimbursement associated with inpatient neuropsychological assessment services. In our setting, we collect only one fifth of what is billed, in large part as a result of a considerable self-pay medicaid population. Another issue relates to the so called 'incident to' rule, where testing services performed by technicians and students are viewed as incidental to the service that is already paid for by Medicare payments to the medical center. This means that only the time spent by the neuropsychologist on assessment activities can be billed. Accordingly, inpatient work becomes even less cost effective. One form of dealing with the problem of poor inpatient reimbursement has been to re-direct inpatient referrals to outpatient clinics whenever appropriate. This approach cannot be applied to all referrals, however, as some referral questions need to be answered in order to direct treatment or disposition planning while patients are still hospitalized. In addition to achieving the potential reimbursement benefits, the strategy of re-routing patients to outpatient clinics has the advantage of affording the clinician some control over the evaluation procedure. For example, patients can be evaluated in the absence of distractions (as is often the case on medical units), and resources (e.g. space, personnel, students) can be allocated for these assessments in advance. For many of the remaining inpatient referrals, evaluations are conducted with the expectation that reimbursement will likely be minimal. Another changing aspect of practice that has been driven by economics has been the tendency to provide fewer services to public aid and pro bono recipients. Additionally, there is an increasing role for involvement in forensic neuropsychological work to offset declining reimbursement from other payers. Finally, consistent with the realization that payers are less willing to reimburse for lengthy and extensive neuropsychological evaluations, we are also faced with the substantial challenge of streamlining assessment procedures without compromising the validity and the quality of the evaluation.

Perspectives and Future Directions

In a closing note, it is hoped that a balanced description of what it is like to work as an adult neuropsychologist within a University affiliated medical center has been provided. The clear advantages of working in this setting include the opportunity to provide a range of clinical services to a variety of different patients, to pursue research and teaching interests, to establish professional and collaborative relationships with medical colleagues, and to continue learning by being a part of an academically stimulating environment. The challenges primarily center on interacting with medical colleagues with varying degrees of sophistication about the potential contributions of neuropsychology. Because of this, it is important for the neuropsychologist working within this setting to understand and anticipate that a significant amount of energy will be required to educate our colleagues about what we do. It is important to remember that in large part the actual value of any service is intimately tied to the perceived value to the person asking for the service. The understanding of the importance of neuropsychology, however, needs to go beyond influencing our medical colleagues. It is quickly becoming apparent that if our field is to survive and hopefully thrive, it is our duty (as a field, and within this setting) to also relay this message to the general public, to insurance companies, and to legislators. Moreover, the most likely means of achieving this will be to stimulate cost effectiveness outcome studies in the same way that Health Psychology has considered these issues in the past (Friedman, Sobel, Myers, Caudill, & Benson, 1995). Therefore, we hope that the current efforts to offset declining reimbursement by increasing forensic work, shortening batteries, seeing more patients, transferring inpatients to outpatient clinics, and turning away public aid patients are only short-term solutions to current trends.

References

Auerbach, S.H., Cicerone, K.D., Levin, H.S., & Tranel, D. (1994). What you can learn from neuropsychologic testing. In H. Schroeder-Mullen (Ed.), *Patient care* (pp. 97–116).

Friedman, R., Sobel, D., Myers, P., Caudill, M., & Benson, H. (1995). Behavioral Medicine, Clinical Health Psychology, and cost offset. *Health Psychology, 14*, 509–518.

Keefe, R.S.E. (1995). The contribution of neuropsychology to psychiatry. *American Journal of Psychiatry, 152*, 6–15.

Proceedings of the Houston Conference on Specialty Education and Training in Clinical Neuropsychology (1998). *Archives of Clinical Neuropsychology, 13.*

Report of the Therapeutics and Technology Assessment Subcommittee of the American Academy of Neurology (1996). Assessment: Neuropsychological testing of adults. Considerations for neurologists. *Neurology, 47*, 592–599.

Sweet, J.J, Moberg, P.J., & Westergaard, C.K., (1996). Five-year follow-up survey of practices and beliefs of clinical neuropsychologists. *Clinical Neuropsychologist*, 10, 202–221.

Sweet, J.J, Westergaard, C. K., & Moberg, P.J. (1995). Managed care experiences of clinical neuropsychologists. *Clinical Neuropsychologist, 9*, 214–218.

Chapter 12

PEDIATRIC PRACTICE IN A UNIVERSITY-AFFILIATED MEDICAL CENTER

Keith Owen Yeates, Andrew N. Colvin and John T. Beetar

In this chapter, we describe the Pediatric Neuropsychology Program at Children's Hospital in Columbus, Ohio. The program came into being in September 1989, when the senior author was hired as a staff psychologist. Over the next decade, in response to a growing demand for neuropsychological services, the program has gradually evolved to include four staff neuropsychologists, two postdoctoral neuropsychology fellows, and one full-time and one half-time psychometrist.

With this growth have come significant changes in our practice. Indeed, although the current chapter provides a snapshot of our practice patterns, professional practice in neuropsychology is a moving picture that is affected by myriad forces, including those that govern health care in the United States. Hence, although we intend this chapter to describe our current practice, we also hope that it illustrates how the program has evolved over the years and indicates how we believe it will do so in the future.

Evolution of the Program

The Pediatric Neuropsychology Program had its genesis in 1989. At that time, the senior author accepted a position as a staff psychologist at Children's Hospital, with an appointment as a Clinical Assistant Professor in the Department of Pediatrics at The Ohio State University. Although the position was not initially expected to entail exclusively neuropsychological services, those services were in such demand that they quickly became the sole focus of the position.

During the next year, the senior author obtained a contract for neuropsychological services from a local psychiatric hospital. The contract provided initial funding for a postdoctoral training program in pediatric neuropsychology, which began with one postdoctoral fellow in 1990. The number of fellows was increased to two in the fall of 1993, based on the growing demand for neuropsychological services. The postdoctoral training program, which joined the Association of Postdoctoral Programs in Clinical Neuropsychology in 1994 (Hammeke, 1993), is now fully funded by Children's Hospital. The original contract with the local psychiatric facility lapsed because of budgetary constraints imposed by changes in insurance reimbursement for inpatient psychiatric services.

In 1994, again in response to the demand for neuropsychological services, a second clinical faculty position in neuropsychology was approved by the hospital, and the new faculty member began work in the fall of 1995. The addition of a second clinical faculty member allowed the senior author to share supervisory responsibilities in the postdoctoral training program, and he was therefore able to move to a tenure-line faculty position as an Assistant Professor in the Department of Pediatrics. The move permitted him to devote more time to research, based on a reduction in expectations for clinical service.

In 1997, a third clinical faculty position was authorized by the hospital, and the new staff member began work in the fall of 1998. Around the same time, the administrative responsibilities entailed by the growth of the Pediatric Neuropsychology Program were recognized by the hospital administration via the creation of an official title for the Director of Pediatric Neuropsychology, which is the position now held by the senior author.

In 1998, a fourth faculty position was authorized. The fourth faculty member was recruited and began working in March 1999. A fifth position, for a tenure-line faculty member, was authorized early in 2002, in hopes of expanding the research programs in the Pediatric Neuropsychology Program. Recruitment for that position is underway.

Program Setting

The Pediatric Neuropsychology Program is situated within Columbus Children's Hospital, which is a private, non-profit institution. The hospital houses the Department of Pediatrics for the College of Medicine and Public Health at The Ohio State University. The hospital has three primary missions: clinical service, teaching, and research. More than 270,000 patients visit the hospital each year, ranging in age from newborns to young adults. Teaching activities involve more than 1,800 students in medicine, nursing, and allied health professions. Research is coordinated through the Children's Research Institute, which is housed in a separate facility, the Wexner Institute for Pediatric Research.

The Pediatric Neuropsychology Program is located within and administratively responsible to the Department of Psychology at Columbus Children's Hospital. The Director of Pediatric Neuropsychology reports to the Director of Psychology, who also is Chief of the Division of Psychology within the Department of Pediatrics at The Ohio State University. The Department of Psychology consists of nine full-time doctoral-level faculty, all of whom also hold faculty appointments in the Department of Pediatrics. Two additional faculty positions have recently been authorized. Several of the faculty hold tenure-line academic positions, with the rest holding adjunct clinical positions.

In addition to a postdoctoral training program in pediatric neuropsychology, the Department of Psychology supports a predoctoral internship in pediatric psychology that is accredited by the American Psychological Association (APA), as well as several postdoctoral fellowships in pediatric psychology and developmental disabilities. Graduate students from the Department of Psychology at the Ohio State University also complete practica on site. More broadly, Children's Hospital provides training in pediatrics for medical students from The Ohio State University College of Medicine and Public Health, has a residency program in pediatrics, is a major rotation for other residency programs located at the Ohio State University Medical Center (e.g., physical medicine and rehabilitation; neurosurgery; neurology), and supports fellowships in numerous pediatric sub-specialties. The multiple training programs in psychology and medicine provide substantial opportunities for professional socialization for the postdoctoral neuropsychology fellows.

Staff Background

Dr. Yeates obtained his graduate training in child clinical and developmental psychology at the University of North Carolina at Chapel Hill. As part of his graduate work, he completed a predoctoral research fellowship in mental retardation and child development, as well as an APA-approved predoctoral internship in child clinical psychology at Judge Baker Children's Center and Children's Hospital in Boston. After obtaining his doctorate in 1984, Dr. Yeates completed a postdoctoral research fellowship in social and behavioral sciences in the Department of Psychiatry at the Harvard Medical School. Dr. Yeates obtained training in clinical neuropsychology during both his internship and postdoctoral fellowship.

In 1986, Dr. Yeates began working as a neuropsychologist at a state psychiatric hospital for children and adolescents outside Boston. He subsequently accepted a position as a staff member in the Neuropsychology Program and Learning Disabilities Clinic at Boston Children's Hospital. During this time,

Dr. Yeates also was a co-principal investigator on a study of a school-based intervention program designed to promote children's interpersonal development. The study was based at the Harvard Graduate School Education, and Dr. Yeates held a position as an Instructor in the Department of Psychiatry at Harvard Medical School.

In 1989, Dr. Yeates accepted a position as a staff psychologist at Columbus Children's Hospital, with an initial academic appointment as a Clinical Assistant Professor. In 1993, he obtained his Diplomate in clinical neuropsychology from the American Board of Clinical Neuropsychology/American Board of Professional Psychology. He is currently Director of Pediatric Neuropsychology in the Department of Psychology at Columbus Children's Hospital, and was promoted to Associate Professor in the Department of Pediatrics of The Ohio State University in 1999.

Dr. Colvin completed his graduate training at the University of Florida in the Department of Clinical and Health Psychology. His initial interests were in child clinical and pediatric psychology, but he later changed his area of emphasis to neuropsychology. Dr. Colvin completed an APA-approved predoctoral internship in clinical psychology at Columbia-Presbyterian Medical Center in New York, where he participated in the neuropsychology track. From 1996 to 1998, Dr. Colvin completed a 2 year postdoctoral fellowship in pediatric neuropsychology at Columbus Children's Hospital. Following the fellowship, Dr. Colvin accepted his current staff position as a pediatric neuropsychologist at Columbus Children's Hospital. He holds the academic rank of Clinical Assistant Professor in the Department of Pediatrics, and is also Director of Internship Training.

Dr. Beetar worked as a teacher for ten years before obtaining a masters degree in educational psychology and becoming certified as a school psychologist. He received his doctoral training at Hahnemann University in Philadelphia, where he participated in the neuropsychology specialty track in the clinical psychology program. He completed an APA-approved predoctoral internship in the neuropsychology track of the Brown University Clinical Psychology Internship Consortium. He remained there for a one-year postdoctoral fellowship in clinical child neuropsychology at Emma Pendleton Bradley Hospital. In 1995, Dr. Beetar began working as a staff neuropsychologist at Bradley Hospital, and he was appointed a Clinical Assistant Professor in the Department of Psychiatry and Human Behavior at the Brown University School of Medicine. In 1999, Dr. Beetar accepted his current position as a staff neuropsychologist at Columbus Children's Hospital. He holds the academic rank of Clinical Assistant Professor in the Department of Pediatrics.

Referral Patterns and Mechanisms

Over the years, referral patterns for the Pediatric Neuropsychology Program at Children's Hospital have shifted. The shift reflects a substantial increase in the number of outpatient evaluations that the program is able to complete each month, as compared to the relatively stable number of inpatient consultations that the program receives (see Table 1). The shift also reflects a substantial increase in the size of the Division of Pediatric Neurology at Children's Hospital, which has grown from two to six neurologists over the past decade.

On average, the program receives between four and six inpatient referrals each month, a rate that has held relatively stable from 1989 to the present. Most inpatient consultations are requested by Physical Medicine and Rehabilitation (PM&R), for children who are admitted to the hospital's Rehabilitation Unit, which is accredited by the Commission on the Accreditation of Rehabilitation Facilities. PM&R accounts for about 75% of all inpatient referrals, with the percentage increasing somewhat over the years. Most of the remaining referrals come from Neurology. In earlier years, Neurosurgery and Pharmacology/Toxicology also made frequent referrals. The decline in referrals from Neurosurgery is attributable in part to a decline in the rate of hospitalization for children with milder head injuries, as well as to a shorter length of stay for those who are hospitalized (Thurman & Guerrero, 1999).

The most common referral diagnosis for inpatients is head injury, which accounts for about 55% to 65% of all consultations. Other common referral diagnoses include seizure disorder, stroke, infectious disease (e.g., encephalitis, meningitis), lead intoxication, anoxic insult, and brain tumor.

The number of outpatient evaluations that are conducted by the program each month has increased by nearly 100% over the past ten years. Referral sources for outpatients are much more diverse than for inpatients, and have changed more over the years. Within the hospital, five medical services have consistently accounted for the largest percentage of outpatient referrals. They

Table 1. Number of inpatient and outpatient referrals for neuropsychological evaluation, 1990–2001.

Year	Inpatient	Outpatient
1990	48	93
1991	49	161
1992	46	153
1993	44	129
1994	41	147
1995	66	174
1996	62	180
1997	69	196
1998	42	221
1999	70	311
2000	61	284
2001	60	277

are Hematology/Oncology, Infectious Disease, Neurology, Neurosurgery, and PM&R, each of which makes about 5% to 15% of the total referrals.

Over the past ten years, the total percentage of outpatient referrals accounted for by those services has declined from around 65% to 40%. The decline reflects a relative increase in the number of referrals received from community sources, who have become familiar with the program largely by word of mouth. Community pediatricians account for about 10% to 15% of outpatient referrals, community behavioral health professionals make about 7%, and direct parent referrals comprise about 7%. In recent years, referrals for forensic evaluations also have increased, and now account for approximately 5% of all outpatient referrals. Requests for forensic evaluations are typically directed to the senior author, for whom they account for approximately 15% to 20% of all evaluations.

Referral diagnoses for outpatients are similarly diverse. Medical and neurological diagnoses account for the majority of referrals, with neurodevelopmental and psychiatric disorders accounting for the remainder. Because of an increase in referrals from community sources, the proportion of outpatient referrals accounted for by medical and neurological diagnoses declined somewhat in the mid-1990s, but it has increased recently because of difficulties obtaining insurance reimbursement for neurodevelopmental and psychiatric disorders. The most common medical and neurological diagnoses among outpatient referrals are head injury, seizure disorder, brain tumor, perinatal complications (e.g., low birthweight, prematurity, intraventricular hemorrhage), leukemia, and infectious disease, including HIV. The most common developmental diagnoses are specific learning disability and attention deficit/hyperactivity disorder.

Because of the sustained high demand for neuropsychological services, until recently we had made little effort to solicit additional referrals from sources that are not familiar with the program. Indeed, because of the lengthy wait that our outpatient referrals typically endured before being seen, we had occasionally considered closing referrals to all but hospital medical staff. However, hospital administrators did not consider this desirable, in part because Children's Hospital, as the major provider of pediatric services in central Ohio, wants to be responsive to community needs.

By adding staff positions, we have reduced the outpatient waiting list substantially, and have made specific efforts to increase our stream of referrals. We have contacted our major referral sources, both within the hospital and in the community, to announce the addition of new staff members and associated reductions in the outpatient waiting list. We have also sought to establish closer relationships with certain Sections within the hospital (e.g., Hematology/Oncology) by having our faculty and fellows participate in relevant clinics and engage in other activities that increase our visibility. Fortunately, the ability to provide more services often seems to bring a corollary increase in demand for those services.

Practice Mechanics

Inpatient consultation

As noted earlier, most inpatient referrals come from PM&R for children admitted to the Rehabilitation Unit. Our program is consulted for all admissions to the unit that involve disorders of the central nervous system. Patients are admitted to the unit after being stabilized medically. For example, most patients with head injuries have progressed at least to Ranchos-Los Amigos Level IV (Hagen, Malkmus, & Durham, 1979).

Consultations are called into the Psychology Department by unit clerks, and are distributed by our secretarial staff to the neuropsychology postdoctoral fellows, who are responsible for completing the neuropsychological evaluation prior to the patient's discharge. In general, the fellows complete all testing for inpatient consultations. The psychometricians are not typically used for inpatient evaluations. The two postdoctoral fellows are responsible for keeping a written log of all inpatient consultations.

The neuropsychology fellows monitor the patient's progress on the Rehabilitation Unit through weekly staff rounds, as well as through informal contacts with rehabilitation team members. The fellows work closely with team members such as the classroom teacher, speech/language pathologist, occupational therapist, and physical therapist, who can provide the fellows with estimates of a patient's cognitive functioning and their readiness for formal testing. As a general rule, testing is not begun until the patient is oriented and no longer demonstrates any post-traumatic amnesia, although this general rule is increasingly coming into conflict with the demands associated with reduced lengths of stay.

As a patient nears discharge, the fellow who is responsible for that case schedules the evaluation. The test battery used varies according to the patient's age. A typical inpatient battery for school-age children is shown in Table 2. All test batteries include measures of general intellectual functioning. Measures of language and nonverbal skills are also administered, as are measures of verbal and nonverbal memory, executive functions, and sensorimotor functions. Single-word reading ability is also measured, and is often used as an estimate of premorbid functioning.

In most cases, the test batteries are fixed, so that the same tests are typically administered to all children in a given age range. The tests were selected to provide information about the functional domains listed above in a reasonable amount of time. For most children, the testing can be completed in a total of about three hours. Testing is typically spread across two or more sessions, to reduce fatigue and maintain motivation. If clinically indicated, the battery can be modified, so that it does not become too demanding. For example, children with profound deficits may complete a brief screening, instead of the entire battery.

In addition to formal testing, inpatient evaluations also include a review of medical records and a parent interview. When children are admitted to the

Table 2. Typical inpatient test battery for a school-age child.

Test name
Wechsler Abbreviated Scale of Intelligence
NEPSY (Language, Visuospatial, Attention/Executive Functions, and Sensorimotor core subtests, and Sentence Repetition and Verbal Fluency subtests)
Boston Naming Test
California Verbal Learning Test—Children's version
Children's Memory Scale (Stories and Faces subtests)
Hooper Visual Organization Test
Rey–Osterrieth Complex Figure
Trail Making Test
Wisconsin Card Sorting Test
Abbreviated Sensory-Perceptual Examination
Grooved Pegboard
Wide Range Achievement Test–Third Edition (Reading subtest)

Rehabilitation Unit, parents are also asked to complete a history questionnaire, as well as rating scales that assess behavioral adjustment (e.g., Child Behavior Checklist; Achenbach, 1991) and adaptive functioning (e.g., Scales of Independent Behavior-Revised; Bruininks, Woodcock, Weatherman, & Hill, 1996). For the two rating scales, parents are asked to make their ratings retrospectively, in order to provide estimates of children's premorbid functioning.

After completing testing and obtaining supervision, fellows are responsible for providing feedback to parents about their child's neuropsychological functioning, the risks they face upon community re-entry, and recommendations for clinical management. Fellows are also responsible for sharing this information with rehabilitation team members and with school personnel. The findings and recommendations resulting from the evaluation are often discussed with school personnel at a meeting that occurs at the hospital prior to discharge.

Because formal testing is not usually performed until shortly before discharge, the postdoctoral fellows are usually required to provide feedback to parents and staff within a day or so after they complete the evaluation. The written report of the evaluation also needs to be completed relatively quickly, so that it can be placed in the patient's chart before discharge. If the report cannot be completed prior to discharge, a detailed progress note that documents the findings and recommendations is placed in the chart, and the written report is added to the patient's medical record soon thereafter.

Inpatient consultations are also received from other services, including neurology, neurosurgery, and pharmacology/toxicology. In these cases, the fellows are usually required to begin the evaluation within 24 hours after the consult is received, because the patients are usually discharged within one or two days. The test batteries are the same as those used with inpatients on the rehabilitation unit. Because most of these patients are discharged immediately after testing is completed, the fellow usually provides verbal feedback to the referring physician as soon as possible after testing, and places a brief progress note regarding the findings in the medical record. A written report is then prepared, and copies are sent to the referring physician and to parents.

Verbal feedback is also provided to the parents. Whenever possible, feedback is given prior to discharge. When feedback cannot be completed until after discharge, fellows arrange to discuss the findings with parents, either by telephone or in person. Telephone consultations are often more convenient for families, especially those that reside a long distance from the hospital. Unfortunately, telephone consultations cannot be billed to insurance companies and are not ordinarily billed to families, so that the service usually is not reimbursed.

Occasionally, inpatient consultation is requested when there is not sufficient time to complete testing before discharge or when the patient is not judged to be testable. For instance, patients who are hospitalized for extended video EEG monitoring may be having multiple seizures and hence be unsuitable for testing. In these cases, the fellows schedule the evaluation on an outpatient basis, as soon after discharge as possible. The appropriate inpatient test battery is then administered to the children. After completing testing and receiving supervision, the fellows prepare a written report, which is distributed to the referring physician and the patient's parents. A feedback session with the parents is also scheduled.

Outpatient assessment

Outpatients are referred by a variety of sources, as described earlier. All referrals are processed by the Psychology Department secretarial staff, who collect intake information that is entered into a computer database. Outpatient evaluations are scheduled by a secretary specifically assigned to make appointments for neuropsychological evaluations.

In the past, the high demand for services resulted in a waiting list of approximately six months for outpatient evaluations, but evaluations were scheduled only about one month in advance. We found that parents often forgot or needed to reschedule appointments that were scheduled any further in advance. In addition, we were then able to arrange appointments on an emergent basis if necessary, as is sometimes requested by referral sources, although patients were typically seen on a 'first come, first served' basis. More recently, the waiting list has been reduced to about two to three months. In many cases, therefore, parents are now given appointments when they first call to request an evaluation. In addition, if a parent requests it, a patient can be placed on a cancellation list. If an appointment is canceled with at least 24 hours warning, we are usually able to fill the slot using the cancellation list. When an evaluation is scheduled, the secretary sends the child's parent or caregiver an 11-page history questionnaire, along with parent and teacher forms of the Child Behavior Checklist for children of the appropriate age. Ideally, the questionnaire and rating scales are completed and returned prior to the evaluation. However, parents often bring the forms on the first day of testing. In most cases, we also obtain pertinent information from other sources (e.g., school and medical records).

Outpatient evaluations are usually scheduled for two sessions of about three hours each, although the duration of each session varies depending on the patient's age and level of functioning. For example, preschool children usually are seen for about one to two hours each session. Sessions are scheduled for either the morning or afternoon. Morning sessions generally begin at 9 AM, and afternoon sessions begin at 1 PM. We prefer to see younger patients in the morning.

Our practice supports a full-time psychometrician who has ten weekly time slots available for testing outpatients (morning and afternoon, Monday through Friday), and another half-time psychometrist who has four weekly slots available. Each staff member and postdoctoral fellow is assigned one or two of those slots. The psychometricians administer a portion of the neuropsychological test battery for each outpatient evaluation. The psychometricians also complete a standardized behavioral observation checklist, and frequently confer with the clinicians regarding children's test performance and behavior.

Typically, on the first day of an evaluation, the clinician conducts a brief interview with the child and his or her parent before accompanying the child to the psychometrician. Then, while the psychometrician completes the initial testing, the clinician conducts a comprehensive interview with the parent and any other family members or caregivers who accompany the child. The goal of that interview is to review the referral question and to collect additional information regarding the patient. The second testing session typically occurs within a week of the first session, and is conducted by the staff member or fellow assigned to the case.

Our outpatient test batteries are largely fixed, so that the same tests are usually administered to all children in a given age range. A typical outpatient test battery for a school-age child is listed in Table 3. The batteries reflect the availability of tests and norms at certain ages, and were selected to assess the relevant neurobehavioral domains: overall cognitive ability; language and nonverbal skills; verbal and nonverbal memory; attention and executive functions; sensorimotor functions; and academic achievement. We also obtain standardized ratings of behavioral adjustment, and often of adaptive functioning. Tests may be added or deleted from the battery, depending on the referral question, the child's overall functioning, and other relevant factors. For instance, we typically add tests of phonological processing when the referral question raises concerns about a possible reading disability.

Table 3. Typical outpatient test battery for a school-age child.

Test name
Wechsler Intelligence Scale for Children-Third Edition (WISC-III)
NEPSY (Language, Visuospatial, Attention/Executive Functions, and Sensorimotor core subtests, and Sentence Repetition and Verbal Fluency subtests)
Boston Naming Test
California Verbal Learning Test—Children's version
Children's Memory Scale (Core subtests)
Hooper Visual Organization Test
Rey–Osterrieth Complex Figure
Gordon Diagnostic System
Trail Making Test
Wisconsin Card Sorting Test
Children's Category Test
Sensory-Perceptual Examination
Finger Tapping Test
Grooved Pegboard
Wide Range Achievement Test—Third Edition

Tests are scored both by the psychometrician and by the individual clinician. The psychometrician typically scores the measures administered during the first testing session, and the clinician is responsible for scoring most of the tests administered during the second session. Qualitative analysis of all test data by the clinician is also an integral part of each case formulation.

Following each evaluation, the clinician prepares a detailed report describing the reason for referral, data sources, relevant history, direct behavioral observations, and test results. The report concludes with an integrative summary of the findings, a discussion of etiology and differential diagnosis, a description of the risks faced by the child in light of their neuropsychological profile, and associated recommendations for educational assistance, psychosocial intervention, and medical follow-up. The typical report is six to seven pages long. Each report is accompanied by a one page cover letter that summarizes the major findings and recommendations. Reports for outpatient evaluations are required to be produced no more than four weeks after testing is completed.

Several copies of the report are sent to the child's parents, and a copy is also sent to the referral source. Thus, the family has copies they can share with school personnel and other health care providers. In most cases, we prefer to provide parents with reports prior to conducting informing sessions. Informing sessions can be conducted in a more focused fashion when parents read the reports beforehand. This procedure also helps to limit the telephone calls that parents make to ask questions about the report if they receive it after the informing session. The sessions are therefore scheduled approximately one month after testing is completed.

Office Environment

The Department of Psychology occupies the entire fourth floor of one of the professional office buildings at Children's Hospital. All faculty, fellows, and interns have individual offices, as well as personal computers that are connected to the hospital's computer network, which has a direct connection to the Ohio State University computer facilities. The floor also contains office space for three secretaries, two psychometrists' offices, conference room, file room, mail room, and waiting room. Additional office space for research is located on the second floor of the same building.

The Pediatric Neuropsychology Program does not have a separate budget. Its expenses are included in the Psychology Department budget. Personnel expenses account for more than 90% of the budget. The budget also includes expenses for equipment and supplies, but does not include overhead. Items costing more than a predetermined amount are considered capital expenses, and require special budgetary approval. The budget also includes academic support funds. Each faculty member is allocated a yearly stipend for conference travel, continuing education, professional membership fees, book and journal purchases, and related purposes. Limited academic support funds are also available for interns and postdoctoral fellows.

The hospital administration expects the Psychology Department to cover its budget expenses through a combination of clinical revenue and grant funding. The emphasis on clinical productivity has increased in recent years, in response to greater demands for fiscal accountability across the entire hospital. All clinicians are expected to bill a specific number of hours each week. The number of hours differs for clinical-line and tenure-line faculty.

Clinical revenue for the department as a whole is assessed by multiplying total billings by the overall reimbursement rate, which is estimated by the hospital's Accounting Department. Unfortunately, the Accounting Department does not provide timely information regarding reimbursement for individual outpatient evaluations, and reimbursement rates for inpatient evaluations are difficult to estimate accurately, because the bills are rolled into patients' inpatient charges. Thus we cannot readily affect the revenue stream by attempting to increase reimbursement. Fortunately, the combination of estimated clinical revenue and grant funding does cover the budget, as long as all clinicians meet their productivity expectations.

Coding and Billing

Clinicians assign diagnoses after completing evaluations. The hospital uses ICD-9 diagnostic codes. We prefer to use non-psychiatric codes whenever possible. For example, children with seizures are diagnosed using the appropriate codes for epilepsy, and children with closed-head injury are diagnosed using the appropriate codes for intracranial injury. Psychiatric codes equivalent to those in DSM-IV are used when children do not have any specific medical or neurological disorder. Relevant diagnoses include learning disorders, communication disorders, attention-deficit/hyperactivity disorder, pervasive developmental disorders, mental retardation, and Tourette's syndrome. On rare occasions, psychiatric diagnoses such as major depression are used.

A billing specialist in Patient Accounts reviews the assigned diagnostic codes and, when necessary, discusses their suitability with the clinicians. In addition, when clinicians are uncertain what code to use for a particular case, the billing specialist can be consulted regarding possible diagnostic codes.

Billing is handled by Patient Accounts. Virtually all neuropsychological evaluations are billed using the CPT code 96117. On average, inpatient evaluations are billed for approximately 6 hours, and outpatient evaluations are billed for approximately 9 hours. The informing sessions that are held following most outpatient evaluations are billed separately. The hospital sets the hourly billing rate for psychological services, and it is currently (as of February 2002) approximately $152. Inpatient evaluations are not itemized, but are included in the patient's inpatient charges. Outpatient evaluations are billed as facilities charges, rather than professional services, so that bills are generated on behalf of Children's Hospital rather than on behalf of the clinicians. This procedure reduces the effective reimbursement rate for patients with Medicaid, but also avoids difficulties associated with "incident to" regulations.

The hospital does not currently provide any formal support for pre-certification by insurance companies. Parents are expected to contact their insurers directly to request pre-certification, although the secretaries in the Psychology Department assist parents in this process. We have boilerplate letters that clinicians can individualize that describe the reason for referral, underscore the specialized nature of neuropsychological assessment, provide a list of the tests to be administered, and summarize the amount of time needed to complete the evaluation, including report-writing time.

None of the staff neuropsychologists are currently listed on any insurance provider panels. We have deliberately chosen not to join any panels, because we are reluctant to have insurers dictate our methods of practice and because we have evidence that it would reduce our reimbursement rates. In recent years, the average reimbursement rate for outpatient neuropsychological evaluations is approximately 70% of total billings. Traditional fee-for-service insurance plans provide about 80% reimbursement, and private managed care plans average about 50%. Medicaid has a much lower reimbursement rate, which is about 25%. Less than a third of our patients are covered by Medicaid. Reimbursement rates are typically higher for children with medical or neurological rather than psychiatric diagnoses, because in many cases the evaluation will be paid for by medical component of the patient's insurance, rather than by the behavioral health component.

Billing for forensic evaluations is handled separately by the hospital's Accounting Department. Billing is done in 15-minute increments. The current hourly rate for forensic services, including consultation, evaluation, and testimony, is $250 per hour. We do not require attorneys to provide retainers in advance, but we do ask that they provide us with a letter of guarantee that indicates they will assume full responsibility for payment.

From the Past to the Future

The Pediatric Neuropsychology Program continues to evolve. The rapid growth that has occurred over the past decade is likely to slow, but with the increased stability comes the opportunity to seek new referral sources, build relationships with existing ones, and otherwise enhance the services offered by the program. The faculty, fellows, and interns who are part of the program will need to work together to develop a shared vision of our clinical service, research, and training missions.

The program's future looks promising. Although we cannot foresee how changes in the United States health care system, and particularly trends in insurance coverage and reimbursement, will affect the delivery of neuropsychological services nationally, the robust local demand for our services is unlikely to abate. Funding for research in pediatric neuropsychology and related areas has become more readily available, at least for now, because of substantial budget increases at the National Institutes of Health, and we will continue to active seek grant funding for our research programs. Our program's vitality also will continue to be enhanced by the steady stream of students seeking postdoctoral residences in pediatric neuropsychology, and by the faculty's participation in the development of guidelines for education and training (Hannay, 1998). We hope that the future will bring continued growth and integration of our clinical service, research, and training activities.

References

Achenbach, T.M. (1991). *Manual for the Child Behavior Checklist/4-18 and 1991 profile*. Burlington, VT: Department of Psychiatry, University of Vermont.

Bruininks, R.H., Woodcock, R.W., Weatherman, R.F., & Hill, B.K. (1996). *Scales of Independent Behavior—Revised comprehensive manual*. Chicago: Riverside Publishing Company.

Hagen, C., Malkmus, D., & Durham, P. (1979). Levels of cognitive functioning. In

Rehabilitation of the head injured adult: Comprehensive physical management (pp. 8–11). Downey, CA: Professional Staff Association of Rancho Los Amigos Hospital.

Hammeke, T.A. (1993). The Association of Postdoctoral Programs in Clinical Neuropsychology (APPCN). *The Clinical Neuropsychologist, 7*, 197–204.

Hannay, H.J. (1998). Proceedings of the Houston Conference on Specialty Education and Training in Clinical Neuropsychology. *Archives of Clinical Neuropsychology, 13*, 157–249.

Thurman, D. & Guerrero, J. (1999). Trends in hospitalization associated with traumatic brain injury. *Journal of the American Medical Association, 282*, 954–957.

Chapter 13

MANAGEMENT OF A UNIVERSITY-BASED ATTENTION DEFICIT DISORDER AND LEARNING DISORDERS CLINIC

David C. Osmon and Yana Suchy

Introduction

Among clinical neuropsychologists, a college or a university as a primary work setting is a relatively uncommon occurrence. In fact, in a recent large-scale survey of practicing clinical neuropsychologists, fewer than 5% reported having such an affiliation (Sweet, Moberg, & Suchy, 2000). The demographic, economic, and practice characteristics of the individuals who comprise this group are not well known, as any such characteristics have likely been subsumed in prior professional surveys by the overwhelming non-academic majority. This lack of understanding became clear in preparing this chapter and being faced with a dearth of knowledge about not only what type of clinical work neuropsychologists in academia typically practice, but also whether they practice at all. In order to rectify, at least in part, this gap in our knowledge, a brief survey was e-mailed to neuropsychologists with primary academic affiliations ($n = 114$). Basic information was gathered from academic neuropsychologists who were identified by addresses from the current membership directories of the National Academy of Neuropsychology

Table 1. Responses to survey of academia-based clinicians.

Survey Question	Percent
Type of clinic (n=34)	
Training Clinic	65
Professional Service Clinic	17
Other	26
Type of work (n=34)	
Student Supervision	65
Billed Institutional work (institution collects fees)	53
Pro-bono Institutional work	41
Private Practice (clinician collects fees)	41
Other	12
Compensation available for institutional clinical work (n=28)	
None	64
Supplies & expenses	21
Merit	10
Direct Monetary Reimbursement	07
Salary Bonus	04
Client type (n=34)	
General neurologic patients	44
ADA protected clients	41
General psychiatric patients	32
General university students	18
Other	21

Note. Percents are calculated using the number of respondents for whom a given question was relevant (presented in parentheses). Percents add to more than 100 because respondents often endorsed more than one item.

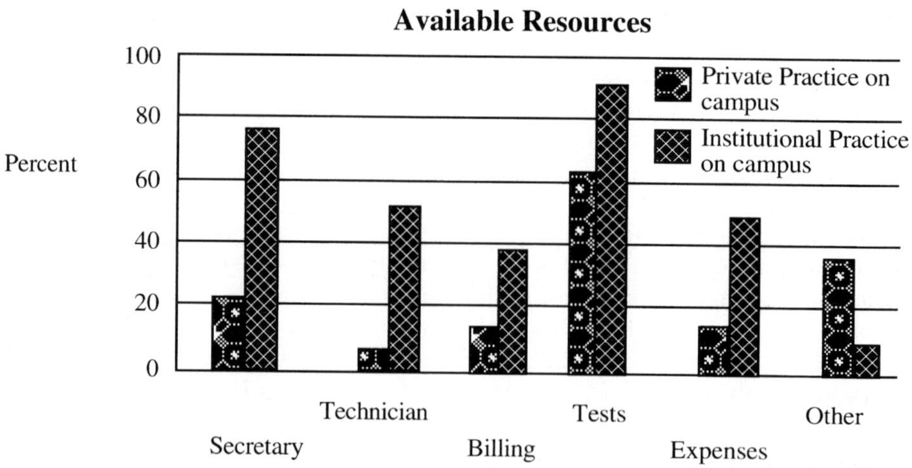

Figure 1. Resources available for clinical neuropsychologists in academia (n = 54).

and the American Academy of Clinical Neuropsychology. Responses were received from 54 colleagues (47%), and of these 34 (62%) indicated that they practice clinical neuropsychology on campus. These responses are summarized in Table1 and in Figure 1.

As can be seen in the Table, the typical clinical neuropsychology practice in academia appears to be based on humanitarian and academic principles, with minimal emphasis on economic concerns. The modal neuropsychologist in academia serves both as a clinical supervisor and as a direct service provider, with the majority of the clinical work being conducted without direct monetary compensation to the clinician. The most typical form of reimbursement appears to be access to a 'supplies & expenses' account, which may be used for journal, book, and software purchases, convention expenses, etc. The most typical resources that are made available to clinicians in academia include testing materials, secretarial support, and technicians (the availability of space is assumed, as only those neuropsychologists who conduct clinical practice within the walls of their academic institutions were included in this group). Finally, the most common populations serviced by these clinicians included general neurologic patients and individuals seeking protection under the Americans with Disabilities Act. This latter finding is consistent with prior research that has shown an increase in the availability of clinics that provide services for college students in line with the requirements of the Americans with Disabilities Act (ADA; Satcher, 1992).

The adult learning disorders assessment service which is the focus of this chapter (hereafter referred to as 'LD Clinic') is in a university-based training clinic within an academic department of psychology at the University of Wisconsin-Milwaukee (UWM). The primary goal of the clinic is to provide affordable service for university students, while also meeting secondary goals of training and research. Business concerns were eschewed by virtue of an emphasis on the goals of service, research, and training. Expenses were minimal because the costs of evaluations were built into the LD Clinic director's academic duties and the neuropsychometrist's training and research needs. Additionally, the research opportunities afforded by this structure provided further compensation for participating faculty. The secretarial support needs were minimal due to the overlap with secretarial needs of the department's training clinic. The end result was a cost effective means of providing service for learning disordered students that, on the one hand, discharged the responsibility of the university to those students and, on the other hand, enriched graduate clinical and research training.

Historical Perspective

The historical context of the current practice model is limited, given that the LD Clinic has been in existence for a short time. Furthermore, the legislative history that forms the basis for the existence of such clinics is of recent origin.

Added to the short history is the rapidly changing marketplace of professional psychology. These factors make it difficult to provide a past context and a map of future clinical endeavors in an adult learning disorders clinic. However, the sheer number of disabled individuals and the great need for services on today's university campuses suggest that adult learning evaluation services will be a permanent fixture for some time to come.

The certain future of these services is suggested by Federal Bureau of the Census statistics, where 48.9 million persons were estimated to qualify as disabled subsequent to enacting the ADA in 1990. That number represented an astounding19.4% of the total U.S. population at the time (see http://www.cdc.gov/epo/mmwr/preview/mmwrhtml 00038522.htm#top). Subsequent estimates suggest an increase in the ranks of the disabled. For example, Mellard (1990) found that only 1% of the student body were enrolled for learning disability accommodations in the California community college system. However, only four years later, the American Council on Education (ACE: www.acenet.edu/home.html) reported a figure that was three times higher than the 1990 data. Similar figures were reported by HEATH Resource Center, which found that in 1998 one in every elf new college freshmen reported a disability. While this figure has been stable since 1991, it represents a three-fold increase from when disability questions were first asked in 1978, when only 2.6% of freshman self-reported a disability (US Department of Education report entitled *Students with Disabilities in Postsecondary Education: A Profile of Preparation, Participation, and Outcomes*, available free: 1-877-4ED-Pubs). Many believe this increase represents a greater personal acceptance of, and societal tolerance for, disability.

In addition to increasing numbers of disabled individuals, students with learning disabilities have been the fastest growing group among disability self-reporters, growing from 25% of the total disability population in 1991 to 41% in 1998, according to the Department of Education report mentioned above. Among the 3.8 million persons under age 18 who qualified as disabled (7.9% of this segment of the population), the most frequent category was learning disability, accounting for 29.5% of the diagnoses. Speech problems (13.1%) and emotional disorders (6.3%) were also large contributors to the ranks of disability in this age group.

Coincident with the need for services due to the growing ranks of disabled individuals, other factors suggest a need for assessment services to distinguish learning disability from alternate learning styles. For example, the surge in emphasis upon lifelong learning, the rise in the frequency of undergraduate and post-graduate education, and the trend toward more flexibility in changing paths late in one's occupational career all suggest that issues in adult learning will become more and more important. In addition, the increasing diversity of cultural representation, as well as the addition of many new venues for an education upon university campuses (e.g., paradigm of discovery and distance learning), may necessitate better preparation for and tolerance of alternate learning styles. It is thus conceivable that one of the main future endeavors in a learning disability clinic might be to distinguish learning disability from alternate and unique learning styles. In fact, learning disability clinics may be best able to take the lead in exploring the nature and implementation of alternate learning styles. Certain styles may be better suited to particular venues of learning and subject matter. The relationship between learning style and venue may ideally be studied and understood in a learning disorder clinic within research-focused academic departments. Again, it is found that practice models that are not profit-based serve unique purposes. It is up to those involved in such models to creatively implement and develop that uniqueness and further define their niche.

A Learning Disorders Clinic in Academia

Thorough evaluation of learning disorders is commonplace in today's elementary and secondary educational institutions. A vast research literature on the subject has accumulated over the latter half of the 20th century, providing guidance for the clinical management of these disorders. Psychologists and learning disorder specialists who work in elementary, secondary, and post-secondary levels of education make use of both this guidance and legal precedents. Such precedents were developed to insure both an adequate educational experience and freedom from discriminatory practices against learning disordered individuals.

Awareness of these legal and political foundations for evaluating and accommodating learning disorders is crucial for individuals running LD clinics. Likewise, training across a number of areas is relevant to the clinical responsibilities in such clinics. The training requirements are often beyond that of one individual, such that a multidisciplinary clinic is often a necessity.

The remainder of the chapter details the workings of 'A Learning Disorders Clinic in Academia,' and highlights several dimensions important to consider in beginning such a clinic. A brief summary concludes the chapter.

Experiences Relevant to the Position of LD Clinic Director

The senior author (DCO) is the director of the learning disorders clinic at UWM, and his background consists of an integration of the science and practice aspects of clinical psychology leading to a healthy respect for both basic and applied aspects of the field. This background results in a style that makes use of a moderately lengthy flexible battery and combines actuarial and process approaches to clinical judgment. This professional style was influenced through graduate training at the University of South Dakota during the early stages of Dr. Charles Golden's career.

The senior author's graduate training occurred during the mid to late 1970s, a period of great growth for clinical neuropsychology. The training featured a close integration of science and practice and saw the development of the Luria–Nebraska Neuropsychological Battery (then known as the Luria South Dakota Neuropsychological Battery). This approach to assessment served to integrate the scientific rigor of neuropsychology's actuarial/ psychometric approach and the theoretical power of neurology's clinical process approach to evaluating brain-behavior relationships.

In addition to the training and practice philosophy mentioned above, other experiences in the senior author's background proved important to the LD Clinic's director's role. For example, working with a developmentally disabled population and chronic, diffuse neurological patients (e.g., alcohol rehabilitation patients), was helpful in understanding the more subtle and less focal nature of learning disability presentations. Finally, the decision to establish a non-business oriented clinic can be understood from the standpoint of the senior author's private practice of 20 years. His practice has evolved from outpatient evaluations to predominantly forensic work in the past ten years. This evolution can be largely attributed to the decrease in outpatient assessment referrals from the influence of managed care. Experiencing this change in professional role was formative in the dawning recognition that alternative practice models which are not based upon business concerns have a role in health care's future.

Practice Setting

In 1997, in an effort to comply with the spirit of the Americans with Disabilities Act of 1990 (ADA; PL 101-336), section 504 of the Rehabilitation Act of 1973 (PL 93-112), and the guidelines of the Association on Higher Education and Disability (AHEAD, 1997) for documentation of learning disability, the Student Accessibility Center of the University of Wisconsin-Milwaukee joined forces with the Psychology and Education departments in founding a Learning Disorders Clinic. The LD Clinic is situated within the Psychology Training (PT) Clinic of the APA-approved doctoral program in Clinical Psychology at UWM. The PT Clinic's primary goal is to provide support for the training and research of doctoral-level graduate students, with the secondary goal of service provision. In contrast, the primary mission of the LD Clinic is to provide evaluations for the Student Accessibility Center (which administrates accommodations for students with learning disorders at UWM), with training and research occupying a secondary role. Despite this difference in primary interests, merging of resources of the two Clinics has worked out well, as both the PT Clinic and the LD Clinic have benefited.

The PT Clinic resources

The PT Clinic occupies most of the ground floor of a building, fostering a confidential and comfortable milieu. Its ample resources include:

a) a large reception/waiting area with an adjacent smaller room where cabinets with client charts are kept;
b) several testing/therapy rooms, equipped with two-way mirrors and adjacent observation rooms with audio and video capability;
c) one larger room for group therapy or family meetings, also equipped with a two-way mirror;
d) offices for faculty/clinical supervisors and for the PT Clinic director;
(e) area dedicated to research;
(f) storage area for testing materials;
(g) one full-time support staff;
(h) IBM personal computer with clinical practice software

LD Clinic advantages of resource-sharing

The above resources lend themselves well to the LD Clinic's primary objective of service provision. Clients are scheduled and received by the PT Clinic secretary, whose duties are dedicated on a full-time basis to the smooth running of the PT Clinic. Clients are received in the large and comfortable reception area. Clinical interview and testing take place in therapy/testing rooms, while feedback sessions with LD Clinic clients, family members, and the Learning Disability Specialist from the Student Accessibility Center take place in a larger group therapy/meeting room. At the time of the feedback, clients make payment in full to the PT Clinic secretary, or arrange for an installment plan with her. The PT Clinic has recently purchased practice software with the goal of tracking and cross-referencing client appointments and payments.

The availability of PT Clinic resources is conducive to the LD Clinic's secondary objective of training. The two-way mirrors that are available in all testing and feedback rooms are important for training of new technicians, as well as for Learning Disability Specialist trainees. Technician trainees benefit by observing test administration techniques to see the range and idiosyncrasies of performances that can be expected from LD Clinic clientele. Learning Disability Specialist trainees benefit by becoming familiar with the tests that are used, and observing first hand the types of difficulties LD clients have on these tests. This experience adds to their ability to translate results and recommendations made by a neuropsychologist into meaningful accommodations tailored to the specific learning issues of each particular client.

Finally, resources available in the PT Clinic also facilitate the LD Clinic's research goals. Specifically, the practice software recently purchased by the PT Clinic designed to track appointments and payments can also be used for tracking client outcome and should develop into outcome research once a sufficiently large database is gathered.

PT Clinic advantages of resource sharing

While the LD Clinic benefits from having access to all PT Clinic resources, the PT Clinic also benefits from this arrangement. When ample resources were not previously fully utilized, the PT Clinic was under frequent scrutiny because of perennial competition among University departments for space. Loss of some of its space/resources to other departments whose primary activities and objectives would be unrelated to the PT Clinic's goals of training, clinical research, and service provision could be disruptive to the PT Clinic's milieu. This threat was diminished by the 'double occupancy' of the available space, leading directly to a significant increase in the volume of clients seen. This not only improved the utilization of resources, but also provided new opportunities for students in the clinical program. Students in the clinical practica now have additional opportunities to observe client testing, as well as an exposure to previously virtually unavailable populations. Additionally, LD Clinic evaluations have been the source of presentations in the Clinical Program's case conferences, supporting general training of graduate students in the specialty practice of neuropsychology and learning disability.

Referral Sources

As a university service that is not financially dependent on client revenues, the LD Clinic has no need to cultivate multiple referral sources. Our referrals come almost exclusively (i.e., about 90%) from the Student Accessibility Center (the campus disability office). Consequently, only occasional referrals come through other sources on campus, including the student health center. As campus demand for evaluations matches closely the LD Clinic's resources, in order to ensure timely evaluations for campus-based clients, outside referrals are discouraged. Off campus referrals, including those from Vocational Rehabilitative Services and the local Veterans Administration Hospital, are also rare.

Because the overwhelming majority of the referrals come from the Student Accessibility Center, the remainder of this section will focus exclusively on the relationship with the Learning Disability Specialist, who is the primary contact person for the LD Clinic, as well as serves as one of the LD Clinic personnel.

Learning disability specialist

The Learning Disability Specialist at a university typically resides in a student support office (at UWM known as the Student Accessibility Center). This office and the LD Specialist position have been developed specifically to provide accommodations to students with alternate needs (i.e., LD and/or other disabilities), and are ultimately responsible for justifying a student's need for protection under the Americans with Disabilities Act. An extensive involvement of the LD Specialist with the LD Clinic facilitates tailoring of the clinical services to the needs of this important referral source. At UWM, the LD Specialist is involved in virtually all levels of the LD Clinic's operation.

The LD specialist was involved in the early planning stage of the LD Clinic. During this stage, the Specialist's thorough knowledge of the Americans with Disabilities Act and of the guidelines for documenting learning disability in adults (AHEAD) was particularly helpful. Understanding these guidelines was crucial for the development of a test battery that was both clinically appropriate and legally sound for comprehensive evaluation of learning disabilities in adults. The Specialist's familiarity with the disability population also ensured a sensitive approach to the human aspects of the evaluations, such as considering the length of individual testing sessions and considering appropriate fees for the evaluation.

Once the LD Clinic was in operation, frequent and thorough communication between the neuropsychologist and the Specialist continued. Because the LD specialist works closely with students who seek help in the Student Accessibility Center, she is able to provide helpful consultation before and after the evaluation, participate in feedback sessions, interface with clients' social supports (parents, significant others, etc.), generate specific ways in which the evaluation's recommendations translate into accommodations, coordinate follow-up services, and gather client outcome data.

University administrative officials

The Provost/Vice Chancellor's office serves as the prime administrative support of the LD Clinic. This office specifically, supports the testing technician's income and provides for some supplies and expenses of the LD Clinic. Continuation of this support is contingent upon adequate justification of the LD Clinic's financial and administrative needs, outlined in an annual report of the LD Clinic's activities, which is prepared by the director and submitted to the Provost/Vice Chancellor's office. This report consists of a yearly description of the clientele seen in the LD Clinic, the volume of clients, the cost of providing the service including capital equipment, supplies and expenses, the revenue generated by the LD Clinic, and measures of program evaluation and client outcomes.

Although successful justification of the LD Clinic's existence in the annual report is crucial for continued support by the Provost/Vice Chancellor, the initial impetus for providing support to the LD Clinic was provided by recent developments in the legal arena (e.g., 'somnolent Samantha' speech by Boston College Provost: Lewin, 1997). While the Provost at UWM was well aware of the potential legal ramifications of these developments for university campuses that do not proactively attend to the needs of LD students, this might not be the case at all campuses. Faculty who consider starting an LD Clinic may need to prepare a report that outlines these issues and communicates the need for a clinic persuasively to their appropriate administrator.

Consumer

Because recommendations typically include accommodations that impact on the faculty and the ways in which they teach their courses, maintaining open communication and healthy professional relationships between the LD Clinic staff and faculty on campus is crucial to the successful implementation of recommendations for individual LD clients. Some accepted types of reasonable accommodations include: (1) alternative instructional methods, such as using advanced organizers, overhead transparencies, and PowerPoint slides, (2) auxiliary aids, such as taped textbooks and notetakers, and (3) alternative course evaluation methods, including different exam formats and different written products (Scott, 1994). Given the disruption to the classroom and the burden on the teacher often associated with such accommodations, it is necessary that university faculty understand the nature of the student's learning disabilities and the requirements of the Americans with Disabilities Act. While it is primarily the job of a Disability Service Administrator to educate the faculty in this manner, it is not uncommon for university faculty to speak directly with the LD Clinic director about a given student's accommodations. Such communications can be greatly enhanced if the director is thoroughly familiar with the following:

1. The distinction between the requirements of an entitlement statute, such as the Individuals with Disabilities Education Act (IDEA), versus a civil rights statute, such as the Americans with Disabilities Act,
2. The rigorous procedure for determining a disability, as set down in Title II of the Americans with Disabilities Act Technical Assistance Manual (US Department of Justice, 1992),
3. Association on Higher Education and Disability (AHEAD, 1997) guidelines for documenting a learning disability, as well as accepted types and specific instances of accommodations that are reasonable to require at the university level (Keiser, 1998).

LD Clinic personnel

Learning disabilities and Attention Deficit Disorder in adults represent a gray area of study that does not categorically fall under the purview of any one discipline. Rather, for optimal assessment and intervention, multiple competencies are needed. Primary among these are a clinical background in adult clinical neuropsychology. This qualification assumes familiarity with administration, scoring, and interpretation of the instruments used for assessment, as well as a good theoretical grasp of functional neuroanatomy, and an understanding of the theoretical models of etiology and pathophysiology for LD and ADD.

A theoretical and clinical background in Attention Deficit Disorder (ADD) and Learning Disability (LD) in children is also useful for diagnosing these conditions in adults. Experience with the clinical presentation of these conditions in children, along with an understanding of the natural history of ADD and LD, can significantly improve a clinician's efficacy. As an example, such experience facilitates the clinician's ability to focus on the relevant information in clients' educational and psychosocial history needed for a reasonable and defensible diagnosis. Familiarity with the developmental literature is therefore critical, as the largest body of research literature about learning problems exists in the pediatric/developmental arena.

Clinical experience with adult and pediatric populations is uniquely useful if it is supplemented with certain types of interpretive strategies. Specifically, making a diagnosis of learning disability that is both *legally* and *clinically* defensible in the context of the current ADA laws requires that individual performances be interpreted *both* relative to a given client's overall profile *and* relative to the client's peers. Hence, both level-of-performance and non-linear, pattern-of-performance methods of interpretation (e.g., disjunctive and conjunctive interpretation: Ganzach, 1995) are important.

An additional required area of expertise is an advanced knowledge of psychometrics. Since the interpretation of psychological instruments naturally relies upon actuarial data, the ability to interpret meaningful statistical and clinical discrepancies is the cornerstone of effort for a neuropsychologist working in such a clinic. Unfortunately, practicing clinicians have been notoriously poorly informed in these areas. For example, Ross (1992) found that only 8.7% of 287 school psychologists accurately evaluated whether aptitude-achievement discrepancy scores represented reliable, non-chance differences. Likewise, Gaudette (1992) demonstrated in a meta-analysis study that although neuropsychologists achieve high diagnostic hit rates (84%) that are above chance, they have a difficult time using base rate information to improve upon their diagnostic accuracy. Finally, as LD and ADD clients undergo repeated assessments in order to document continued qualification for protection, familiarity with the latest methods for estimation of retest gains (e.g., Reliable Change Index: Sawrie, Chelune, Naugle, & Lueders, 1996) is necessary.

Finally, familiarity with federal, local, and institutional *laws and guidelines*, as they relate to LD and ADD issues, facilitates the generation of realistic and meaningful recommendations.

Since few clinicians can claim such extensive expertise, the UWM LD Clinic was developed as a multidisciplinary and interdisciplinary service. As a result, the professional staff included the following individuals: Two adult neuropsychologists, one child neuropsychologist, one Learning Disability Specialist, one counseling psychologist with expertise in intervention and program evaluation, and a neuropsychometrician. Such a diverse group of experts was culled partly out of common interest, and partly out of the complexity, uniqueness, and newness of the professional evaluation of learning disability. Each of these professionals played a unique role in establishing the LD Clinic service by contributing to the design of the test battery, conceptualizing the nature of the test report, and structuring the organization of the LD Clinic. Each of these professionals are described below in terms of their contributions and their professional credentials.

The LD Clinic Director, also serving as chief clinician, is an adult-oriented, board certified neuropsychologist with extensive past clinical experience and a considerable interest in psychometrics and advanced interpretive strategies. This neuropsychologist conducts all of the clinical evaluations and oversees the LD Clinic's daily operation.

A second adult-oriented neuropsychologist with a research focus was also included in the original inception of the LD Clinic. This person was included to develop the LD Clinic's research goals and to design a rigid core set of tests to facilitate the development of a database of subjects used for large-scale psychometric studies, including construct validity and longitudinal outcome studies. Another research goal that was considered in developing LD Clinic procedures was the distinction between genetic/biologic contributions versus environmental/family variable contributions to the development of learning difficulties. Furthermore, relatively few studies exist that explore the long-term outcome of childhood learning disability, and variables to include in the LD Clinic evaluation relevant to these issues had to be considered. The unique nature of the LD Clinic lends itself to such research goals, and a professional dedicated to this issue was important in forming LD Clinic procedures.

A child neuropsychologist, serving as a consultant both during the Clinic's inception and during regular meetings in which cases are discussed, is an individual with both clinical and research experience. This individual provided expertise in the state-of-the-art literature relevant to the field (e.g., Teeter & Semrud-Clikeman, 1997) and made contributions that were key in developing the test battery and conceptualizing the format of test reports.

A counseling psychologist with expertise in outcome research and intervention was originally included in the planning stages of the LD Clinic. This individual was seen as an important component of the team because of the need to make recommendations for remedial strategies for both the primary and secondary effects of learning disabilities. Having expertise in intervention strategies was helpful in conceptualizing the structure of the evaluation and test reports.

The Learning Disability Specialist was a key member of the team, serving a unique administrative and political role in the LD Clinic. In addition to the contributions mentioned earlier, the LD Clinic relies on this individual for updates on continuing developments in the field. Such updates are important because of the constant flux surrounding criteria for documenting disability and the interpretative aspect associated with eligibility criteria for disabilities.

Finally, it was decided that student training goals could best be served by including a neuropsychometrician in the LD Clinic. This individual was chosen from among those students in the Clinical Psychology program who have both completed basic training in general psychological assessment and gained experience in administration and scoring of neuropsychological instruments. In addition, didactic and clinical experience with neuropsychological syndromes is helpful, as the examiner needs to be able to recognize those signs of brain dysfunction that do not lend themselves easily to quantification, but may influence test performance and interpretation (e.g., word-finding hesitancies, subtle paraphasic errors, motor impersistence, dysprosodia, right-left confusion, echopraxia, and perseverative tendencies). Thus, the person serving this role in the LD Clinic tends to be a doctoral-level clinical psychology student with a focus in neuropsychology.

Clientele

The University of Wisconsin-Milwaukee (UWM) is an urban university servicing both traditional and nontraditional students. The nontraditional student population is reflected in the fact that 42% of the student body attend school part-time, and 44% are employed while attending school. Nontraditional students tend to take evening classes (40.2% take only evening classes compared to only 8.2% of traditional students), and are older than traditional students, averaging 34.2 years. This segment of the student body may also include individuals who have the drive and general aptitude to attain college education, but learning disability or attentional disorder may have discouraged them from pursuing or completing higher education immediately after graduating from high school.

Clients seen within the LD clinic match the demographics of the student body as a whole. Table 2 shows demographic characteristics of the first 40 cases seen in the LD Clinic's first year of operation. As can be seen from the Table, a diversity of both traditional and non-traditional college students are served in the LD Clinic, and the racial composition of the LD Clinic clientele represent the diversity of the UWM student population (see Figure 2).

Approximately 3% of the UWM student body seeks consultation at the Student Accessibility Center (university's office for handling all manner of disability claims), and of that number approximately 75% receive actual classroom accommodations. A segment of that number are clients with LD-related complaints, many of whom are referred to the LD Clinic because of a need for up-to-date documentation of an LD diagnosis. The LD Clinic sees clients at a rate of approximately one case per week throughout the entire year. Figure 3 shows the breakdown of diagnoses seen in the LD Clinic, with a preponderance of clients with learning style issues or no disorder compared with the actual number of disability diagnoses made. In addition, written language disorder and inattentive varieties of ADD make up the majority of disabilities seen in the LD Clinic.

General Assessment Considerations

Evaluations conducted for the purposes of documenting a disability that is protected under ADA have similar requirements of rigorousness and exhaustiveness of documentation, as do medicolegal evaluations, necessitating the use of a highly comprehensive battery. In addition, a comprehensive battery

Table 2. Demographic characteristics of the first 40 clients seen in the LD Clinic.

	Age		IQ	IQ	IQ	Race			%LD
	<26	>26		Estimate 1	Estimate 2	White	Black	Other	DX
Males									
Traditional	8	0	97.4	104.5	102.3	7	0	1	62.5
Nontraditional	1	8	93.5	109.2	107.8	8	0	1	33.3
Females									
Traditional	13	0	99.9	96.2	103.5	12	1	0	53.8
Nontraditional	1	9	96.3	108.2	108.8	9	1	0	30.0

Note. IQ=Woodcock–Johnson-Revised Cognitive battery Broad Cognitive Ability-standard, Estimate 1=Barona demographic estimate of premorbid intelligence, Estimate 2=Vanderploeg demographic estimate of premorbid intelligence, % LD DX=percent receiving a diagnosis of LD.

is made all the more important due to the need to address a wide range of diagnostic, prognostic, and treatment recommendations. For example, learning problems might result from learning disability, attention deficit disorder, learning style issues without diagnosable conditions, or psychological disor-

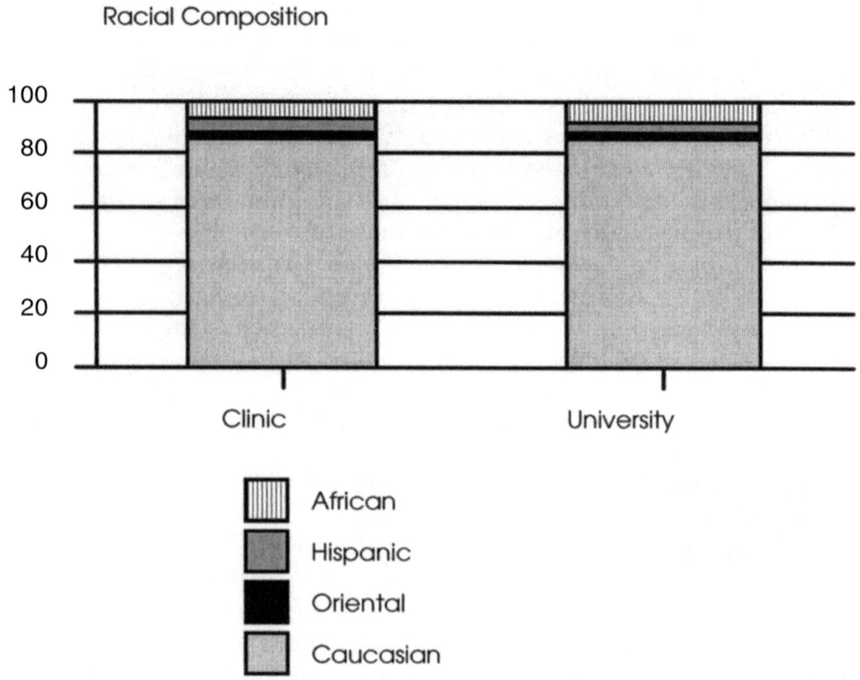

Figure 2. Racial composition of clients seen in the LD Clinic.

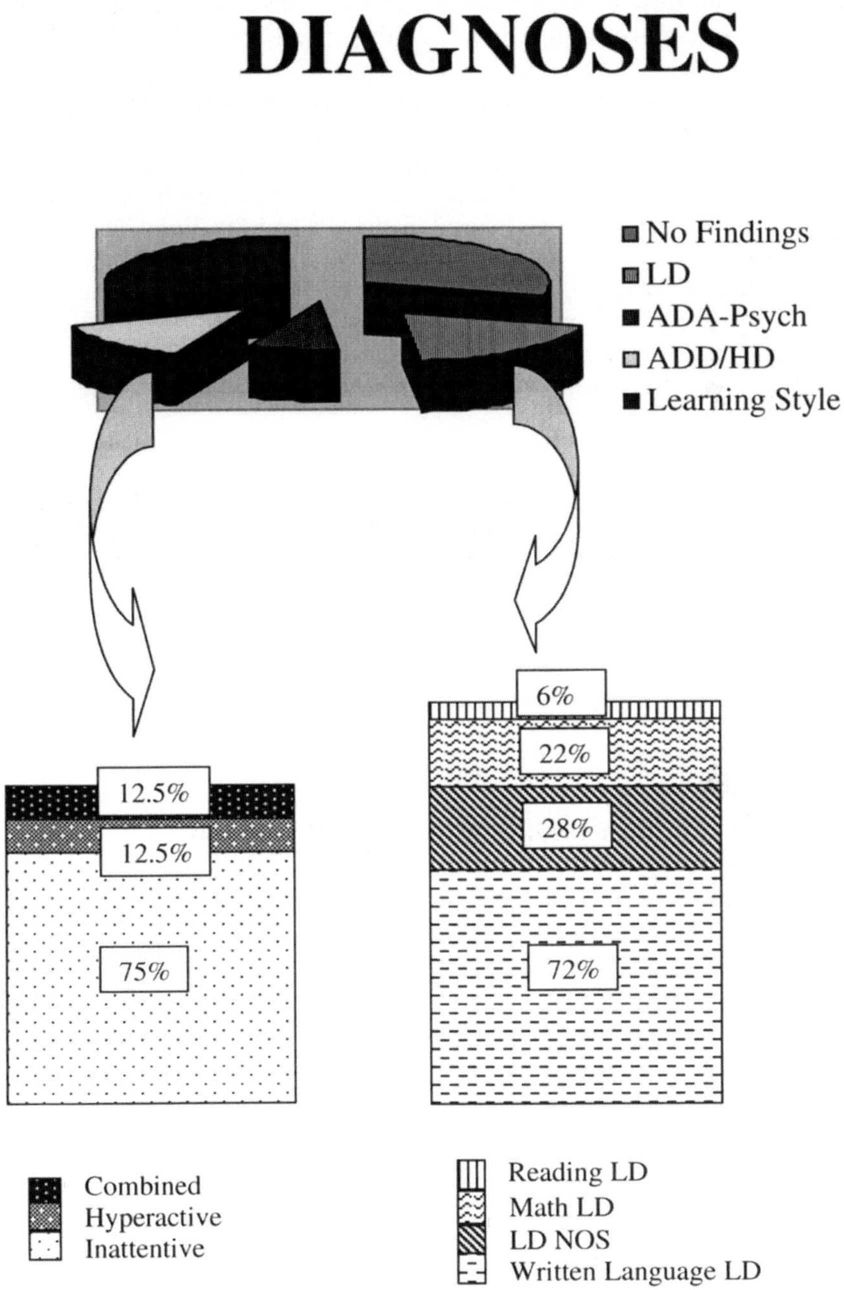

Figure 3. Varieties of diagnostic outcomes in the first year of operation of the LD Clinic.

ders. Finally, because of the rather recent entry of neuropsychology into the professional assessment of learning disability, there has not been a consensus or clear-cut recommendation as to what constitutes an accepted assessment battery. This lack of guidelines again necessitates a comprehensive assessment of neuropsychological and psychological strengths and weaknesses.

In order to address the complex diagnostic issues discussed above, a relatively long battery of tests that can be completed in two half-day sessions and lasts a total of 9–10 hours is used in the UWM LD Clinic. The battery is designed to identify core deficits on the one hand and the success with which compensation has taken place on the other. To that end, both 'specific' and 'global' neurocognitive instruments are used (see Table 3). Specific neurocognitive measures generally reflect the current biological integrity, irrespective of prior learning and compensatory strategies. A global measure of intel-

Table 3. Tests in the UWM Learning Disorders Battery.

Intelligence and Achievement:	
	Woodcock–Johnson Tests of Cognitive Ability-Revised
	Woodcock–Johnson Tests of Achievement Ability-Revised
Mental Speed:	
	Gordon
	Stroop Color-Word Test (Golden version-given at start and end of longest session)
	Trail Making, Part A/B
	Digit Span
Visuospatial:	
	Judgment of Line Orientation
	Facial Recognition
	Rey Complex Figure
Motor/Sensory:	
	Finger Oscillation (Halstead–Reitan)
	Grip Strength (Halstead–Reitan)
	Finger Localization (Benton)
Executive Functions:	
	Ruff
	Controlled Oral Word Association (Benton)
	Category Test (Halstead–Reitan)
Memory:	
	Buschke Selective Reminding
	California Verbal Learning Test
	Rey Figure-delayed recall
Motivation:	
	Category Errors-subtest 1 &2
	CVLT Recognition hits, Long delay-cued, List A Trials 1-5
	Reliable Digit Span
Personality/Psychopathology:	
	NEO
	MCMI-2

lectual function, on the other hand, provides a score that reflects both the biological integrity (or a lack thereof) of the brain as a whole, and the brain's ability to adaptively interact and learn in the environment, over a long period of time.

Additionally, a standardized measure of achievement is used so as to assess the pretesting learning context. However, rather than providing a picture of the overall adaptation of the brain reflected by intelligence, such achievement measures are used to reflect the specific amount of information acquired and retained at different stages of learning (e.g., Frith, 1985).

Finally, as is the case with most neuropsychological evaluations, the possibility that personality and emotional issues factor into achievement and ability development, as well as into current performance on neurocognitive measures, needs to be considered. Thus, personality and psychopathology measures are included in the battery, allowing diagnosis of current and premorbid psychopathology (Putnam, Ricker, Ross, & Kurtz, 1999).

Training and Research Mission

A university-based clinic has other roles, besides offering service to clients; namely, serving as a training clinic for the Clinical Program, as well as a fertile ground for clinical research. Each is discussed in turn below.

Student *clinical* training needs served by the LD Clinic revolve around both learning a neuropsychological test battery and practicing case interpretation. All students learn to administer the basic test battery used in the LD Clinic as part of their first year practicum course. Various levels of case conceptualization skills are acquired, depending upon a given student's training focus in the Clinical Program. For example, those without a neuropsychological focus are somewhat tangentially involved, largely through case conference in which cases from the LD Clinic are occasionally presented. On the other hand, those with a neuropsychological focus typically benefit from the LD Clinic more extensively through additional exposure to LD cases in formal coursework, as well as by having the opportunity to serve as the Clinic's neuropsychometrician.

Student *research* training needs are served by the LD Clinic's database that contains client test results. The policy of administering a core fixed set of tests in the battery allows development of this database and completion of large sample studies. As an example, a construct validation study relating neuropsychological measures and the WJC-R is currently being completed (see Table 3 for abbreviations). Additionally, contractual agreement with clients allows that tests used for specific research projects be added to the battery. A current structure-of-cognition study is looking at the twin constructs of interference and inhibition using experimental reaction time measures. In addition to theoretical research, the service setting of the LD Clinic allows practice-oriented research, such as outcome-based and service utilization types of projects. One project is attempting to demonstrate that interventions for learning problems improve both retention of students at the university and their eventual outcomes (e.g., graduation and job), a topic with much administrative support.

Business Aspects of the LD Clinic

Humanitarian and academic concerns influenced the business decisions that shaped the structure of the LD Clinic. In forging that structure, care was given to develop incentives for faculty involved in the LD Clinic to focus on service, training, and research, rather than monetary gains. These incentives (described in the "Faculty Compensation" section below) encourage faculty to provide a low cost assessment, involve students in the clinical activities, and contribute to a data pool for research in learning problems. Likewise, pro bono work is not punitive, as faculty are not expected to generate clinical income to cover Clinic expenses. In the subsections that follow, several aspects of this model are laid out, including: LD Clinic budget, assessment cost, fee collection, pro bono work, faculty compensation, and marketing and contractual agreements.

LD Clinic budget

Costs of the LD Clinic are minimal and include the technician' s salary, general overhead contributions to the Psychology Training Clinic, test equipment, supplies and expenses, and student help for database management. The technician' s salary is provided by the Provost's office as part of the designated obligation of the university's learning disability services. The other expenses mentioned above are paid out of the fees charged for the evaluations. Fees are dispersed to separate accounts set up to handle five different budgets. The first account is for general overhead paid directly to the Psychology Training Clinic at a rate of 25% of collected fees. Second, 10% of the budget is allotted to an account for purchasing test equipment and software, replacement equipment for the clinical test battery, and supplemental experimental tests and instruments that are used for research purposes. Third, 15% of the budget is allotted for supplies and expenses, consisting largely of ongoing purchasing of test forms and photocopying for research articles and consent forms, among other sundry items. Fourth, 20% of the budget is allotted for student assistance consisting of various research functions, including database management and analysis. Finally, 30% of the budget is set aside for faculty compensation, which is discretionary money for faculty members, as described later in the Faculty Compensation section.

Assessment cost

Full price for an assessment is based upon separate charges for the technician's time and the neuropsychologist's time. The technician's time is billed at a rate based upon what is needed to cover the technician's salary per year; figuring one assessment completed every week. One assessment includes ten hours of face-to-face contact with the client, two hours for test scoring, and one-hour for entry of test data into the database and for time to schedule the client's assessment appointments. The technician's salary is equivalent to that of a university 50% Full-Time Equivalent extrapolated to a twelve-month contract, and is equivalent to a UWM teaching assistantship. The neuropsychologist's time is calculated as an hourly fee equivalent to going market rates, figuring six hours per assessment. The neuropsychologist's time is spent roughly in the following activities: 1) a one-hour interview of the client at the beginning of the assessment, 2) three hours checking the technician's scoring, interpreting the case data, and writing a report, 3) one hour in a feedback session with the client, explaining the assessment results and recommendations, and 4) one hour in administrative and consultative activities. Less than one percent of the clients seen in the LD Clinic are charged full price for the assessment, although the above accounting for time is an accurate model of the time spent with the modal client.

Three levels of discount are available and consist of various accommodations made for the majority of clients seen in the LD Clinic. Students attending the university comprise over 90% of the LD Clinic's clientele and are given a discount as a service of the university. The modal client chooses the most favorable discount, a price that is less than one-fifth of the full price of the assessment. In exchange for this discount, the client agrees to serve as a subject for graduate students in the Clinical Psychology program's assessment practica. As a participant, a 2–5 hour battery of tests is administered by a graduate student in one of the two assessment practica. This testing is in addition to the 9-10 hour battery of tests taken in the LD Clinic evaluation, and is not used as part of the client's clinical evaluation for learning problems. The assessment practicum battery consists of objective and/or projective testing, as required by the protocol of the particular assessment practicum.

If the client does not wish to engage in the extra testing, the second level of discount is given, consisting of a charge for the clinical evaluation which is greater than the above mentioned discount by a factor of approximately 1.5. The third level of discounting is reserved for governmental agencies that occasionally refer clients to the LD Clinic (including the Department of Vocational Rehabilitation and the Veterans Administration Medical Center). This discount is approximately half the cost of the evaluation's full price. All other paying clients are charged full price for the assessment, and the LD Clinic is not set up to bill insurance companies. Thus, all referrals pay out-of-pocket for the assessment.

Fee collection

Fees are collected from clients at the time of the feedback session. If a student is unable to pay the full amount at that time, a payment plan is arranged. Collection rate is high because of the low cost of the assessment and because the cost of the assessment is considered a university fee. University fees, like those for overdue library books, can delay awarding of a diploma if unpaid.

Accounting procedures are computerized, using practice management software (e.g., OPTAIO from The Psychological Corporation at 1-888-4-OPTAIO) to track client fees and to provide an easy procedure for maintaining outcome data. The software allows tracking for scheduling, billing, reporting, as well as pre-and post-measures for use in doing outcome projection, quality of service, and utilization review studies. Such functions streamline business aspects of the LD Clinic and are useful for quality control. Toward that end, the LD Clinic is currently tracking client educational outcomes, payment statistics, client and referral characteristics, and test report response times.

The advantages of a university-based clinic that does not bill to insurance companies are many. Ease of organization of the LD Clinic is perhaps the largest advantage. Since billing is out-of-pocket, great clerical effort is avoided and secretarial needs are minimized. All billing and payment tracking are automated via the practice management software. The expense of training in third party billing practices is also not necessary, and one full-time program assistant staffs the entire Psychology Training Clinic with the LD Clinic accounting for only a small fraction of the secretary's total duties.

Unfortunately, some disadvantages are also present, the largest being meager working capital due to the discount pricing. Currently, there are limited financial benefits to the neuropsychologist as detailed later in the Faculty Compensation section.

Pro bono services

Pro bono work is seen as an ethical obligation of the LD Clinic, currently accounting for 5-10% of the clients evaluated. Typical pro bono clients include economically disadvantaged referrals from outside the university. These clients typically learn of the LD Clinic by informal means, such as word-of-mouth. They seek services, often for family members, who are pursuing self-improvement.

Decisions about which cases qualify as pro bono are made by the LD Clinic director. Referrals are screened by the director, allowing a discussion with the client to determine if the criteria apply and if alternate sources of funding are available to the client. This initial discussion is used to determine whether the client is appropriate for evaluation in the Clinic and what level of charge is made for the services. Those clients who are not evaluated in the LD Clinic are referred to other agencies or professionals.

Faculty compensation

The major distinguishing feature of the current practice paradigm is the ability to circumvent a profit model of practice. That ability issues largely from finding alternate sources of compensation for one of the largest costs of such a LD Clinic, faculty salary. Such an alternate source is feasible because faculty handle LD Clinic evaluations as part of their university duties.

At present, no personal expenditures or salary options are possible since no mechanism is available for fee-for-service work, and regulations preclude university reimbursement beyond the contract salary. However, faculty have other sources of compensation available to them. One compensation is supplies and expenses monies. As noted before, a separate account for the faculty member is funded with 30% of the evaluation fee as it is collected. That money is available to the faculty member to spend at his/her discretion within the limits of allowable university supplies and expenses. These generally include expenditures associated with the faculty member's research and conducting LD Clinic business. As an example, a faculty member might buy a computer, computer supplies, or neuropsychological test equipment. Another form of compensation includes having a built-in research population, using the test battery data generated in the assessment of the LD Clinic clientele. Finally, course buy-outs (i.e., release from duties of teaching a course) are available for work done in the LD Clinic.

Marketing and contracting issues

No formal arrangements, contracts, or attempts to publicize the service are made, although approximately 10% of referrals are accepted from the Department of Vocational Rehabilitation, the Veterans Administration Hospital, and self-referrals. The lack of marketing strategies and attempts to secure contracts is purposeful because of two considerations: 1) the LD Clinic exists foremost as a service to the university student body; 2) the LD Clinic's low fees are well below market value, and as such, if offered more extensively would undercut the private sector.

Summary

An alternative health care delivery service for adult learning problems was presented. This service is university-based and has the advantage of being built upon training and research goals, rather than business necessities. Such basis allows a service mission that can provide low cost care to disability clients by combining training needs of doctoral students with research goals of both university faculty and students. An exhaustive, 9–10 hour, state-of-the-art neuropsychological battery of tests applies current psychometric standards to the diagnosis of adult learning problems (e.g., the Gf-Gc theory of intelligence: McGrew & Flanagan, 1998). Intelligence and Achievement batteries are combined with neuropsychological tests of specific neurocognitive abilities, personality and psychopathology measures, and motivation in an attempt to research the etiology and clinical presentation of adult learning problems.

This model of service delivery is seen as a minority alternative to current private sector service delivery models, and one that serves a useful and complementary role in the health care marketplace. Being free of business concerns of the marketplace allows experimentation with various training models and the pursuit of research goals applicable to clientele who fall under the protective coverage of the Americans with Disabilities Act. New training models and research goals, which may not otherwise be pursued in profit-based models of service delivery, may extend the range of applicability of assessment techniques, thereby enhancing the quality of service for that clientele.

The future of such service models seems assured, given the proliferation of university-based assessment services for student learning problems since the "somnolent Samantha" speech. This proliferation has fostered a zeitgeist in which accommodations for all manner of occupations, entrance tests, and training programs are being provided (see Banks, Guyer, & Guyer, 1995 for an example in medical school). The certain future of these service models is also suggested by the projection of individuals eligible for coverage under the Americans with Disabilities Act, as mentioned in the Historical Comments section.

Thus, universities are in a unique position to address the sociopolitical mandate of the ADA, a mandate that challenges our ability to understand adult learning issues. This can be accomplished by linking university interests and resources for training and research with the public's need for services. In this way, it seems apparent that multiple models of service delivery are important in satisfying the need to both serve and learn.

References

AHEAD (1997). *The AHEAD guidelines for documentation of a learning disability in adolescents and adults.* Columbus, Ohio: The Association on higher Education and Disability.

Banks, S. R., Guyer, B. P., & Guyer, K. E. (1995). A study of medical students and physicians referred for learning disabilities. *Annals of Dyslexia, 45*, 233–245.

Frith, U. (1985). Beneath the surface of developmental dyslexia. In K. E. Patterson, J. C. Marshall, & M. Coltheart (Eds.), *Surface dyslexia.* London: Lawrence Erlbaum Associates.

Ganzach, Y, (1995). Nonlinear models of clinical judgment: Meehl's data revisited. *Psychological Bulletin, 118*, 422–429.

Gaudette, M. D. (1992). *Clinical decision making in neuropsychology: Bootstrapping the neuropsychologist utilizing Brunswik's lens model* (Doctoral dissertation, Indiana University of Pennsylvania, 1992). Dissertaton Abstracts International, 53, 2059B.

Keiser, S. (1998). Test accommodations: An administrator's view. In M. Gordon & S. Keiser (Eds.), *Accommodations in higher education under the Americans with Disabilities Act (ADA): A no-nonsense guide for clinicians, educators, administrators, and lawyers* (pp. 46–69). New York: The Guilford Press.

Lewin, T. (1997). Suit focuses on rights of learning disabled. *The New York Times*, April 8, A9–10.

McGrew, K. S. & Flanagan, D. P. (1998). *The intelligence test desk reference (ITDR): Gf-Gc cross-battery assessment.* Needham Heights, MA: Allyn & Bacon, Inc.

Mellard, D. F. (1990). The eligibility process: Identifying students with learning disabilities in California's community colleges. *Learning Disabilities Focus, 5*, 75–90.

Putnam, S. H., Ricker, J. H., Ross, S. R., & Kurtz, J. E. (1999). Considering premorbid functioning: Beyond cognition to a conceptualization of personality in postinjury functioning. In J. J. Sweet (Ed.), *Forensic neuropsychology: Fundamentals and practice*. Lisse, Netherlands: Swets & Zeitlinger.

Ross, R. (1992). Accuracy in analysis of discrepancy scores: A nationwide study of school psychologists. *School Psychology Review, 21*, 480–493.

Satcher, J. (1992). Community college faculty comfort with providing accommodations for students with learning disabilities. *College Student Journal, 26*, 518–524.

Sawrie, S. M., Chelune, G. J., Naugle, R. I., Lueders, H. O. (1996). Empirical methods for assessing meaningful neuropsychological change following epilepsy surgery. *Journal of the International Neuropsychological Society, 2*, 556–564.

Scott, S. S. (1994). Determining reasonable academic adjustments for college students with learning disabilities. *Journals of Learning Disabilities, 27*, 403–412.

Sweet, J. J., Moberg, P. J., & Suchy, Y. (2000). Ten-year follow-up survey of clinical neuropsychologists: Part I. Practices and beliefs. *The Clinical Neuropsychologist, 14*, 18–37.

Teeter, P. A., & Semrud-Clikeman, M. (1997). *Child neuropsychology: Assessment and interventions for neurodevelopmental disorders*. Boston: Allyn and Bacon.

US Department of Justice (1992). *The Americans with Disabilities Act title II Technical Assistance Manual*. Washington, DC: US Government Printing Office.

Chapter 14

THE PRACTICE OF CLINICAL NEUROPSYCHOLOGY IN A VA SETTING

Richard C. Delaney

Introduction:

It is probably important to stress at the outset that this chapter will present the practice of clinical neuropsychology in *a* VA setting rather than to imply that all Veterans Administration Medical Centers (or Healthcare Systems, as they are increasingly being designated) operate in an identical manner. The author has had sufficient exposure through his training, work experience, site visits to numerous VA settings, and professional contacts with other 'VA neuropsychologists' to discuss some of the consistencies across settings. However, I generally agree with the aphorism "If you've seen one VA, you've seen one VA." This has never been truer than in recent years as important changes and pressures occur within both larger VA subsections, which are now designated as Veterans Integrated Service Networks (VISNs), and individual medical centers themselves. A few pieces of historical background may be helpful at the outset to place VA Neuropsychology in perspective.

World War II had a tremendous impact on the developing field of applied psychology. In 1944 over 200 clinical psychologists were commissioned by the Army to serve in military hospitals and rehabilitation centers. The following year the Veterans Administration appointed George A. Kelly as a consultant to initiate a new clinical psychology program that was then instituted in 1946 with approval of the American Psychological Association. That year the VA met with representatives of 22 universities to encourage the development of training of clinical psychologists who were needed for the care of veterans. These events, which are recognized as landmarks in the history of clinical psychology (Nawas, 1971), established a relationship between the Veterans Administration and the practice of clinical psychology that has continued to this day. Among the obvious effects of this relationship have been the growth of applied psychology, including clinical neuropsychology, and the continued strong support for the doctoral degree with well-defined clinical training as necessary for the independent practice of psychology. For example, since the early 1980s, the VA (now the Cabinet level Department of Veterans Affairs) has required that its psychologists have matriculated through APA-accredited graduate programs in clinical or counseling psychology and have successfully completed APA-accredited internships. The fact that the Psychology Services in VA settings were established as administratively independent services under the Chief of Staff (rather than a subsection of a Psychiatry or Neurology services) also afforded opportunities. Of course, these opportunities for change and development would certainly not have been possible without the support of the medical services and the often-close working relationships with affiliated medical school/hospital programs.

Comprising at one point over 150 hospitals with psychology programs, the VA medical system clearly represented the largest extant healthcare system, providing organized support in clinical, research, and training endeavors for such specialized fields as clinical neuropsychology. In 1975 there were a total of approximately 36 psychologists assigned to the practice of neuropsychology in VA settings while by 1980 that number had grown to 64 (Mancusi, 1981). At this time nearly every VA setting has state of the art neuropsychology services and many are involved at graduate practicum, internship, and/or postdoctoral training of clinical neuropsychology following the model of the Houston Conference (Hannay et al., 1998). VA neuropsychologists have been leaders in developing neuropsychology training and in contributing to the establishment of clinical neuropsychology as a specialty in psychology. While the Boston VAMC has often been justly singled out as a center for the field (e.g. Meier, 1992), notable programs exist and have existed 'coast to coast', including those in Albuquerque, Ann Arbor, Iowa City, Los Angeles, Memphis, Miami, New Orleans, Portland, and Salt Lake City, and San Diego to list only a few. The Pittsburgh VAMC can also boast a long and distinguished history of neuropsychological service and research. While the focus and practice at that setting has differed somewhat from that at West Haven, readers may find of interest a comparison of a current VA neuropsychology practice with the description of Gerald Goldstein's Neuropsychology Laboratory at the Pittsburgh VAMC nearly two decades ago (Matthews, 1981). Despite the many changes occurring currently within the Department of Veterans Affairs medical system, clinical neuropsychology continues to have a strong presence in nearly all VA settings.

About the Author:

I was not actually born in a VA but my first clinical experience was in a VA Medical Center in a practicum at the Hines VAMC outside Chicago. Until that point, late in 1972, I was one of several strange ducks (interested in Clinical Psychology and Physiological Psychology) in a newly APA-accredited, relatively traditional, graduate training program in Clinical Psychology (then University of Illinois Chicago Circle, now simply University of Illinois, Chicago). Neuropsychology at the Hines VA, as at the West Side, Chicago VA where I subsequently obtained training, operated essentially as a consultant service, primarily to the Neurology and Neurosurgery Services. Referrals came down, and we went out; or patients came down to us, and then returned to their units. The work was primarily assessment. Communication with referral sources in these settings included brief conversations and reports that were written on standard forms and placed into the Medical Record. Certainly by this time several VA settings had established more prominent research and training programs that included clinical neuropsychology as important contributors to such processes as Grand Rounds with broad involvement of medical and surgical services.

After completing all of my doctoral requirements except the dissertation, I elected to pursue an additional, specialized year of training in Clinical Neuropsychology at the VAMC, West Haven, CT. This program was just getting started under the direction of Dr. Robert Novelly and with the strong support from both the VA Psychology and Neurology Services and the Neurology Department at the Yale School of Medicine. The primary work was based in the Epilepsy Center, a prototype for a number of similar units later developed within the VA system, where we functioned less as peripheral consultants and more as members of a multidisciplinary team. Consultant services were also provided to General Neurology and other hospital services. There was opportunity to provide brief treatment and limited rehabilitation work with neuropsychology patients. There were also weekly Neurology Grand Rounds and other inter-service teaching experiences. After taking advantage of a second, advanced training year at West Haven — one that afforded enough research time to complete a dissertation — I accepted a position to establish neuropsychological services on a Stroke Unit. This was a second multidisciplinary specialized Neurology Unit that was adjacent to the Epilepsy Center. In that setting, taking advantage of the flexibility afforded by the VA position, I was able to develop additional group and family work, to develop services throughout the Medical Center, and to become increasingly involved in training and research. If neuropsychology flourished at West Haven, it is in no small part due to contacts and influences of neuropsychologists in other centers and to the student interns who have since matriculated.

While my own training pre-dated the INS-Div. 40 guidelines, I believe that it matches well with those recommendations as well as those of the Houston Conference. I took advantage of training/education and research opportunities afforded specifically by the VA healthcare system. These opportunities included conferences that brought together VA neuropsychologists from widely disparate VA settings for discussions on various practice topics (e.g. Salt Lake City, 1981 and Northport, N.Y., 1982). I sat for the ABPP-CN as soon as it was offered (and before I could forget too much!) in 1983. Research opportunities included involvement with the VA Merit Review, a grant process similar to that coordinated by NIH but with federal monies directed toward the VA. In addition, I was able to gain experience with the VA Cooperative Studies, a program that affords an excellent basis for research that involves multiple settings addressing a topic; thus, increasing the number of subjects and the generalizability of results. In these efforts I was fortunate to be able to work with Richard Mattson, M.D., who established and for many years headed the Yale-West Haven VA Epilepsy program, and neuropsychologists Mary Prevey, Ph.D. and John Beauvais, Ph.D.

A VA Practice Setting

Administration

By 1997 both the inpatient Epilepsy and Stroke Units had faded into history with the unfortunate pragmatics of fiscal constraints, and the West Haven VAMC had been merged with the Newington VAMC to form the VA Connecticut Healthcare System. This consolidation reduced the number of administrative positions and continued a process of reducing staff costs, but the practice of neuropsychology proceeded as established. At the time of this writing the Psychology Service at VA Connecticut Healthcare continues to function as an independent service with a Chief of Psychology who reports to the Chief of Staff and the Healthcare System Director. That individual is responsible for the administration of psychology at the West Haven Campus, the Newington Campus, and at the affiliated outreach and satellite clinics; clinical neuropsychology also functions under the directions of Chief of Psychology. At those VA settings where psychologists have been absorbed into what may be termed a Product Line or a Service Line (a matrix of clinicians often administratively headed by a psychiatrist — though occasionally by a psychologist) the actual practice of neuropsychology may not be significantly altered, but the administrative ‘chain of command’ differs.

Space and facilities

The West Haven Campus of VA Connecticut Healthcare System (henceforth, West Haven) is fairly typical within the VA. Each professional psychologist is provided an office, and there is shared space available for interns and for clinical assessments with conference rooms shared and scheduled among many services. Additional space for research, research assistants, or post-doctoral students is ‘earned’ through the successful application for external funding, including granting agencies specifically established for supporting research within the VA (e.g. Merit Review, Cooperative Studies). For historical reasons, most of the space utilized by Clinical Neuropsychology is in close proximity to the inpatient unit to which neurological patients are admitted. However, as discussed further below, the work itself has shifted rather dramatically to a greater outpatient than inpatient caseload. Moreover, because my time has for many years been split between clinical neuropsychology responsibilities and those of the Director of Clinical Training, my office has been adjacent to the Chief of Psychology to allow a centralized administration of the Psychology Service. Thus, the space available for the work of clinical neuropsychology includes two offices shared by the two neuropsychology interns and the office of the neuropsychologist. Additional office space has been utilized in conjunction with research projects.

In addition to the usual array of testing materials, which are regularly updated or replaced through justified order requests, VA clinical services now operate with an increasingly utilized and fairly sophisticated electronic medical record. The DHCP system, which will soon be superceded by a 'windows' based state of the art software package, is actually a quite reasonable medical documentation procedure (Kolodner and Douglas, 1997). While the author is aware that its implementation has not been uniformly smooth throughout the VA system, at West Haven it has afforded an increasing ease of communication and a marked decrease in the problem of lost or missing neuropsychology reports. Through this system staff and interns have access to the bulk of the patient's current medical file (including clinic visits for the past several years, radiological reports, medications, and other pertinent material). Local and external e-mail messaging are built in. Each clinical office has either a terminal to access this system or a PC that can operate with other office type software as well. It is through this system that most communication flows, from referral through neuropsychological report.

Affiliations

An important facet in many VA medical centers is the designation and function as a Dean's Committee facility, which reflects a formal linkage between the medical center and the affiliated medical school. At West Haven this has meant a close involvement with the Yale School of Medicine. Residents from various departments (including Medicine, Neurology and Psychiatry) rotate between Yale-New Haven Hospital and West Haven and a considerable amount of training at all levels of healthcare is the routine. The attending physicians at West Haven are typically an important part of the faculty at Yale (thus, answering to two masters: Chief of Staff/Director and Department Chair), and most of the staff psychologists are reviewed during the hiring process for appointment as faculty in an appropriate department at Yale. For neuropsychology, medical school involvement has historically been through the Neurology Department, though there have also been close connections within Psychiatry. The psychologist who elects a 'full-time' rather than a clinical appointment is typically more committed to conducting research as a major portion of his/her career, and, if involved with outside practice, does so through some component of the Yale School of Medicine system. This has benefits (space, letterhead, etc.) and costs (a percentage of the income goes back to Yale). Most psychology staff, including those who have practiced in neuropsychology, elect the clinical track; thus, consulting or outside clinical work becomes a separate 'private practice' separate from the tour of duty at West Haven. However, in either case the everyday experience is a close involvement with the larger system comprising the Yale Medical School Community for the purposes of research planning and consultation, shared opportunities for continuing education, and expectations for contributing to the teaching functions related to the affiliated department.

Referrals/Professional Relationships

In the days of multidisciplinary clinical research units like the Epilepsy Unit and the Stroke Unit, nearly all patients were seen without the need for referral, and some patients would be seen on multiple occasions if there were long hospital stays. Epilepsy admissions would range from several days to several weeks (and with multiple admissions within the year for the Epilepsy Surgery Program). Patients in the Stroke Unit or General Neurology would not infrequently have stays of 25–30 days, with some patients staying considerably longer. Obviously, under these circumstances the opportunities for extensive or repeat evaluations (considering the process of change) and for research were many. It has been rather fascinating over the past few years at West Haven to participate in a major change in VA healthcare delivery, one that is also reflected in the nation as a whole. The patients and the reasons for referral have changed relatively little, but the model of care has changed from an inpatient, specialist directed approach to an outpatient-based, primary care system. Thus, at West Haven there are now relatively few inpatient beds and fewer Neurology beds. Referrals of outpatients for evaluation on a scheduled, outpatient basis have become nearly 80% of the workload. It is most typical for referrals to be made by the Primary Care physician, who may be simultaneously referring to other services including Neurology. Outpatient Psychiatry is also a major source of referrals, since there remain a rather large number of patients who are followed by the VA primarily for mental health rather than for all medical care. In addition, longer term care patients in Geriatrics or the Blind Rehabilitation Center, who may be at the setting for 3–6 months are often seen for questions related to progress, prognosis, or placement. Consult requests are not rare from 'external' sources such as the VA Regional Office in Hartford (Vocational Rehabilitation), the Groton Naval Base, or the Coast Guard Academy.

Certain facets of the work remain unchanged. Although in some respects Clinical Neuropsychology has returned to an operation more like a consulting service, it remains quite closely involved with medical services for both the clinical work and research. Communication with referring sources in order to understand the specific nature of the question in many cases is quite important. This does not necessarily limit or even focus the assessment undertaken, but it does assure that the clinician making the referral obtains the information requested in a clearly stated form in our report. The practice of neuropsychology is well-established at West Haven, as at many VA settings; however, each year it is typical to provide orientation presentations to new residents in order to teach the types of issues best addressed by a neuropsychological assessment and to minimize the number of purely psychodiagnostic referrals which are typically handled by other psychologists in the setting. However, in recent years the neuropsychologist has not been involved to any significant degree in recruiting referrals. As new problems or issues arise, as has been the case in the past 10–15 years with the rise of AIDS and the Persian Gulf Syndrome, it is usual and expected that the Psychology Service and the Clinical Neuropsychology subsection would be involved in the planning and implementation of appropriate contributions to clinical care. Acute inpatient referrals will nearly always have priority, since discharges are nearly always imminent. However, in some instances an inpatient referral made late in a patient's stay that is not critical for discharge planning can be deferred to outpatient follow up.

Personnel

The author worked for many years with Dr. Novelly in sharing the clinical and teaching responsibilities in neuropsychology at West Haven. For several years after Dr. Novelly's departure, the work was coordinated with Dr. James Sullivan and subsequently Dr. Alexandre Bennett. At the present time there is one neuropsychologist with the chief clinical responsibility for the West Haven neuropsychology services. A very important aspect of the clinical neuropsychology program has been the interns who are completing their APA-accredited training in psychology. It is typical for two of the seven interns at West Haven to be 'majoring' in neuropsychology, which means a significant amount of their clinical training is devoted to neuropsychology — perhaps 75%. In addition, there are quite often one or two practicum students and/or an additional intern who are 'minoring' in neuropsychology during the training year. There are many VA settings that have utilized the practice of technician or neuropsychometrist testing, though West Haven has not. The students do a considerable amount of the actual testing, especially once they have become familiar with the approach and the instruments (which clearly takes longer with those having had less prior experience, such as the practicum students). The approach is an apprenticeship model rather than a technician model at West Haven. That is, students may work in conjunction with the staff neuropsychologist or will at least interact with their supervisor rather closely before, during, and after the actual testing. Neuropsychology can make use of a fraction of the Psychology secretary, but typically handles its own scheduling, computerized workload documentation, and report writing with either PC or hospital computer terminal. There have been postdoctoral students in the past, and many VA are moving in that direction during Fiscal Year 2000 with a centralized push and encouragement toward postdoctoral opportunities through funding.

Mechanics/Conduct of Practice

Consult flow

With the exception of referrals from outside agencies, which usually come through telephone or mail, consult requests are entered by the referring clinician into the DHCP computer. These are simultaneously printed centrally at the Psychology Service secretary's printer and flashed into an 'alert' message on the neuropsychologist's DHCP terminal. The neuropsychologist 'logs in' that the consult has been received and begins the process of triage. For many routine referrals, the triage process simply involves a perusal of the details of the consult; for others, contact with the referring source is essential. Priorities are established and patients are contacted by phone and/or letter to be scheduled for the examination. Inpatients are almost invariably seen within a day or three of receipt of the consult; outpatients are seen within 3–4 weeks in most cases. Reports are intended to follow shortly the completion of the clinical work (one to two days from draft to entered report). These are typically generated and corrected through standard word processing on PC and then entered into the DHCP computer system where they become immediately available for all appropriate clinicians. A computer system 'alert' is automatically generated to the referring source when the case is logged in and the report is completed.

Assessment approach

The nature of the work and breadth of the types of referrals at West Haven has always mitigated against a fixed battery approach. Indeed, during the span of time (1975–1993) when the Yale-West Haven VA Epilepsy Program functioned with a highly utilized sharing agreement, children and adolescents were seen as well as the adult veteran age range (20-90+). The approach that has worked best has been a flexible battery approach that has made use of a quantitative core of well-standardized procedures that have been studied for utility with neurological populations. Additional testing instruments and procedures are brought to bear to either follow-up and further define deficits or to answer more specific questions. Typical referral questions include 1) Dementia vs. Depression, 2) Identify or define possible deficits secondary to a disorder (e.g. cerebrovascular disease, epilepsy, head trauma, multiple sclerosis, Parkinson's Disease, or substance abuse), 3) Contribute to the differential diagnosis (e.g. psychiatric vs. neurological process, residual learning disability or ADD in adults, subtle manifestations of a seizure disorder, delirium vs. dementia with competency issues etc.), and 4) Contribute to questions of change with and without treatment (which might include anticonvulsant toxicity, progress of a dementing process, or changes related to drug trials or neurosurgical interventions). Over the years, various adaptations have been necessary to answer essentially the same types of questions with patients who have profound sensory limitations (e.g. rehabilitation planning for Blind Center patients or cochlear implant candidates).

At West Haven, the neuropsychological assessment is defined as an approach that considers Attention and Executive Control, Motor Integrative, Sensory Perceptual, Cognitive-Intellectual, New Learning and Memory, Speech and Language, and Personality/Emotional factors as overlapping areas of functioning requiring specific consideration. Tools selected for a bedside exam of a 78-year-old patient referred for issues of competence or delirium vs. dementia would certainly be quite different than those utilized to consider problems associated with Persian Gulf Syndrome. The former might involve the Mattis Dementia Rating Scale buttressed with a few WAIS-III subtests (such as Comprehension), the Hooper Test of Visual Organization, the Babcock Story Recall, the Boston Naming Test, and a clinical interview (perhaps including the Geriatric Beck Scale), while the latter would more typically entail a more extensive assessment that could include a complete WAIS-III, Logical Memory and Visual Reproduction (possibly the complete Wechsler Memory Scale-III), the Complex Figure Test, the California Verbal Learning Test, the Halstead–Reitan Battery, Controlled Oral Word Association, the Boston Naming Test, the MMPI-2, and perhaps the Test of Memory Malingering. Where visual perceptual problems emerge, the Benton measures have proven useful (e.g. Visual Form Discrimination, Judgment of Line Orientation, Facial Discrimination). For elderly patients with clearly impaired processing, the Fuld Object Memory Test is likely to replace the CVLT. With a referral question or provisional diagnosis raising certain questions, the initial interview is critical in helping the clinician select tasks appropriate to the individual patient. This neuropsychologist has always found it helpful to observe the patient both succeeding and failing in functional areas in order to understand the presentation. An hypothesis testing approach generated after a baseline core assessment is accomplished determines the final spectrum of testing procedures employed. While inpatients these days are likely to be quite acutely ill or dysfunctional, the basic approach is the same for both inpatients and outpatients. The results of any single measure may raise more questions than it answers, and efforts are made to observe the patient both pass and fail tasks in a given functional area in order to have the most complete impression of the individual.

Forensic issues

One area from which clinical neuropsychology at West Haven, as in most VA settings, has been sheltered is forensics. The Department of Veterans Affairs has budgeted for clinicians to be available to provide for the healthcare needs of its constituents, and there is no interest in having staff getting over-involved up in legal activities that can take up considerable time and effort. While there are many instances where the medical record, which includes the neuropsychology report, becomes a part of a court proceeding, the test protocols and the neuropsychology personnel typically do not. Subpoenas, which have been rare events, are simply turned over to the federal district counsel who assists in providing medical record information to those appropriate to receive them and explains the limits of involvement of staff when necessary.

Training

The training of clinical and counseling psychologists in general and clinical neuropsychologists in particular has been an important facet of the work at West Haven. At VA settings training is typically restricted, with a few exceptions, to the clinical teaching of individuals who might one day be able to be employed through the VA system; i.e. American citizens who are matriculating through APA-accredited university programs in clinical or counseling psychology. VA settings are required to maintain individual APA-accreditation in order to maintain funding for the training program, though the nature of the training programs can vary quite widely. At West Haven, the training has been on a 'track' basis, with students electing Clinical (Mental Health), Health Psychology, or Clinical Neuropsychology as their major focus. In the latter two tracks, a training minor is also selected to complement and broaden the experience. The neuropsychology training program has been identified as an apprenticeship in model, scientist-practitioner in philosophy, and in full compliance with the International Neuropsychological Society-APA, Division 40 Task Force Guidelines on training (1987) (though actually predating them). It would be impossible to over-estimate the importance of the student-interns to the service, research, and esprit of neuropsychology at West Haven.

Research

Conducting research is not a necessary component of the mechanics of practice within VA neuropsychology; however, it is not only a common one but also a very sensible one. It is sensible for many reasons, including the following most central purposes: 1) The VA system has always supported research, as suggested above; and staff can be afforded a significant portion of work time in its pursuit; 2) there are multiple opportunities to conduct research; 3) research can invigorate and improve the clinical work and the individuals conducting it; 4) a successful research program helps to build the clinical service, through the acquisition of space, personnel, and equipment and by helping to recruit excellent students; and 5) research involvement maintains a neuropsychology program's connection with one of the major missions of the university and the medical center. Therefore, at West Haven, as at many VA settings, a considerable amount of time has been spent by staff and students in research. Among the primary areas of interest have been epilepsy (with special attention to memory functioning and behavioral toxicity to anticonvulsants), cerebrovascular disease, post-traumatic stress disorder, and cocaine abuse.

Business

VA settings vary considerably in how certain budgetary issues are handled and the federal budget process is, of course, a public and political one. Currently, VISNs are run by a CEO who determines budgets for individual healthcare settings. VA psychology staffing is then determined by the medical center or healthcare system director through consultation with the Chief of Psychology or the Chief of the Mental Health Service Line. There is competition with other services or service/product lines in a climate of fluctuating but generally declining resources. Nonetheless, VA settings have generally been quite stable in terms of staffing and have been considered relatively 'secure' positions. In recent years, staff reductions have been handled through attrition (e.g. retirement), though the federal government has the option of the equivalent of lay-offs through the complicated RIF (Reduction in Force) procedure. Budgeting for students is entirely separate and is handled through a centralized request made each year for training funds. This too has been relatively stable, though changes occur periodically — as in FY 2000 when settings have the option of giving up an intern training slot in return for the funding of two postdoctoral slots.

In some settings there is a specific budget that is provided to the Psychology Service for equipment, materials, and continuing education. West Haven Psychology has always had a small CE budget, and one staff meeting each month is devoted to continuing education. In recent years the availability of training conferences for VA settings has increased. Funding for external training is currently quite limited, and may only cover tuition, though an individual's research budget can expand opportunities for reimbursement. Neuropsychology equipment and supplies have in recent years been obtained through requests with written justifications. These requests are then reviewed through channels (Fiscal and Supply Services), and the materials have been obtained as prioritized in each quarter of the fiscal year. This has not been particularly problematic and has worked well, though staff has always recognized that there are clear financial constraints. For example, it would be difficult (read impossible) to purchase the 50-100 computer generated personality reports each year, which could arguably be clinically helpful, through the National Computer System on the MMPI-2 or the Millon Scales. On the other hand, these scales can be computer scored with scales available for the clinician's interpretation as a part of a fairly extensive psychological testing package on the DHCP computer system. Liability insurance is not an issue, since clinicians are institutionally 'covered' for their 'in-house' activities.

Many psychology staff, of course, must handle liability insurance for their outside private practice work separately.

Coding/Billing

For many years billing was not an issue that neuropsychologists thought about in VA settings, and it is one that is only very peripherally considered at present. Recently, VA medical settings have become competitive for health-care business and non-service connected veterans or their third party carriers are now billed for services. This is a process in its relative infancy and has not affected service delivery to date in ways it might in managed care settings where clear limitations on hours and procedures have been developing. On the other hand, with the advent of the electronic medical record, coding for both diagnosis and clinical procedures has become routine. Neuropsychologists also indicate the amount of time (or number of times) that a procedure was performed with each patient. This process is handled entirely by the neuropsychologist at the completion of the work, and is used primarily as a methodology of workload monitoring in West Haven at present. Nonetheless, it is also a mechanism that is likely to be increasingly utilized for budget and billing of patients under developing circumstances. Thus, it is easy to predict that within a few years VA neuropsychologists will need to be as familiar with the authorization process prior to the clinical work and the collections process after as are their counterparts in the 'real world'. At such time, analyses of reimbursement rates and contract appropriateness will become important for the neuropsychologist, for the lead psychologist, or for business managers who may begin to question clinical approaches from a cost-effectiveness perspective.

Overview and Comments Regarding the Future

It should be evident that clinical care and the operations of neuropsychology within a VA setting have undergone considerable change over the past 20 years, and this process of change continues. Without question many of the changes are similar if not identical to the types of changes experienced in other large medical centers, public and private throughout the United States. Changes must continue; for example, because the demographics of the veteran population shift, and the process of priorities within the federal system tend to become complicated by political considerations. However, for many of us working within this complex system, the VA maintains several real advantages that should be underscored: 1) Research and training opportunities abound and are supported by a system closely connected to yet not dominated by solid academic environments; 2) while fiscal concerns have increased markedly, most neuropsychologists within this system are able to practice according to their training model without over-concern or considerable administrative time spent in gaining approval to provide service from external agencies; 3) even within these times of change, a stability of practice has been the rule; and 4) in most VA settings there is an atmosphere of collegiality with other psychologists and with professionals of other services with whom we work.

References

Hannay, H.J., Bieliauskas, L.A., Crosson, B.A., Hammeke, T.A., Hamsher, K., & Koffler, S. (1998). Proceedings of the Houston Conference on Specialty Education and Training in Clinical Neuropsychology. *Archives of Clinical Neuropsychology, 13,* 157–250.

INS-Division 40 Task Force on Education, Accreditation, and Credentialing (1987). Guidelines for doctoral training programs in clinical neuropsychology. *The Clinical Neuropsychologist, 1,* 29–34.

Kolodner, R.K. & Douglas, J.V. (Eds.) (1977). *Computerizing large integrated health networks: The VA success.* New York: Springer-Verlag.

Mancusi, J.L. (1981). *Introductory remarks.* In Perspectives in Veterans Administration Neuropsychology and Rehabilitation: Proceedings of the Mental Health and Behavioral Sciences Conference, Salt Lake City.

Matthews, C.G. (1981). Neuropsychology practice in a hospital setting. In S.B. Filskov and T.J. Boll (Eds.), *Handbook of Clinical Neuropsychology* (pp. 645–685). New York: John Wiley and Sons.

Meier, M. J. (1992). Modern clinical neuropsychology in historical perspective. *American Psychologist, 47,* 550–558.

Nawas, M. N. (1972). Landmarks in the history of clinical psychology from its early beginnings through 1971. *Journal of Psychology, 82,* 91–110.

Chapter 15

THE PRACTICE OF CLINICAL NEUROPSYCHOLOGY IN A GENERAL HOSPITAL SETTING

Michael McCrea

Introduction

This chapter is based on the recent history of a hospital-based Neuropsychology Service in the suburban area of a large mid-western city. A formal Neuropsychology Service was founded in 1996, at the request of physicians and administrative staff recognizing the need for such a specialty, both within the hospital and throughout the continuum of outpatient care provided by the comprehensive health system affiliated with the hospital. Clinical psychologists on staff at the hospital had previously provided minimal neuropsychological services amounting to perhaps a dozen evaluations per year, but neuropsychology had not been recognized as a specialty of its own. The historical perspective outlined herein is intended to provide some insight into the building of a hospital-based Neuropsychology Service, as well as to point out some of the growing pains experienced throughout its early development. This chapter is not intended as a perfect recipe for success, but the author now recognize certain strategies that may or may not be advantageous to the development and growth of a Neuropsychology Service in a non-academic, general hospital setting.

About the Author

The author completed his graduate doctoral training in clinical psychology at the University of Wisconsin-Milwaukee, followed by an APA-approved pre-doctoral internship in clinical psychology and neuropsychology at the Vanderbilt University Medical School in Nashville, Tennessee. My internship training was somewhat unique, with approximately 50% of clinical time devoted to neuropsychological assessment, 40% to psychological assessment, and 10% to psychotherapy and intervention methods. The author then completed a two-year post-doctoral fellowship in clinical neuropsychology at Northwestern University Medical School and Northwestern Memorial Hospital in Chicago. Fellowship training consisted of inpatient and outpatient neuropsychological assessment, research collaboration, and involvement in teaching and supervision within the neuropsychology track of the graduate program affiliated with the medical school.

The author was hired directly out of fellowship to establish the hospital-based Neuropsychology Service on which this chapter is based, which at that time consisted of only the author. The Neuropsychology Service has since grown to include a second adult neuropsychologist, two part-time technicians, one full-time secretary, and several graduate and undergraduate research assistants. Plans are in place to now develop a pediatric component to the Neuropsychology Service. The author now heads up the Neuropsychology Service and is responsible for its daily clinical operation, budget considerations, managed care contract negotiations, human resource issues, and other aspects critical to the success of the service. The author also remains active in clinical research in the areas of concussion, traumatic brain injury, dementia, and neurocognitive test development. He currently holds an academic appointment as adjunct clinical professor within an APA-accredited graduate program in clinical psychology at a local university.

Framework of the Neuropsychology Service in a General Hospital Setting

Practice setting

The Neuropsychology Service is based within a 275-bed tertiary care medical center in suburban Milwaukee, Wisconsin, with a service area population of approximately 350,000 people. The hospital is the main provider of inpatient medical services in the outer west suburban area, with more than 12,000 hospital admissions per year. In addition to general medical-surgical units, specialty care units serve patients from pediatrics, obstetrics, cardiology, oncology, orthopedics, neurology, physical medicine and rehabilitation, and psychiatry. The Level II emergency department also responds to more than 33,000 visits per year. The radiology department conducts over 86,000 procedures per year, including CT, MRI, and SPECT, and has recently gone to completely 'filmless' studies that allow the radiologist to view digital scans on a monitor or computer screen and eliminates the need to manually transport conventional films. The hospital medical staff is made up of approximately 725 physicians, including approximately 18 neurologists, 10 neurosurgeons, 20 psychiatrists, 10 radiologists, 3 physiatrists, 15 emergency medicine physicians, 2 addiction specialists, and more than 150 primary care physicians.

The larger health system affiliated with the hospital includes 12 off-site primary care clinics staffed by member physicians from the hospital medical staff who are responsible for approximately 200,000 office visits per year. Various specialists also hold offices in several of these clinics. Specialty programs affiliated with the hospital and relevant to the practice of neuropsychology include: the Senior Health Center, a hospital-based geriatric evaluation clinic; the Lawrence Center, a stand alone inpatient and outpatient chemical dependency treatment facility; the Regional Cancer Center, providing comprehensive cancer diagnosis and treatment; and, a Family Practice Residency Program affiliated with the local medical school. The Neuropsychology Service also provides consultation throughout a large network of nursing homes and eldercare facilities formally affiliated with the hospital and health system.

Administrative structure

The Neuropsychology Service is configured within the Center for Behavioral Health, a comprehensive outpatient mental health clinic on the hospital campus. The clinic is physically situated within a professional office building, sometimes referred to as a medical arts building, directly adjacent and connected by enclosed walkway to the hospital. In addition to the neuropsychologists on staff, the Center for Behavioral Health is comprised of psychiatrists, addictionologists, psychologists, psychotherapists, and chemical dependency counselors. The Division of Psychology is administratively a subspecialty within the Section of Psychiatric Medicine. The author currently serves as the Head of the Neuropsychology Service and the Chair for the Division of Psychology. Staff neuropsychologists are categorized as members of the paramedical hospital staff, which entitles each to various medical staff privileges, including access to computerized medical records system, extensive medical library services, transcription support for inpatient dictation, mailbox, parking, and participation in various medical staff events.

Neuropsychology service personnel

The Neuropsychology Service currently consists of two full-time adult neuropsychologists, with plans to expand with a pediatric specialist in the near future. Both neuropsychologists have similar training, including completion of an APA-accredited doctoral program and predoctoral internship, as well as a two-year post doctoral fellowship in clinical neuropsychology meeting the standards set by various governing bodies within neuropsychology (Hannay et al., 1998). There are essentially two sets of minimal requirements to be eligible for hire as a neuropsychologist within the current setting. The first requirement consists of essential or preferred background as outlined by the

Neuropsychology Service itself and pertains more directly to the neuropsychologist's training within the specialty, including:

1. Completion of doctoral degree from APA-accredited program.
2. Completion of APA-accredited predoctoral internship.
3. Completion of formal post-doctoral fellowship in clinical neuropsychology.
4. Eligibility to pursue board certification in clinical neuropsychology (obtaining board certification is preferred, but not required for hire or continued employment).

Additionally, each neuropsychologist must meet all medical staff requirements for hire and hospital privileges as a clinical psychologist. Historically, members of the Division of Psychology and Section of Psychiatric Medicine established these guidelines in order to ensure minimal standards of training, competence and practice. In addition to items 1 and 2 listed above, specific medical staff requirements for clinical psychologists include valid licensure, inclusion in the National Register of Health Service Providers in Psychology, and clearance on a state mandated criminal background check. All candidates must also be approved through an interview process with representatives from the Division of Psychology and Section of Psychiatric Medicine.

Two part-time neuropsychological technicians each work approximately 15–20 hours per week to support the outpatient practice of each neuropsychologist. Technicians administer and score neuropsychological and psychological tests, as well as assist with day-to-day operations of the service and various ongoing research projects directed by each neuropsychologist. Technicians do not participate in testing associated with inpatient consultations. Technicians are routinely, and almost exclusively, recruited from a local APA-approved graduate program in clinical psychology with a specialty track in neuropsychology. This approach has proven much more efficient in the training of new technicians, and provides a training element to the Neuropsychology Service. Both staff neuropsychologists hold academic appointments within the graduate program from which technicians are recruited. Graduate students from the program also regularly rotate through the Neuropsychology Service for practicum experience. Several undergraduates from local colleges and universities are also involved as research assistants supporting various ongoing projects directed by each neuropsychologist.

A full-time secretary is employed for patient scheduling, transcription, copying, and other clerical services vital to the efficiency of the Neuropsychology Service. Other staff within the Center for Behavioral Health provide back-up clerical and receptionist support when necessary. An insurance authorization specialist is employed by the Center for Behavioral Health, but each neuropsychologist directly manages this task due to complications often encountered when securing insurance authorization for neuropsychological services.

Physical layout

As noted, the Neuropsychology Service is located within a larger behavioral health clinic with approximately 50 practitioners. Although a seemingly mundane topic relative to other issues discussed as part of this chapter, be assured that the struggle for physical space is often encountered in any hospital-based service. The current Neuropsychology Service is fortunate to have an arrangement in which staff neuropsychologists have a designated area where all offices and testing rooms are directly adjacent to each other. Each neuropsychologist has a testing room directly across the hall from their office where technicians conduct formal testing. This layout has positively impacted the efficiency of the neuropsychologists' outpatient practice and allows for convenient nearby supervision of technicians. The neuropsychologists' offices and testing rooms are equipped with computers so that any computerized testing can be conducted in either location. All offices and testing rooms are also hard-wired for direct access to the hospital network to facilitate electronic transfer of data files and documents. Testing rooms are not equipped with video recording equipment, audio recording devices, or one-way mirrors, although these options are being considered as part of future renovation. Each testing room is large enough to comfortably situate the technician and patient, as well as storage of all testing supplies, research materials, and other items. All patient files containing raw data are maintained by each neuropsychologist and securely stored in the testing rooms. At present, the larger clinic stores a file on each patient seen by the Neuropsychology Service, which contains a copy of the patient registration, insurance information, and neuropsychological report, but no test records or raw data.

Nature of Neuropsychological Practice in a General Hospital Setting

By it's very nature, neuropsychology in a general hospital setting is primarily a clinical service. It is strongly recommended, however, that the service aim for a more diversified approach to include components of research and training. These elements not only enhance the identity of the Neuropsychology Service, but also further the professional development of the practicing neuropsychologist. Research activity within the present Neuropsychology Service has increased the specialty's credibility and proven as an invaluable vehicle for exposure to the larger medical staff, referring physicians outside the hospital system, other local referral sources, and even managed care agencies. In turn, physician exposure to research projects directed by the Neuropsychology Service has definitely resulted in a greater volume of referrals for clinical services.

Although increasingly more difficult to accomplish in a challenging economic health care climate, providing graduate training in neuropsychology via clinical and research experience is also seen as a 'win–win' situation for both the Neuropsychology Service and the trainee. In the particular region

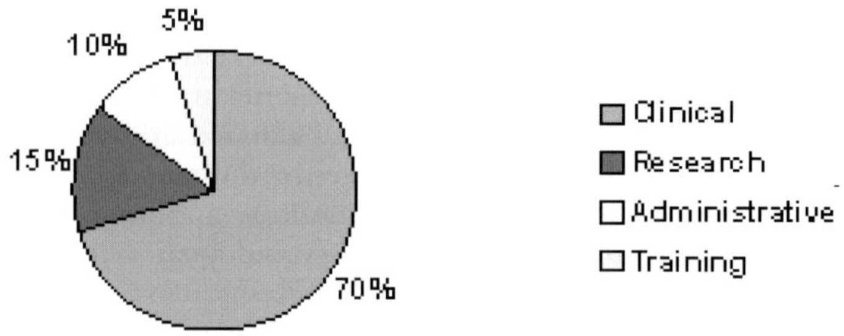

Figure 1. Percentage of time devoted to specific aspects of neuropsychological practice.

of the present Neuropsychology Service, there are few options for training outside the local graduate program, so faculty and students are eager to collaborate. Naturally, a fair amount of administrative activity also comes with the territory of managing an efficient and productive hospital-based service. Figure 1 provides a breakdown of time the head of neuropsychological services devotes to clinical, research, training, and administrative activity. The specific nature of activities within each of these domains is described below in more detail. With the exception of perhaps the administrative duties, it is hoped that the present and future staff neuropsychologists will also follow a similar model of practitioner-scientist activity.

Clinical Service

At present, the Neuropsychology Service sees exclusively adults over the age of 16, as neither staff neuropsychologist is formally trained in pediatric neuropsychology. Like many neuropsychology programs in academic and nonacademic settings, the service is largely assessment-driven. More than 85% of the total clinical service activity is devoted to neuropsychological testing, neurobehavioral assessment, competency evaluations, psychological testing, and forensic consultation. The balance of activity includes a minimal amount of brief psychotherapy, cognitive rehabilitation, and behavioral medicine services. Neuropsychological testing clearly accounts for the largest segment of overall clinical activity.

A diversified practice arrangement is essential to increasing volumes and activity by the Neuropsychology Service in a general hospital setting. A busy conventional outpatient practice is supplemented by clinical service to inpatient medical and psychiatric units, an on-site outpatient dementia clinic, and local geriatric care campuses with various levels of assistance for the elderly (e.g., independent living, assisted living, dementia specialty care units, group homes, skilled nursing).

As is illustrated in Figure 2, traditional outpatient neuropsychological assessment accounts for the largest segment of clinical activity by the Neu-

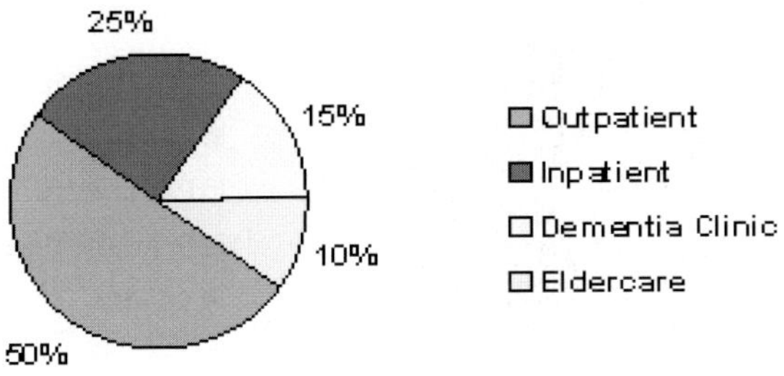

Figure 2. Percentage of clinical activity by setting.

ropsychology Service, but approximately 25% of clinical activity is devoted to inpatient consultation-liaison. A small but significant amount of clinical service is also provided to a dementia clinic and several eldercare facilities affiliated with the hospital and health system. Within the eldercare settings, neuropsychology can be especially valuable in assisting staff on decision-making about the need for a resident to transfer to the next level of care (e.g., independent to assisted living) due to cognitive decline.

At present, two staff neuropsychologists are responsible for approximately 700 patient visits per year, including 350 outpatient evaluations, 175 inpatient consultations, 105 dementia clinic evaluations, and 70 eldercare facility consultations. Involvement in several arms of the larger hospital and health system not only increases the volume and variety of clinical activity, but also serves as a vehicle for exposure to and collaboration with other potential referral sources. The experience of the current hospital-based neuropsychological service indicates that inpatient, dementia clinic, and eldercare facility consultation has also expanded the outpatient referral base.

Examining the pattern of physician referrals and diagnostic classification is also informative as to the nature of clinical activity provided by a hospital-based Neuropsychology Service. Figure 3 indicates that neurologists account for the largest segment of referrals to the Neuropsychology Service, but that physiatrists, psychiatrists, and primary care physicians also regularly depend on the Neuropsychology Service to assist in the diagnosis and treatment of their patients. A small but significant number of referrals are also received from nurse practitioners, unit care coordinators, psychotherapists, social workers, community agencies, and other sources. Finally, patients or their family members will often self-refer because of concerns about changes in cognitive or functional status.

A hospital-based Neuropsychology Service is likely to consult on a wide variety of neurologic disorders, which will vary from service to service based on the nature of practice or expertise by referring physicians and those services directly affiliated with the hospital. Figure 4 illustrates the breakdown of patient volumes within various diagnostic categories for the present Neu-

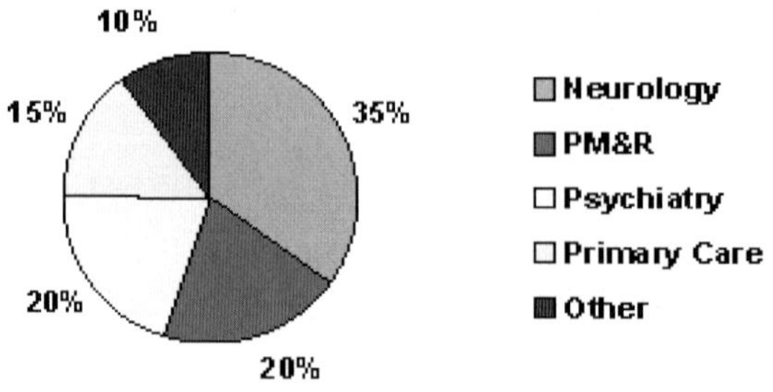

Figure 3. Percentage of patient referrals by specialists.

ropsychology Service. Collectively, dementia syndromes (i.e., Alzheimer's disease, vascular, Lewy body, frontal/frontotemporal, Parkinson's disease, etc.) are the leading diagnostic category seen by the neuropsychologists. This pattern is due to a number of factors, including involvement at the on-site dementia clinic and local eldercare facilities, collaboration with various community agencies serving the elderly, exposure coming from dementia research by the Neuropsychology Service, and demographics of the region in which the hospital is located. A significant number of patients with traumatic brain injury, stroke, and other neurologic disorders (e.g., multiple sclerosis, brain tumor, cerebral aneurysm, epilepsy, etc.) are also consulted on each year. The Neuropsychology Service is also often called in to consult on various medical disorders (e.g., delirium, encephalopathy, meningitis, toxic exposure, CNS lupus, chemical overdose, etc.) with accompanying cognitive or behavioral deficits. Involvement with local neurology clinics, the physical medicine and rehabilitation program, cancer treatment center, and emergency department has increased the volume of non-demented, neurologic patients referred for neuropsychological services.

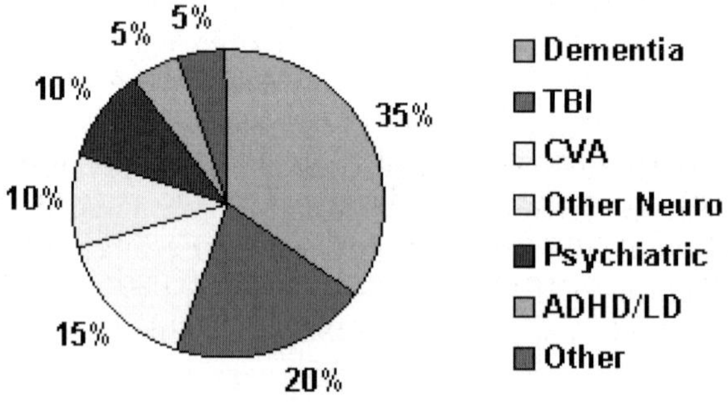

Figure 4. Percentage of referrals by diagnostic category.

By virtue of its location within a comprehensive outpatient mental health clinic and the presence of an inpatient psychiatric unit within the hospital, a significant number of referrals are received from psychiatrists and other mental health providers. The Neuropsychology Service is frequently consulted to assist in differential diagnosis and treatment planning with various psychiatric disorders, including schizophrenia, delirium, dementia, and alcohol and drug abuse. Several adult cases of possible Attention-Deficit Hyperactivity Disorder, Learning Disabilities, and other developmental disorders are evaluated by the Neuropsychology Service. Neuropsychological testing before and after the administration of electroconvulsive therapy (ECT) for treatment of depression has also been requested by the treating psychiatrists in order to establish a baseline level of cognitive functioning, track post-treatment recovery, and correlate cognitive status with depression severity.

Research activity

Although primarily a clinical service, the practice of neuropsychology within a general medical setting may also benefit from many opportunities for research collaboration. The present Neuropsychology Service has numerous ongoing research projects, most of which relate directly to neuropsychological assessment or practice. Time dedicated to research is certainly difficult to secure given clinical demands, but the current Neuropsychology Service has been able to find a balance to allow for research activity. As noted, the exposure and credibility amongst referral sources that results from research activity and publications in turn benefits the clinical service through increased referral volumes. More recently, the staff neuropsychologists have also had reasonable success in securing outside grant funding to support their research efforts. Interestingly, there is some indication in recent years that non-academic sites are becoming more competitive for research funding due to several factors, including lower overhead costs and greater patient availability.

Several factors are key to finding time to mix neuropsychological research with clinical practice in a general medical setting. These include contact with other medical staff with research interests, collaboration with research and statistical experts in formal academic settings, utilization of competent research assistants, securing outside grant funding, and gaining support from the department and hospital administration. Neuropsychologists in both academic and non-academic settings have realized in recent years that computerized records can aid in research productivity generated directly from clinical practice. Use of a computerized database by the current Neuropsychology Service to store all information from the neuropsychologists' clinical practice has created a more efficient way of exploring research ideas through prospective and retrospective exploratory analysis.

Education and training

Frequent interaction and an open line of professional communication with faculty from the local medical school and a graduate program in clinical psychology is very beneficial to the neuropsychologist practicing in a general hospital or other non-academic setting. Staff neuropsychologists regularly attend a weekly journal club organized by the neuropsychology section at the local medical school, and consult faculty members there on several research projects and professional issues. A critical realization for the staff neuropsychologist in a general hospital setting is that those in an academic setting need not be viewed as 'the competition,' but represent experts with whom professional consultation and research collaboration may be very beneficial to both parties. All in all, close ties with those in an academic setting can result in a sense of greater connectedness to the field of neuropsychology for the neuropsychologists in a general hospital setting.

The current Neuropsychology Service provides training opportunities for students from the local graduate program who are planning to specialize in neuropsychology. Graduate students are encouraged to utilize the clinical service to initiate research projects of their interest, with eventual goal of a published work under the supervision of a staff neuropsychologist. Recruitment of paid technicians from that graduate program has also proven as a great benefit to both the students and the Neuropsychology Service. Many undergraduate students from local colleges and universities are also involved as research assistants to support several studies directed by the staff neuropsychologists.

Administrative duties

As Head of the Neuropsychology Service, the author is directly responsible for most administrative duties associated with the service, and report to the Director of Behavioral Health. The Director typically defers issues related to clinical service delivery and the daily operation of the Neuropsychology Service, but is directly informed or involved in collaboration with me on matters related to the budget, human resources, equipment purchases, research grant funding, managed care contract negotiations, and other business-related issues. The author am primarily responsible for hiring technicians, ordering new test equipment, service expansion, public relations, program development, and other aspects, but relies heavily on input from the other staff neuropsychologist and the Director of Behavioral Health. In fact, both staff neuropsychologists now share a great deal of the effort necessary for program development and public relations. The author also monitors revenue-related issues such as billing, reimbursement, hourly rates, payer mix, and collections, all of which is discussed below in greater detail. Each year, the author provide the Director of Behavioral Health with a review of highlights (e.g., financial and productivity data, program expansion, research activity and funding, public relations, etc.) from the previous fiscal year and objectives for the following year.

The Process of Efficient Clinical Practice in a General Hospital Setting

Efficiency is increasingly the name of the game during rather trying economic times for the practice of neuropsychology, regardless of practice setting. The author has made a conscious effort since the inception of the Neuropsychology Service to identify areas of practice inefficiency and continually revise the process to improve overall efficiency. Time devoted to the development of various forms and other methods of streamlining the practice process have reaped returns several fold. Described below is the current stepwise model utilized by the Neuropsychology Service to enhance practice efficiency.

1. Intake/scheduling
All calls for outpatient neuropsychological consultation are directed to the Neuropsychology Service secretary, who utilizes the Neuropsychology Service Intake Registration Form to record all demographic (e.g., patient data), referral (e.g., physician, presenting problems, suspected diagnosis), insurance (e.g., primary, secondary), and appointment information. The secretary then immediately provides the patient or referral source with a scheduled appointment and forwards a copy of the intake form to the neuropsychologist scheduled to see the patient. Computerized scheduling software is now used by the clinic, which not only allows for more efficient patient scheduling, but also stores data for retrospective analysis of various aspects of clinical practice, including referral source volumes, neuropsychologist productivity, services provided, etc. All outpatients are sent a letter requesting that a family member or person familiar with their condition accompany them to the appointment. This letter also confirms the date, time, and approximate length of the consultation. A map is sent with the letter to assist the patient and family members in locating the neuropsychologist's office. All outpatients pre-register through the hospital admitting department prior to the neuropsychological consultation, at which time demographic and insurance information are updated. This information is entered into the computerized medical record system and then forwarded to the Neuropsychology Service secretary.

The hospital-based Assessment and Referral (A&R) service triages all requests for inpatient neuropsychological consultation. The A&R service is notified directly by the unit clerk or nursing staff when physician orders for neuropsychological consultation are entered. The A&R service then generates copies of all relevant documentation (e.g., emergency room report, history and physical, consultation reports, neuroimaging results, insurance information) from the computerized medical records system used by the hospital, and informs the Neuropsychology Service regarding the consultation request. The neuropsychologist covering the inpatient service is then forwarded the information gathered by the A&R service and conducts the consultation within 24 hours of the physician's request, typically on the same day.

2. Obtaining medical records

Soon after the initial contact, the Neuropsychology Service secretary faxes a brief memo to the referring physician's office requesting that relevant records be forwarded before the date of the scheduled neuropsychological consultation. In many cases where the patient's physician is on hospital medical staff or diagnostic procedures were conducted at the hospital, medical records (e.g., neuroimaging results, past inpatient records, etc.) can be accessed directly from the computerized medical records system utilized by the hospital.

3. Insurance authorization

Each staff neuropsychologist is responsible for verifying the patient's insurance coverage and the need for pre-authorization of services. The experience of the Neuropsychology Service indicates that this issue is often too complicated for clerical or support staff to undertake, especially concerning the dilemma regarding whether neuropsychological services should be covered by the patient's medical or mental health benefits. Although often frustrating, this task has become quite manageable for the author and the other staff neuropsychologist. The Neuropsychology Service secretary forwards the intake form containing insurance information to the neuropsychologist scheduled to see the patient and verification of benefits is typically resolved at least one week prior to the patient's scheduled appointment. Seldom is there a need to reschedule or cancel an appointment because of insurance complications, despite a dense market of managed care where the current Neuropsychology Service is located.

For inpatient consultation, the A&R service forwards insurance information from the computerized database and the neuropsychologist attempts to clarify coverage before seeing the patient, but with the goal of completing the consultation within 24 hours. Fortunately, insurance complications are less often problematic for patients already hospitalized for medical reasons. A special note in this regard is that conventional Medicare does not require pre-authorization for inpatient or outpatient services, but an increasing number of HMO Medicare plans are coming into existence which require pre-authorization much like traditional managed care plans for younger patients.

4. Patient registration

Patients check in at the reception desk just inside the Center for Behavioral Health clinic. The Neuropsychology Service secretary and other support staff then ensure that all relevant paper work is completed by the patient and/or caregiver, including insurance information, informed consent, information releases, and billing notification. The neuropsychologist is then notified that the patient is ready to be seen.

5. Consultation model

The Neuropsychology Service follows the assessment model utilized by many other programs, both in and out of academic settings. The neuropsychologist first typically interviews the patient and family members or others accompanying the patient in order to gather information relevant to the presenting problem, past medical history, current medications, diagnostic test results, psychiatric history, and social/educational/legal background. Records able to be obtained in advance are also reviewed by the neuropsychologist. The neuropsychologist then conducts a portion of the neuropsychological examination before escorting the patient to the adjacent technician's office to complete the balance of testing. The neuropsychologists' offices and testing rooms are equipped so that any computerized testing can be conducted in either location.

Although there is some variability in their overall approach, neuropsychologists utilize a domain-driven approach to neuropsychological testing. None of the staff neuropsychologists adhere to a fixed battery model. Test batteries are flexible and selected measures depend largely on several factors, including the presenting problem, patient demographics, information contained in available medical records, expected outcomes from the evaluation, and time constraints set by insurance or managed care agencies. Domains of function typically assessed as part of a comprehensive neuropsychological battery include: sensory-motor-perceptual functions, premorbid baseline abilities, general intellectual functioning, attention, memory, language, visuospatial skills, executive functions, and activities of daily living.

Staff neuropsychologists typically make use of veteran neuropsychological measures with established norms demonstrating validity and reliability (e.g., WAIS-III, WMS-III, Boston Naming Test, Wisconsin Card Sorting Test, Trail Making Tests, etc.), and which are commonly used in neuropsychological practice (Puente, 1998). Several computerized methods (e.g., continuous performance tests, reaction time measures, response bias/malingering measures, etc.) are also utilized. Screening instruments and short-forms of various neuropsychological tests have recently been employed in instances where clinically appropriate and the neuropsychologist is faced with time constraints for any reason. Various self-report measures (e.g., ADHD symptom scales, post-concussion symptom checklists, etc.) are used to supplement neuropsychological test results. Psychological tests (e.g., depression scales, personality inventories) are also often given to gain insight into non-neurologic factors contributing to the patient's presenting problems.

Comprehensive outpatient neuropsychological evaluations under the current model typically take approximately 4–7 hours to complete, which normally includes one hour for patient interview, 3–4 hours of testing, and 2–3 hours for scoring, interpretation, report generation, and patient or physician feedback. Evaluations may require more testing and overall time depending on the complexity of the case. The neuropsychological technician completes the scoring of tests administered, which is then double-checked by the attending neuropsychologist. The technician and attending neuropsychologist then typically discuss the case upon completion of the testing, including the behavioral observations made by the technician. The neuropsychologist is solely responsible for interpretation of test data and formulating the neuropsychological report. The attending neuropsychologist typically provides direct feedback to the referring physician soon after seeing the patient, prior to the written report arriving at the physician's office. Feedback to the patient and relevant family members is routinely relayed within 1–2 days of the evaluation. Direct and prompt physician and patient feedback has been an effective strategy for marketing the value of the Neuropsychology Service.

Because of situational constraints, brief neuropsychological tests and other bedside assessment methods are routinely used for inpatient neuropsychological consultation. Inpatient assessments are typically designed to address a specific referral question relevant to the immediate clinical picture (e.g., competency, discharge plan, appropriateness for rehabilitation, return to work issues, etc.). Inpatient consultation is often followed by more extensive outpatient follow-up to more precisely clarify the nature and extent of residual neurocognitive or neurobehavioral deficits, and provide helpful treatment recommendations accordingly.

6. **Report generation**

The Neuropsychology Service utilizes a computerized database to generate evaluation reports. The program combines the ability to enter most information via check boxes or text fields and transcription entered by the secretary from the neuropsychologist's dictation. Separate windows allow for entry of data on several variables relevant to:

- patient identifying information
- referral source information
- presenting symptoms
- history of present illness
- past medical history
- past psychiatric history
- developmental history
- family history
- social history
- laboratory/diagnostic test results
- current medications
- behavioral observations
- neuropsychological test results
- diagnostic classification
- clinical impression
- recommendations
- consultation/practice/billing
- information

All information entered is then archived for later statistical analysis. The hospital information systems department was instrumental in applying the neuropsychologists' ideas for such a package and making it a reality for actual application. The computerized method greatly minimizes the amount of text dictated and significantly reduces the time required by the neuropsychologist and secretary to complete a neuropsychological report. This model also allows for efficient storage of all information collected from a clinical consultation, which can then be archived and analyzed for the purpose of research, either pertinent to neuropsychological topics or other aspects of clinical practice (e.g., billing and reimbursement, productivity, referral patterns, etc.). Physicians have also provided favorable feedback on the structured report, especially the use of tables and check boxes instead of extensive text. The neuropsychologist's report regularly arrives at the referring physician's office within 5–7 days after the evaluation.

Reports for inpatient neuropsychological consultation and evaluations in the hospital-based dementia clinic are telephonically dictated on the hospital dictation system and transcribed by the health information management department. A written consultation note is entered in the patient's chart by the neuropsychologist at the time of the consultation, and a full report is dictated by the neuropsychologist within 24 hours. Turn around time for dictation is typically about 24 hours, at which time the report is automatically printed on the unit where the patient is hospitalized and a hard copy is deposited in the medical staff mailbox of the neuropsychologist, attending physician, and any other physicians consulting on the case.

7. Database management

The neuropsychological technicians are responsible for data entry and management, with some support from the Neuropsychology Service secretary. Each neuropsychologist uses a hard copy of the patient database form while interviewing and examining a patient. All test results and appropriate normative values for a particular patient from the assessment are also recorded in a table within this hard copy, which will eventually serve as a backup in case of any failure in accessing the electronic database. All information recorded on this hard copy is then entered by the technician into the computerized database, known as the Neuropsychology Service Consultation Database. This database can then be used to generate assessment reports or analysis of all variables related to the Neuropsychology Service, including practice-related issues (e.g., productivity, billing, reimbursement, referral patterns, etc.) or clinical research topics (e.g., validity and reliability of measures, diagnostic variables, etc.).

8. Record storage

All patient files containing raw data are maintained and securely stored by each neuropsychologist. At present, the larger clinic stores a file on each patient seen by the Neuropsychology Service which contains a copy of the patient registration, insurance information, and neuropsychological report, but no test records or raw data.

The Business Side of Clinical Practice in a General Hospital Setting

The Head of the Neuropsychology Service, in collaboration with the Director of Behavioral Health, is directly responsible for overseeing the financial management of the service. The two parties have regular meetings to discuss issues related to billing rates, reimbursement patterns, managed care contract negotiations, staff salaries, equipment costs, and other financial matters. The Director assembles the formal budget for approval by the larger hospital and health system administration, with input from me regarding anticipated revenue and costs for the upcoming fiscal year. Major categories contained in the Neuropsychology Service budget include staff salaries and benefits, technician and secretarial salaries and benefits, equipment and supplies, and general hospital overhead (e.g., physical space, public relations, etc.). At present, approximately 70% of the total budget goes toward neuropsychologists' salaries and benefits, 15% to technician and secretarial salaries, 10% to general hospital overhead, and 5% to equipment and supplies. This distribution closely parallels that reported in national surveys of neuropsychology practice patterns (Puente, 1998). Annual costs will vary to some extent from year to year, based on start-up associated with a new staff member joining the service, as well as the need for updating equipment (e.g., computers) and test supplies.

The author works closely with the Director of Behavioral Health in developing a fair and competitive salary package for neuropsychologists. Data from national surveys on neuropsychologists' salaries is used as a benchmark for staff compensation based on the practice setting, years of experience, geographic region and other relevant factors (Putnam & Anderson, 1994; Putnam, DeLuca, & Anderson, 1994). Staff neuropsychologists are currently compensated via a salary plus incentive plan, which includes a base salary with benefits and a bonus system based on a percentage of their total revenue collected during each fiscal quarter or year. This package allows the neuropsychologist some degree of security, especially when starting a new practice. On the other hand, it also provides the incentive of greater earning power based on productivity, which reduces the overall financial risk of the hospital and avoids the neuropsychologist's perception of a 'ceiling' on their earning capacity regardless of their workload. The neuropsychologists' expenses related to malpractice/liability coverage, medical staff membership dues, and other professional fees are covered by the hospital each year. Each neuropsychologist is also granted a stipend and paid time off each year for continuing education.

The Neuropsychology Service secretary is paid an hourly wage with benefits, while neuropsychological technicians are considered part-time 'pool' employees and are paid an hourly wage without insurance or other benefits.

Billing process

The Neuropsychology Service is fortunate to be supported by the same billing service used by the larger hospital and health system. A designated representative from the billing service is directly responsible for managing all patient accounts for the Neuropsychology Service and the Center for Behavioral Health. This representative provides the author with a monthly, computerized report of billing and reimbursement information for the entire service, as well as a separate report for each neuropsychologist. A separate database of practice-related variables (e.g., patient contacts, hours of service, amount billed, revenue collected, etc.) is maintained by the head of the neuropsychology service to compare against quarterly and annual figures posted by the billing service. The author also meets regularly with the billing service representative to discuss billing procedures, reimbursement patterns, payer mix, delinquent accounts and other financial matters.

Each staff neuropsychologist is responsible for submitting a billing invoice for all services delivered. The Neuropsychology Service uses a standardized billing form to record the patient's name, date and place of service, patient status (inpatient, outpatient, etc.), procedure code, diagnostic codes, hours of service, total amount billed, and pre-authorization insurance codes (if applicable). This form is completed by the attending neuropsychologist and submitted to secretarial staff who then attaches all patient registration and insurance information before forwarding to the billing service representative. The billing service is then responsible for processing and the submitting the claim to the identified payer, as well as monitoring payment of the claim and keeping the neuropsychologist informed of any billing problems.

All neuropsychological services are billed hourly according to established practice standards (Dalton, 1995; National Academy of Neuropsychology, 1998; Puente 1998), including time for clinical interview, test administration, scoring, interpretation, and report generation. Hourly fees are set according to national and regional estimates on usual and customary rates for neuropsychological services (Practice Management Information Corporation, 1999). Websites and various publications generated by the National Academy of Neuropsychology (NAN), International Neuropsychological Society (INS), American Psychological Association (APA) Division 40, and the combined work of experts (Puente, 1996, 1998) on the topic of neuropsychology billing and reimbursement have been very helpful in the financial management of the present Neuropsychology Service. In line with recommendations from these respected sources, every attempt is made by the current Neuropsychology Service to adhere to the following principles related to billing for neuropsychological services:

1. Neuropsychologists should only use medical diagnoses.
2. Neuropsychologists should use appropriate Current Procedure Terminology (CPT) codes for billing (American Medical Association, 1998).
3. All neuropsychological services should be billed on an hourly basis.
4. Neuropsychologists should bill for all time devoted to a particular patient.
5. Neuropsychologists should always verify patient benefits before delivering services.

Because assessment accounts for the largest segment of clinical practice, the current Neuropsychology Service most often bills under CPT codes 96117 (Neuropsychological Testing) and 96115 (Neurobehavioral Examination). CPT code 96100 is used when the assessment more closely resembles a psychological evaluation. CPT codes for individual psychotherapy (90804, 90806, 90808) are indicated for intervention-related services, with the specific code dependent upon the length of the therapeutic session. The International Classification of Diseases, Ninth Edition, Clinical Modification, Fifth Edition (ICD-9-CM) is used to reference specific diagnostic codes for billing purposes. Again, medical rather than mental disorder diagnoses are routinely used to bill for neuropsychological services. The National Academy of Neuropsychology Membership Directory also includes an appendix containing helpful references on CPT procedure codes and ICD diagnostic codes commonly used by neuropsychologists.

Market variables and payer mix

Like in any business, familiarity with market factors that affect the rate of reimbursement for services is vital to the financial survival of a hospital-based Neuropsychology Service. In the current age, knowing the extent of managed care penetration within the respective service area is especially critical. The current Neuropsychology Service is fortunate to consult with hospital representatives who are directly responsible for monitoring these variables within the regional market. During the early development of the current Neuropsychology Service, the author relied heavily on the leadership of these experts in establishing provider privileges with various insurance carriers, managed care panels, Medicare, and Medicaid. Information from hospital representatives was also helpful in forecasting gross estimates of reimbursement by these payer groups for neuropsychological services. Figure 5 below illustrates the percentage of reimbursement by various payers for services provided by the current Neuropsychology Service.

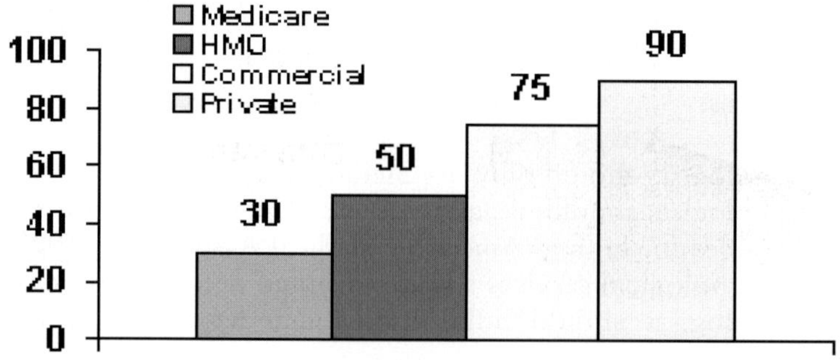

Figure 5. Percentage of reimbursement by payers for neuropsychological services.

Monitoring the mix of payers for neuropsychological services within a hospital-based practice is very informative not only in terms of reflecting reimbursement patterns, but also in identifying the potential need for a shift in nature of clinical practice. The regional market for the current Neuropsychology Service is rather heavily saturated with HMO's and other managed healthcare entities, which will ultimately affect the Neuropsychology Service 'bottom line.' Having a sense of the service area demographics is also beneficial, particularly in estimating the percentage of overall clinical practice that will be devoted to Medicare patients. Knowing the approximate percentage of Medicare patients with a supplemental secondary insurance plan is also informative.

Figure 6 provides a breakdown of the percentage of all neuropsychological services delivered to patients covered by commercial, managed care (HMO), and Medicare/Medicaid benefits, as well as those who pay privately. Comparing the rate of reimbursement by these payer groups (Figure 5) with the percentage of services delivered to patients within each payer group indicates that this is not an ideal mix from a reimbursement standpoint. The large percentage of Medicare patients is due to several variables, including involvement at the on-site dementia clinic and local eldercare facilities, collaboration with various community agencies serving the elderly, exposure coming from dementia research by the Neuropsychology Service, and demographics of the region in which the hospital is located. Additionally, perhaps somewhat distinct from a private practice arrangement, a hospital-based Neuropsychology Service is a bit more inclined to serve patients with all forms of benefit coverage, including commercial, managed care, Medicare, Medicaid, and sometimes even those with no coverage at all. After closely monitoring the payer mix over time, efforts are now being made to increase the volume of referrals within the higher reimbursement categories (e.g., commercial).

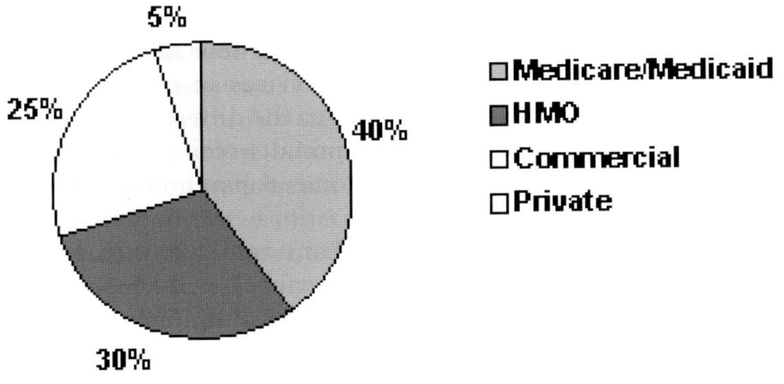

Figure 6. Mix of payers for neuropsychological services.

- *Print marketing efforts*: The Neuropsychology Service has been highlighted in several forums, including Center for Behavioral Health publications, Medical Staff newsletters, hospital media coverage, and correspondence directed to managed care representatives or third party payers.
- *Public speaking*: Neuropsychologists have been invited to delivery medical staff grand rounds, specialty conferences, local seminars, and other lectures which have resulted increased exposure, both within the hospital system and larger metropolitan area.
- *Research Publicity*: Various research projects directed by the Neuropsychology Service have been publicized and enhanced the overall image of the service throughout the hospital and community.
- *Hospitality*: The Neuropsychology Service annually distributes holiday offerings (e.g., fruit baskets, bakery goods, etc.) in appreciation of patient referrals throughout the year. Gestures are personally delivered by the neuropsychologists to referral sources just before the holidays, of which the cost is minimal in comparison to the benefits. An increase in referrals is often the case soon thereafter.

Advantages to a hospital-based neuropsychology practice
The Neuropsychology Service in a general hospital setting benefits from several amenities related directly to clinical service and other aspects of maintaining a professional practice, including:

- Frequent contact with medical staff physicians and referrals sources.
- Inpatient care units and on-site programs with natural links to neuropsychology: physical medicine and rehabilitation, neurology, geriatrics, psychiatry, emergency medicine, radiology, etc.
- Financial/Administrative assistance: Billing service, regional market information, managed care contract negotiations, more natural justification of medical rather than mental health coverage for neuropsychological services, etc.
- Professional practice support: Medical library, malpractice/liability coverage, legal counsel, computerization and information services, institutional review board (IRB) and research committees, grand rounds and other educational programs .

In closing, the author has attempted to identify the key ingredients to the success of the current Neuropsychology Service and the satisfaction of practicing in a general hospital setting. The short list in Table 1 marks those strategies that have been most effective, and which would be implemented first if the author were to, as they say, *do it all over again*.

Table 1. Ten helpful strategies for a Neuropsychology Service in a General Hospital setting.

1.	Establish an identity for Neuropsychology as a unique, valued specialty.
2.	Emphasize a diversified practice model to include outpatient, inpatient, and off-site clinical consultation, as well as elements of research and training.
3.	Stress efficiency throughout the entire practice model by staff neuropsychologists, technicians, and support staff.
4.	Utilize direct physician contact and any form of visibility or exposure (e.g., lectures, correspondence, public relations, etc.) to build a referral base.
5.	Provide competent *and timely* consultation in order to maintain and increase the referral base.
6.	Closely monitor the business side of professional practice, especially reimbursement patterns, market variables, and payer mix.
7.	Attempt to secure additional revenue (e.g., program stipends, research grants) for non-billable services to offset the practice *bottom-line.*
8.	Turn to hospital-based experts for direction (e.g., administrative, financial, public relations, legal, library, technological, etc.) and support.
9.	Establish a working relationship with neuropsychologists in other settings (e.g., academic centers) for consultation on research and professional issues.
10.	Utilize modern technology (e.g., email, computerized databases, computerized reports, internet resources, on-line professional exchange forums, etc.) to enhance practice efficiency and stay connected to the larger field of neuropsychology.

References

American Medical Association (1998). *Physicians' Current Procedural Terminology (CPT) Manual.* Chicago, IL: American Medical Association.

Ball J.D., Archer R.P., Imhof E.A. (1994). Time requirements for psychological testing: A survey of practitioners. *Journal of Personality Assessment, 63*, 239–249.

Chelune G. (1999). Looking ahead to the 21st century. *American Psychological Association , Division of Clinical Neuropsychology Newsletter*, 17(2), 20.

Cripe L.L. (1995). Special Division 40 presentation: Listing of Training Programs in Clinical Neuropsychology — 1995. *The Clinical Neuropsychologist* 9, 327–398.

Dalton J.E. (1995). Time parameters for Neuropsychological Testing. *Wisconsin Psychological Association Newsletter, 19*, 9.

Hannay H.J., Bieliauskas L.A., Crosson B.A., Hammeke T.A., Hamsher K. deS., Koffler S.P. (1998). Proceedings of the Houston Conference on Specialty Education and Training in Clinical Neuropsychology. *Archives of Clinical Neuropsychology, 13.*

International Classification of Diseases, 9 ed., Clinical Modification, 5 ed. (ICD-9-CM), Vol. 1, 2. 1996. Salt Lake City, Utah: PMIC.

National Academy of Neuropsychology (NAN). *1998–99 Membership Directory.* Neuropsychological CPT codes and ICD diagnostic codes commonly used in Neuropsychology, pp. 268–291. Denver: NAN.

New York State Psychological Association (July, 1996). *The Neuropsychological Neurodiagnostic Examination. Statement developed by the New York State Psychological Association's Neuropsychology Division.* NYSPA Notebook.

Practice Management Information Corporation (1999). *Medical Fees in the United States: National Charges for medicine, surgery, laboratory, radiology and allied services* (6th ed.). Los Angeles, CA: PMIC. Document also posted at http://www.medicalbookstore.com.

Puente A.E. (1996). CPT Changes for 1996. Document posted on National Academy of Neuropsychology website at http://nan.drexel.edu.

Puente A.E. (1998). *Reimbursement of Clinical Neuropsychological Services*. Presentation at annual meeting of National Academy of Neuropsychology (NAN), Washington DC.

Putnam S.H., Anderson C. (1994). The second TCN salary survey: A survey of neuropsychologists Part I. *The Clinical Neuropsychologist, 8*, 3–37.

Putnam S.H., DeLuca J.W., Anderson C. (1994). The second TCN survey: A survey of neuropsychologists Part II. *The Clinical Neuropsychologist, 8*, 245–282.

Chapter 16

NEUROPSYCHOLOGICAL PRACTICE IN MEDICAL REHABILITATION

Joseph H. Ricker

About the Author

The author of this chapter, Joseph H. Ricker, Ph.D., ABPP, received his Ph.D. in clinical psychology from Wayne State University in 1992, and completed his internship at the Department of Veterans Affairs Medical Center in Allen Park, Michigan (now the Detroit DVAMC). Subsequently, he completed a combined postdoctoral fellowship in clinical neuropsychology and rehabilitation psychology at the Rehabilitation Institute of Michigan (RIM). Following this fellowship, Dr. Ricker joined the faculty of the department and worked for the next six years as a clinical neuropsychologist at RIM and Wayne State University School of Medicine in Detroit, and is the former Director of Training in the Department of Rehabilitation Psychology and Neuropsychology at RIM.

Since 1999, Dr. Ricker has been the Associate Director of the Neuropsychology Laboratory at the Kessler Medical Rehabilitation Research and Education Corporation in West Orange, New Jersey, and an Associate Professor in the Department of Physical Medicine and Rehabilitation at the University of Medicine and Dentistry of New Jersey. In addition, he maintains a small private practice. He is licensed in the practice of psychology in New Jersey and New York. He is board-certified by the American Board of Professional Psychology in two specialty practice areas: Clinical Neuropsychology and Rehabilitation Psychology.

Introduction

Neuropsychological practice in the context of medical rehabilitation involves the application of psychological principles and procedures (i.e., standardized testing, measurement, structured observation, behavioral intervention, psychotherapy) in the evaluation and treatment of persons with neurologic and /or orthopedic compromise. Neuropsychological services can provide both a unique and necessary component to the evaluation and rehabilitative treatment of the multitude of potential cognitive and emotional compromises following stroke, traumatic brain injury, brain tumor, and other types of central neurologic dysfunction.

Traditional medical tests and examinations provide information on gross anatomic structure and physiology. Because of its psychometric and comprehensive nature, a detailed neuropsychological evaluation can assist in identifying and quantifying the potential functional effects of central neurologic dysfunction. Such deficits include impairments in attention, language, memory, spatial skills, problem-solving, psychomotor abilities, and emotional functioning. This information is critical in the context of medical rehabilitation because, more often than not, the primary diagnosis (e.g., stroke or brain injury) is already known. The unique contribution comes with providing information that will help an individual regain as much independent functioning as possible.

The practice of neuropsychology in rehabilitation hospitals has a relatively long history. The assessment and treatment of cognitive problems is fundamental to rehabilitation medicine, thus the presence of neuropsychologists in such settings is quite logical. Within the American Psychological Association, a special interest group was formed in 1948, which later develop into Division 22 (Rehabilitation Psychology) in 1956. Of note is the fact that the formation of the rehabilitation division actually pre-dates the formation of a clinical neuropsychology division, (Division 40, which became an APA division in 1984). At the time of this writing, the Division of Rehabilitation Psychology has 1,305 members (65% of whom are men).

Training and Credentials

As with other areas of professional psychology, training in clinical or counseling psychology, while not mandatory, will arguably facilitate the process of becoming licensed and gaining hospital appointment in the most expeditious manner. Obviously, psychologists from experimental psychology programs can be licensed and hired, but the nature of neuropsychological practice in medical rehabilitation quite often necessitates intervention skills that are not readily obtained in many types of programs (e.g., physiological psychology or experimental neuropsychology). Formal training and supervision within a medical rehabilitation setting will also facilitate the process, although only a few training programs offer advanced training in both clinical neuropsychology and rehabilitation psychology. Nonetheless, a significant amount of *supervised* experience in a medical rehabilitation context is required before practicing independently, as training only within psychiatric, neurologic, or neurosurgical settings is insufficient for the competent and ethical practice of rehabilitation neuropsychology.

Typically, a clinical neuropsychologist will earn a doctorate and obtain a state license to practice as a psychologist. Of note, however, is the great deal of variability in training and credentials in the practice of neuropsychology in the context of rehabilitation. Since 1947, the American Board of Professional Psychology (ABPP) has been the primary organization that examines and credentials psychological specialists in a manner comparable to medicine (i.e., the American Board of Medical Specialties, or ABMS). The American Board of Clinical Neuropsychology (ABCN), which was incorporated in 1983, is the board of ABPP that develops and administers the examination for the diploma in Clinical Neuropsychology. Attainment of the diploma in Clinical Neuropsychology designates individuals as Clinical Neuropsychologists who have had their credentials thoroughly reviewed, have been subjected to a rigorous examination of their knowledge and practice by their peers, and have been found competent to practice (see Chapter 2). In recognition of the fact that psychological practice within the context of medical rehabilitation constitutes a separate specialty, the American Board of Rehabilitation Psychology was incorporated in 1994, and it is the specialty board of ABPP that is responsible for examinations and credentialing in rehabilitation psychology.

Practice Issues and the Clinical Work Environment

Inpatient neuropsychological practice

In an inpatient rehabilitation setting, the efficient provision of clinical services is critical. This is an important issue not only for patient care (patients and families, having already gone through an acute care hospitalization, do not want an unnecessarily long rehabilitation stay), but also for third party payers. Within inpatient rehabilitation, neuropsychologists are commonly faced with the requirements of the 'three-hour rule.' Essentially, this is a policy of the Health Care Finance Administration (HCFA), stating that if a patient is in an inpatient rehabilitation facility, they must receive one-hour each of physical therapy, occupational therapy, and/or speech-language therapy. Because no aspect of psychological or neuropsychological services is included in this three-hour provision, neuropsychologists and rehabilitation psychologists find themselves competing with other disciplines and consultants for patient time and access, even though they may not be reimbursed for these services.

Extensive neuropsychological testing in the acute care setting immediately following the onset or exacerbation of cerebral impairment may be of minimal or no benefit given the possibility of delirium, post-traumatic amnesia, psychological shock, agitation, anxiety, transient aphasic presentations, or significant motoric compromise. Brief, focused testing (to be followed-up later with a more comprehensive neuropsychological evaluation) can, however, be of benefit in identifying and quantifying residual impairments, as well as in making appropriate recommendations. This is critical for effective rehabilitation programming given the need to determine the individual's functional capacities that are available for compensatory strategies, as well as those areas that may need to be targeted for improvement. Neuropsychological testing can help in formulating plans for community re-integration following cerebral compromise, such as return to work or school. It is also useful in identifying and quantifying areas of improvement, which may be required for certain aspects of re-integration after brain impairment (e.g., re-establishing legal independence following appointment of a guardian). Documentation of improvement is likely to be of comfort to individuals (and to the families of these individuals) who have sustained central neurologic dysfunction. Formal assessment is also useful when formulating individual behavioral management plans, given the fact that such plans rely heavily on an individual's ability to learn and follow directions. Neuropsychological assessment can also, in some instances, be utilized as an index of efficacy for some types of treatment, such as interventions designed to improve or compensate for cognitive impairments (sometimes referred to as cognitive rehabilitation, remediation, or re-training). Neuropsychological testing may also be used to index changes following certain medical interventions (e.g., pharmacotherapy).

Documentation within a medical rehabilitation context is likely to differ from a traditional neuropsychiatric setting. Given the treatment and ongoing assessment orientation of most accredited rehabilitation programs, reports are likely to be briefer, more frequent, and functionally based with recommendations for treatment (rather than simply listing a series of impaired test scores). In addition, greater emphasis may be placed on daily assessment reports and treatment notes. Given the interactive and multidisciplinary nature of medical rehabilitation, it is critical that the neuropsychologist have excellent consultative and interactive skills.

Consultation to the rehabilitation team

In medical rehabilitation, much of the assessment and treatment planning process is multidisciplinary. Findings from evaluations are increasingly described in terms of uniform functional status ratings (e.g., the Functional Independence Measure, or FIM; Hamilton, Granger, Sherwin, Zielzny, & Tashman, 1987), and treatment/discharge plans are frequently presented within a group context (e.g., team rounds or chart rounds).

Within the context of a rehabilitation medicine setting, psychologists may typically be viewed as the primary 'mental health' professionals. This may represent a different relationship when compared to psychiatric settings. In such settings, the psychiatrist is more likely to be seen as the senior mental health professional, and other professionals (e.g., social workers) may be seen as equivalent to psychologists.

For neuropsychologists, however, there may be a different phenomenon in the rehabilitation setting of having to deal with individuals from other allied health professions (e.g., speech–language pathologists) who also assess domains of functioning such as memory, language, problem-solving, and so forth. Furthermore, in some settings, neuropsychologists (along with other professionals, such as speech-language therapists and occupational therapists) provide services focused upon ameliorating acquired cognitive problems. Services may also be provided to assist patients with learning new strategies to compensate for acquired cognitive impairments. These interventions are provided under a variety of names, such as cognitive rehabilitation, neuropsychological rehabilitation, cognitive remediation, and cognitive retraining. These approaches, although in wide use, vary greatly from facility to facility, and have only recently been subject to more rigorous empirical research. Although there are certainly procedures that have demonstrated effectiveness in well-controlled, well-designed, and suitably monitored programs, it is incorrect to assume that anything that is done under the broad rubric of cognitive rehabilitation is thereby also effective. In addition, many activities and procedures that are conducted within the context of rehabilitation may not be uniquely 'rehabilitative' in the most literal sense. For example, training someone to use a personal calendar or planner may certainly increase his or her time management skills, but this is not cognitive rehabilitation per se. When considering a referral for such services (regardless of the discipline that offers the service), it is important to consider the empirical basis for the intervention, the likely improvement in cognition from the passage of time alone, the rationale for the intervention, (e.g., retraining vs. teaching compensatory strategies), the effects of practice, and the qualifications and experience of the provider.

Accurate assessment of cognitive functions becomes difficult with populations who may not have the same level of requisite skills or experiences required to perform adequately on tests. Although there are many available tests and measures, most are normed and standardized on samples of educated, middle-class, Caucasians (e.g., the Boston Diagnostic Aphasia Examination, Boston Naming Test, Ross Information Processing Assessment). Furthermore, there may be a 'clash' between clinicians' values and those of the patient and/or family (e.g., not everyone thinks that reading is important; not everyone values competitive employment).

Although all rehabilitation specialties are unequivocally different disciplines, it is critical that clinicians from all fields make every effort to approach cases from 'the same page,' both conceptually and practically. In other words, it may cause unwarranted confusion and conflict if one discipline views a patient from a strict score-based or numeric 'cut-off' perspective, while another discipline views the same patient in the context of the patient's education, life experience, effort, personal goals, and values. As important as it is for all disciplines to know their professional limits, it is equally important for referral source, professional colleagues, and interdisciplinary teams to also recognize these limits. For example, to a colleague or payer source not familiar with the differences, an occupational therapy or speech-language evaluation of higher cognitive functions and a neuropsychological evaluation might appear very similar. It is critical that each discipline educate consumers as to the unique contributions of each discipline and form of assessment.

Because clinical neuropsychologists are typically trained as clinical psychologists, they are uniquely qualified to formally assess emotional states and to intervene using applied principles of psychology. This is not to say that other rehabilitation professionals have no input into such issues, as their observations may be of great utility in assisting with the formulation of a hypothesis regarding a patient's status, treatment, or outcome. It is within the scope of practice for other rehabilitation professionals to train and counsel patients, family members, educators, employers, and other rehabilitation professionals in adaptive strategies for managing cognitive-communication disorders. Other rehabilitation professionals also must integrate behavior modification treatment techniques as appropriate for the management of associated problems, such as self-abusive and combative behaviors and agitation.

Psychological treatment within the medical rehabilitation setting

Another area for neuropsychological practice might be more accurately classified under the domain of more traditional rehabilitation psychology. Although rehabilitation psychology is arguably a distinct discipline (that is, in many senses, separate from clinical neuropsychology), there are many practitioners who are appropriately trained and can competently practice within both disciplines. For such individuals, the rehabilitation environment provides a very rich and rewarding opportunity to integrate clinical neuropsychology and rehabilitation psychology activities.

Even as an outside consultant to a rehabilitation team, a neuropsychologist can provide an informative perspective. This may be especially true in the context of a rehabilitation setting that is accustomed to patients without prominent cognitive impairment (e.g., a spinal cord injury or orthopedic setting). In terms of assessment, many events that can lead to other medical rehabilitation conditions (e.g., spinal cord injury, complicated fractures), may also result in traumatic brain injury (e.g., motor vehicle accidents, assaults, and falls). Although moderate and severe TBI are not likely to be 'overlooked' clinically, co-existing mild or mild-to-moderate TBI may be missed upon initial examination of the SCI patient in the acute trauma setting (Ricker & Regan, 1999).

Treating the patient with cognitive compromise may pose special challenges for rehabilitation professionals who are accustomed to working primarily with patients who have sustained non-brain injuries or illnesses. Although the acute rehabilitation process for any individual can be stressful to a patient, family, and team members, the rehabilitation process for someone with multiple conditions (e.g., a spinal cord injury and brain injury) is multiply compounded. For instance, many aspects of medical rehabilitation involve educating patients about self-care procedures (e.g., medication regimen training, bowel training, bladder management, transfers). The team's approach to education and training may have to be modified for the patient who presents with significant cognitive symptoms. Such patients may exhibit multiple difficulties in advancing through the rehabilitation program, including difficulties retaining new information over time, sequencing information during multi-step tasks, making judgments about safety, problem solving in novel situations, and initiating self-care behavior. Thus, neuropsychologists can favorably impact patient care by assisting in the modification of the actual treatment program. For instance, the team may need to emphasize caregiver training more heavily than patient training, at least initially. Patient training may also need to be approached using simple and concrete communication. In addition, the patient with cognitive inefficiencies may become 'overloaded' with new information more easily than non-brain-compromised rehabilitation patients.

Even in the context of an injury or illness that clearly involves the brain, rehabilitation teams may still require significant input from the neuropsychologist. Brain injury is by any definition a catastrophic and life-changing event. Immediately after the injury, medical practitioners and family are often most concerned with the patient's acute medical condition and chances of survival. When the patient's survival appears likely, the patient and family often become more aware of and focused on issues of functional loss. A grieving process often begins during the acute medical stage and continues through the rehabilitation process and beyond. In the case of a patient with TBI, emotional adjustment may take a somewhat different course as compared to non-neurologic rehabilitation populations. Accurate assessment of emotional functioning requires that the patient demonstrate some degree of insight and awareness regarding their recent experiences and their emotional functioning. Unfortunately, patients who sustain significant TBI often experience deficits in these areas. Thus, patients may be truly unaware of their situation and may lack many common symptoms of grief and adjustment. Indeed, these patients may report little or no emotional reaction or changes in functioning. This type of presentation may be misinterpreted by staff as representing a purely psychological process such as denial. As the patient recovers from acute brain injury and self-awareness improves, the patient may develop 'delayed' emotional symptoms or behavior problems that were not present or apparent more proximal to the onset of their injuries.

In contrast to the patient who presents with a lack of emotional symptoms, patients with significant TBI may alternatively present with notable emotional symptoms and personality change secondary to the brain trauma itself. These patients may exhibit a variety of symptoms including increased irritability, impatience, agitation, and fatigue, as well as decreased frustration tolerance and motivation. These symptoms may be misinterpreted by staff as either maladaptive psychological reactions to catastrophic injury or simply as the presentation of a 'noncompliant' patient. Staff who are either unaware of the presence of brain trauma in the patient, or who are not accustomed to working with TBI patients, may become easily frustrated with the level of attention, encouragement, and structure required by these patients in combination with their apparent noncompliance with aspects of the rehabilitation program. Behavioral approaches with patients and staff can often help in these situations.

An accurate understanding, therefore, of the patient's initial presentation in inpatient rehabilitation, including an understanding of the extent to which brain trauma has occurred, can greatly assist staff in understanding aspects of the patient's emotional presentation and in addressing issues related to the course of adjustment. This understanding will also assist members of the rehabilitation team in interpreting and monitoring their own emotional reactions to the patient.

Outpatient neuropsychological practice in medical rehabilitation

Given the nature of training and practice of clinical neuropsychology in the United States (i.e., large batteries of psychometric tests), neuropsychologists involved in rehabilitation may find it easier to practice 'traditional' neuropsychology in an outpatient setting. Of note, however, is the fact that such batteries and approaches were developed irrespectively of known or suspected diagnosis, and were not developed within the context of the needs of contemporary medical rehabilitation. In fact, batteries that are heavily dependent upon sensorimotor input and output functions may be of little incremental utility with many neurorehabilitation populations (Rosenthal & Ricker, 2000). In addition, it is important to note that normative databases are rarely equivalent, and are virtually never identical. For example, one group used to norm one particular test may differ dramatically and in clinically meaningful ways from the normative group used for another test. In clinical psychology and neuropsychology, an excellent example is the Wechsler Adult Intelligence Scale-Revised (WAIS-R). The WAIS-R and the WAIS-III are well standardized in the sense of having large normative databases across age ranges. Beyond the Wechsler scales, however, there is not additional cognitive test data obtained from the original standardization sample. In other words, we know how the standardization sample performs on the WAIS-R or WAIS-III, but we have no idea how these individuals perform in other cognitive domains or on other neuropsychological tests. Clinically, however, psychologists routinely use the WAIS-R/III IQ scores as a 'baseline' for comparison, and then proceed to compare additional tests to these scores as if all scores were comparable.

Furthermore, as the population ages and the number of individuals who experience some period of disability in their lives increases, it will be critical to develop tests and normative data that take normal aging into account. Having said this, however, it should be noted that most practicing neuropsychologists do not utilize a rigid fixed-battery approach (Sweet, Moberg, & Suchy, 2000; see also Chapter 3).

It is clear that neuropsychologists can provide useful information to patients and other professionals. First, clinical neuropsychologists can provide neuropsychometric assessment. This refers to the use of various tests and measures designed to allow for inferences about brain-behavior relationships. This type of data can provide information about a client's cognitive functioning and psychosocial issues. A formal neuropsychological evaluation can provide patients and health-care providers with estimates of a client's abilities across many areas of neurocognitive functioning including attention, language, memory, visuospatial abilities, planning, problem-solving, and emotional status. Comprehensive neuropsychological evaluations may also allow for predictions to be made regarding a client's cognitive capacity to return to work, and about the client's motivation to do so. Clinical neuropsychologists can also assist in estimating a client's actual pre-injury or pre-illness level of functioning or adaptation. Because most clinical neuropsychologists are trained not only in brain-behavior relationships but also in clinical or counseling psychology, they are also able to take into account factors other than a primary brain injury that may contribute to abnormal neuropsychological test findings. Such factors can include emotional disruption, age, premorbid psychiatric history, substance abuse, learning disability, decreased motivation, or secondary gain.

In addition, although many clinical neuropsychologists focus primarily or exclusively on neuropsychometric assessment, many provide direct intervention in the form of behavior management, client education, psychotherapy, or guidance in vocational pursuits. Community re-integration may be cognitively difficult and emotionally stressful for clients, and short-term psychological interventions can be quite useful in facilitating adaptive functioning.

Within the context of outpatient rehabilitation, a major focus of neuropsychological practice for the majority of adults is vocational re-integration. Clinical neuropsychologists may provide consultation to vocational counselors, employers, and state vocational rehabilitation services (referred to as job commissions in some states). This is particularly important in light of the Americans with Disabilities Act of 1990, which, among many things, emphasizes accommodations that can assist individuals with successful return to work. Clinical neuropsychologists can be of great utility in assisting institutions and organizations in fulfilling the spirit and letter of this legislation.

Finally, rehabilitative neuropsychological evaluation has also become of increased importance in the forensic arena, where the opinions of neuropsychologists are often utilized in the determination of causality (although this is restricted to physicians in some states), damages, and potential for recovery in litigated head injury cases. Neuropsychologists who practice in rehabilitation settings may also find themselves more frequently involved with litigated cases, particularly in states where health-care reimbursement involves 'no-fault' or other frequently litigious insurance circumstances. In addition, given an unfortunate but nonetheless real history of fraud and abuse in rehabilitation, particularly within the context of traumatic brain injury rehabilitation (Cope, 1995; Ricker, 1998), it is no surprise that third party payers are more carefully scrutinizing what occurs under the broad rubric of 'rehabilitation.'

Psychotherapy in neurorehabilitation

As indicated earlier, an evaluation to assess for the cognitive and emotional impact of brain trauma is often an important early step in the rehabilitation process. When the neurocognitive sequelae result in significantly decreased self-awareness, the types of psychological supports and interventions typically offered to patients and their families may need to be modified. First, traditional insight-oriented therapy approaches may be hampered by the presence of cognitive deficits in the patient's presentation. Such approaches generally depend upon the patient's ability to understand, at least on a basic level, their recent experience and their current situation, to use abilities such as insight and awareness to monitor their own reaction and communicate their reaction to others, and to use abstraction to think about how their current situation may affect their future. Indeed, the patient's ability to monitor and communicate about their internal states is key to many psychotherapeutic approaches to grief and adjustment counseling. As a result, intervention strategies that rely heavily on behavioral strategies and family participation may be most useful in many (if not most) cases of significant brain injury or illness.

Second, the course of emotional symptoms and adjustment reactions in the patient with cerebral compromise can take a different course. As indicated earlier, a patient with significant brain injury may present initially with emotional symptoms secondary to brain trauma itself, and only later, as they recover some degree of self-awareness, present with emotional symptoms secondary to a sense of loss. As a result, treatment approaches for emotional symptoms in these patients will often differ at various times in the process of their recovery. The patient who presents acutely with emotional and behavioral symptoms of brain trauma, may benefit from a quiet, structured, and consistent environment; whereas, the patient who has recovered some level of self-awareness and begins to verbalize feelings of loss may increasingly benefit from more traditional psychotherapeutic approaches.

A third issue related to the psychological treatment of the brain-injured patient is the fact that patients must deal with loss regarding not only cognitive functions, but also psychosocial functions. The patient's physical trauma and immediate cognitive losses are often the initial focus of grief for both the patient and family. As the patient is encouraged to become increasingly independent on the rehabilitation unit and in the community after discharge, the presence of emotional and personality changes may become increasingly apparent. Intervention aimed at assisting the patient and family to cope with loss must attend, not only to the loss of cognitive function, but also to reports that the patient has somehow 'changed.'

Coding and billing practices

Billing practices will vary across facilities. For facilities where all allied health services are 'bundled' (i.e., figured into the per diem), issues related to billing and productivity may be seen as more administrative rather than fiscal per se. In settings where psychologists contract for services or directly bill payers, however, the situation is quite different. Psychologists in general, and perhaps neuropsychologists in particular, are facing many changes in reimbursement for clinical services. Following the passage of the Balanced Budget Act of 1997 (Public Law 105-33), this becomes especially relevant in the case of Medicare billing and 'incident to' procedures. Essentially, the Health Care Finance Administration (HCFA) has determined that services that are 'incident to' those of the primary health care provider (i.e., the services of technicians) are to be considered part of the hospital per diem and not billable as independent services. In traditional medical settings, these services include routine tests (e.g., blood work). Within the context of rehabilitation neuropsychology, services such as test administration by psychometricians, interns, or postdoctoral residents might be interpreted as being subject to the 'incident to' regulations. Although many routine medical technical services are indeed already paid for by virtue of being included under Medicare Part A, comparable psychometric services are not. Nonetheless, a strict interpretation of the regulation suggests that only services directly provided by the licensed psychologist can be billed under Medicare Part B.

In medical rehabilitation, neuropsychologists are likely to bill under a variety of procedure codes. This is partially a function of the distribution of codes that psychologists can use (i.e., psychologists can utilize CPT codes found under psychiatry, neurology, and physical medicine and rehabilitation), but it is also due to the fact that neuropsychologists in rehabilitation settings are often likely to provide assessment, treatment, and many other services. Most neuropsychological testing in rehabilitation settings can be billed under CPT code 96117 ("Neuropsychological Testing"), although brief or bedside testing may be more accurately billed under 96115 ("Neurobehavioral Status Exam"). Neuropsychologists who provide cognitive rehabilitation services to patients may also bill under 97770 ("Development of Cognitive Skills," under physical medicine and rehabilitation). Although it may seem obvious, it is important that the type of diagnosis and CPT codes for the services provided are consistent. For example, if the presenting diagnosis is psychiatric, then the clinician is advised to use psychiatric CPT codes. Likewise, neurologic codes should be used for neurologic diagnoses. This can help ensure that patients will be approved for appropriate services, and also increases the probability that clinicians will be reimbursed for services.

Recently, there has been concern about the Prospective Payment System (PPS). PPS was introduced in the Balanced Budget Act of 1997 as the result of increased post-acute expenditures affecting Medicare. (Note: PPS is to be fully implemented by January 1, 2001). Currently, many payments are made on a cost-basis. In other words, reimbursement is based upon the cost of services (although this is, if course, no guarantee of full reimbursement). Under PPS, patients who are referred for post-acute (i.e., rehabilitation or skilled nursing) services will undergo an admission examination and will be classified into a Functionally Related Group (FRG) established by Medicare. The amount of payment for services will then be based *a priori* on the FRG in which the patient is classified. Thus, reimbursement is not based on what services are provided, but rather is determined prior to service delivery (hence the "prospective" component of PPS).

Future of neuropsychological practice in rehabilitation

Even with greater external constraints being placed on rehabilitation practice, there may be greater numbers of patients that are referred for services. Recent publications suggest the effectiveness of some physical (e.g., constraint induced therapy; Van der Lee et al., 1999) and cognitive (Cicerone et al., 2000) interventions. As empirical support grows for medical rehabilitation, third party payers may be more inclined to approve longer stays — or to approve referral to comprehensive rehabilitation services in the first place.

A recent NIH Consensus Conference (NIH, 1998) also heavily emphasizes the beneficial role that psychologists and neuropsychologists can play in the assessment and rehabilitation of survivors of brain injury. Such influential support will benefit the 'front-line' practitioner.

None of this is meant to imply that the practice of neuropsychology will flourish unfettered, however. Recent research also suggests that rehabilitation services can have the greatest impact on functional outcomes when they are implemented early. The effect of this is that patients are admitted to rehabilitation settings much earlier than in previous years. Thus, the nature of the neuropsychological services that can — and should — be provided is likely to become increasingly different. The provision of multi-hour standardized testing batteries are more likely to be reserved as an outpatient service, with cognitive screening and behavioral management being the focus of inpatient assessment and intervention.

Conclusions

As with all practice environments for neuropsychologists, the medical rehabilitation setting presents many challenges and rewards. The capacity for neuropsychologists to interact directly and regularly with multiple health-care professionals is, although not unique, almost a cardinal feature of rehabilitation neuropsychology. As advances have occurred in acute medical interventions (e.g.;, improvements in managing acute intracranial pressure in brain injury, or early pharmacologic interventions following stroke) rehabilitation neuropsychology has seen an increase in the number of patients, but has also had to look for ways to continue to make contributions in the face of a very different health-care reimbursement market. A large percentage of one's patients will demonstrate improvement and make meaningful re-integration into their communities. The information that the neuropsychologist can communicate, and the interventions that neuropsychologists can provide, play important or even critical roles in this process.

References

Cicerone, K.D., Dahlberg , C., Kalmar, K. Langenbahn, D.M., Malec, J.F., Bergquist, T.F., Felicetti, T., Giacino, J.T., Harley, J.P., Harrington, D.E., Herzog, J., Kneipp, S., Laatsch, L., & Morse, P.A. (2000). Evidence-based cognitive rehabilitation: Recommendations for clinical practice. *Archives of Physical Medicine and Rehabilitation, 81*, 1596–1615.

Cope, D.N. (1995). The effectiveness of traumatic brain injury rehabilitation: A review. *Brain Injury, 9*, 649–670.

Hamilton, B.B., Granger, C.V., Sherwin, F.S., Zielzny, M., & Tashman, J.S. (1987). A uniform national data system for medical rehabilitation. In M. Fuhrer (Ed.) *Rehabilitation outcome analysis and measurement.* Baltimore: Paul Brookes.

National Institutes of Health (1998). Rehabilitation of persons with traumatic brain injury. *NIH Consensus Statement.* Oct. 26–28; *16(1)*, 1–41.

Ricker, J.H. (1998). Traumatic brain injury rehabilitation: Is it worth the cost? *Applied Neuropsychology, 5(4)*, 137–147.

Ricker, J.H., & Regan, T. (1999). Neuropsychological and psychological factors in the rehabilitation of individuals with both spinal cord injury and traumatic brain injury. *Topics in Spinal Cord Injury Rehabilitation, 5(2)*, 76–82.

Rosenthal, M., & Ricker, J.H. (2000). Traumatic brain injury 3. In R. Frank & T. Eliott (Eds.), *Handbook of rehabilitation psychology* (pp. 49–74). Washington, D.C.: American Psychological Association.

Sweet, J.J., Moberg, P.J., & Suchy, Y. (2000). Ten-year follow-up survey of clinical neuropsychologists. *The Clinical Neuropsychologist, 4*, 479–495.

Van der Lee, J.H., Wagenaar, R.C., Lankhorst, G.J., Vogelaar T.W., Deville, W.L., & Bouter, L.M. (1999). Forced use of the upper extremity in chronic stroke patients: Results from a single-blind randomized clinical trial. *Stroke, 30*, 2369–2375.

Chapter 17

NEUROPSYCHOLOGICAL PRACTICE IN RURAL AND SMALL COMMUNITIES: AN APPALACHIAN PERSPECTIVE

Kristie J. Nies and Bernice A. Marcopulos

Introduction

There is a dearth of literature on neuropsychology in rural areas. With the exception of two articles on service delivery (Peake, McClain, Wilson, & Orrell, 1992; Troster, Paolo, Glatt, Hubble, & Koller, 1995) and several articles on illiteracy and aphasia (Lecours et al., 1987; Lecours et al., 1988) discussion of practice issues relative to neuropsychology is non-existent. The presence of psychology in rural areas is largely due to the efforts of the community mental health movement and much of the information regarding the provision of neuropsychological services for this chapter is drawn from the mental health literature. Ironically, it is this very issue that complicates provision of neuropsychological services to medical populations. Psychologists are typically viewed as mental health providers. The diagnostic and procedure codes used by neuropsychologists, however, are often medical in nature. This discrepancy between type of provider and type of service can result in confusion, wasted time, and ultimately unpaid claims. It appears that the theoretical push for integration between medical care and mental health care has clearly outpaced the understanding of third party payers of the role of the neuropsychologist.

To begin, the term rural is not easily or simply defined. Jordan and Hargrove (1987) stressed the difficulty of operationalizing the term 'rural' for behavioral and social sciences research and policy development for health services. Traditionally, rural areas have been defined by population density, percentage of farmers, and degree of isolation. In recent years, however, rural areas have become less homogeneous because of a decline in farming and an increase in technology. The most common classifications currently used to define geographical areas are urban/rural and metropolitan/non-metropolitan. Urban/rural is the terminology employed by the Bureau of Census and refers to population density. Rural populations have fewer than 2,500 inhabitants. Approximately one-fourth of the U.S. population lives in rural areas with more people living in rural areas in the South and the Midwest. Metropolitan/non-metropolitan terminology is employed by the Office of Management and Budget (1975) and is based on Metropolitan Statistical Areas (MSAs). MSAs have a total population of at least 100,000 (75,000 in New England), comprise one or more central cities with at least 50,000 inhabitants, and include adjoining areas that are socially and economically related to the central city (U.S. Bureau of Census, 1978 as cited in Murray and Keller, 1991). Both definitions are considered arbitrary and unsatisfactory (Murray & Keller, 1991).

Rural Americans are a heterogeneous group with diversity in cultures, occupations, income, and lifestyle. Referring to the group as a whole or by using the terms rural and small community synonymously is in no way meant to diminish this diversity and the distinction between subcultures will be highlighted when clinically relevant. For the purposes of this chapter, 'rural' is defined in terms of low population density and degree of isolation. The rural population is generally poor, elderly, experiences poor health, has a low level of formal education, few white collar occupations, a small percentage of both men and women participating in the labor force, and includes elderly migrant workers and farmers (Murray & Keller, 1991). The underserved populations in rural areas, relative to neuropsychology, include those patients with developmental disabilities, traumatic brain injury, stroke and other neurological illness, dementia, substance abuse, and psychiatric disturbance. From a professional standpoint, the clinical neuropsychologist in rural areas, like his or her clients, may have diminished access to large, university medical centers with the latest medical technologies and clinical drug trials and they may lack ancillary clinical resources (e.g., brain injury support groups, residential treatment, respite care). Pragmatically, it also means that because some of these resources are unavailable, potential clients and referral sources may be unaware of the services that a neuropsychologist can provide.

This chapter will focus on the experiences of the authors in a four state area (e.g., West Virginia, Virginia, Kentucky, Tennessee) of the Appalachian region of the United States which strictly defined includes all of West Virginia and parts of 12 other eastern, Midwestern and southern states: New York, Pennsylvania, Maryland, Ohio, North Carolina, South Carolina, Georgia,

Tennessee, Kentucky, and Alabama, Virginia, and Mississippi. Included are descriptions of two rural neuropsychology practices; a review of some of the research relevant to health care, including epidemiology in rural areas; and some of the literature relevant to an Appalachian perspective. The goal is to challenge the reader to reexamine beliefs regarding brain behavior relationships, within the context of a diverse sociocultural atmosphere, and to understand these beliefs as they affect the clinical, as well as professional, practice of neuropsychology.

About the Authors

Dr. Nies

Dr. Nies obtained a Bachelor's Degree with high honors in Psychology and Art Education from Michigan State University. She completed a Ph.D. in Clinical Psychology, with a specialization in Neuropsychology, at Finch University of Health Sciences/The Chicago Medical School. During her internship, which was completed at the West Haven VA in Connecticut, she was able to obtain training in both Neuropsychology and Geropsychology. She completed her postdoctoral fellowship in Clinical Neuropsychology at Evanston Hospital in accordance with the Midwest Consortium of Postdoctoral Programs in Clinical Neuropsychology, which was the predecessor and founding force for the Association of Postdoctoral Programs in Clinical Neuropsychology (APPCN). She received a Diplomate in Clinical Neuropsychology from the American Board of Professional Psychology in 2000. She currently co-owns a Limited License Corporation with three other psychologists who maintain general psychotherapy and assessment practices.

Dr. Nies has adjunct staff privileges at two acute care hospitals, a rehabilitation hospital, and a psychiatric facility. Additional professional duties include serving as the Chairperson for the Behavioral Health Committee for the local Independent Practice Association (IPA) and serving on the Complimentary and Alternative Medicine task force for a local hospital. She has served on the oral examination committee and the ethics committee for the Tennessee Psychological Association and she is the Past President of the InterMountain Psychological Association. Dr. Nies is a Clinical Assistant Professor in the Department of Psychiatry and Behavioral Sciences at East Tennessee State University James H. Quillen College of Medicine.

Dr. Marcopulos

Dr. Marcopulos attended the University of Florida as an undergraduate and she received a B.A. in Psychology with high honors, with an emphasis on physiological psychology. Her work on her senior thesis (animal models of Parkinson's Disease) led her to pursue the study of brain-behavior relationships in humans at the graduate level. She obtained her Ph.D. in clinical neuropsychology from the University of Victoria, British Columbia, Canada.

She further specialized in geriatrics on her internship at the Philadelphia Geriatric Center and during her postdoctoral experience at the Palo Alto VAMC at the Older Adult and Family Resource and Research Center. She received a Diplomate in Clinical Neuropsychology from the American Board of Professional Psychology in 1995. Dr. Marcopulos' current position is directing the Neuropsychology Laboratory at Western State Hospital, a state funded psychiatric hospital affiliated with the University of Virginia, where she holds a clinical faculty appointment in the Department of Psychiatric Medicine and the Southeastern Rural Mental Health Research Center. She also teaches graduate assessment as an Adjunct Professor in the Psychology Department at the University of Virginia and has a part-time private practice in Staunton, Virginia. A particular research interest for her is how education and culture affect performance on traditional neuropsychological instruments.

Description of Practice

The authors have general geographical location and the diversity of people served in common. While their practices are technically in urban areas, they evaluate and treat patients who live in rural areas in Virginia, West Virginia, Kentucky, and Tennessee.

Dr. Nies

Dr. Nies' private practice is in Kingsport, Tennessee, which is in the northeast corner of the state 275 miles from Nashville. Kingsport is part of the Tri-Cities Region that includes 13 counties and 43 municipalities. The population in Kingsport proper is 41,545. The population within a five-mile radius of the city is 134,892. The population of the Tri-Cities MSA is 464,900. The largest manufacturing employers include Eastman Chemical Company and Quebecor Printing Book Group. The largest non-manufacturing employers include Wellmont Health System and the county school system. Thirty-seven per cent of the residents of Kingsport are over the age of 50 (Kingsport Area Chamber of Commerce, 1998).

Psychological Consultants, LLC, leases office space that contains 5 offices, a conference room, a reception area, secretarial; space, and a break room. Dr. Nies shares the cost of a technician (i.e., a Master's level, state licensed Psychological Examiner), including health and life insurance, with one other psychologist. Each psychologist purchases his or her own test forms and equipment although a very collaborative arrangement exists with regard to test usage. The primary referral sources for Dr. Nies' practice consist of local neurology, neurosurgery, trauma, physiatry, and psychiatry practices. Other referral sources include attorneys, insurance companies, pediatricians/family practitioners, and other psychologists. Exposure, via professional activities (e.g., attendance at hospital conferences), remains the primary 'marketing' tool, although formal contacts (e.g., lunches, brochures, etc.) have been used as well. Advertising, of a sort, has also occurred through announcements about her and her practice, which have appeared in the local newspaper, hospital newsletters, and through appearances on local television news programs. Dr. Nies has worked with the Stroke Center and the Oncology Service by way of newsletter articles and a patient education video, respectively.

Dr. Nies schedules 3–4 neuropsychological evaluations and 25–30 psychotherapy/feedback hours per week. The remainder of her time is spent completing hospital consults (ranges from 0 to 3 hours per week).

Dr. Nies uses a technician for all cases seen in the office. The test battery is flexible (i.e., varies depending on the referral question, age of the patient, and insurance status), but is generally completed in six to ten hours inclusive of interview, scoring, record review, and report writing. Several insurance companies require pre-authorization (including a list of planned tests) and many have restrictions regarding the number of hours that will be authorized. Symptom validity tests are used for most clinical cases and all forensic cases. Hospital consults are completed in 1–2 hours and generally result in a recommendation for additional evaluation. In general, reports are completed within one week. If a report is going to be delayed, a summary letter is sent within two to three days of the evaluation or by the time the patient is seen by the referral source.

Attorney referred cases are considered forensic and require pre-payment at a flat rate. The patient's health insurance company is not billed for these types of cases. Additional time spent on the case (i.e., preparation, deposition, record review, etc.) is billed at an hourly rate. Fees for evaluations, depositions, trials, or meetings, are due one week in advance and are non-refundable. Independent Medical Evaluations and Impairment Ratings are also billed at a flat rate and fees are due one week in advance.

An office manager and one full-time secretary manage the office. They are responsible for the day-to-day operations of answering the telephone, scheduling patients, managing accounts receivable and payable, and verifying insurance, as well as billing/collections. The only outside services employed are those of an accountant (and the lawyer who set up the LLC). Practice members are invoiced bi-monthly for rent, advertising, insurance (medical, malpractice, liability), office supplies, and utilities. This 'overhead' is approximately 30% of collections. Membership dues, journal subscriptions, books, pager, cell phone, supplies, test equipment/forms, disability insurance, and Continuing Education expenses are not included in the office overhead, but, rather are paid by each psychologist independent of the practice. Each member is responsible for paying their own quarterly taxes and funding their own retirements. In total, overhead runs about 45-50%. (It should be noted, however, that using this type of calculation is somewhat deceptive. Some costs are fixed and the overhead percentage, at any one time, varies depending on collections.)

Dr. Nies submits billing information, (i.e. CPT and ICD/DSM codes, number of hours involved), to the office staff for preparation of Health Care

Finance Administration (HCFA) forms or other billing statements (e.g., in the case of attorneys). Forms are expected to be sent out within 72 hours of provision of service. Pro bono cases are seen, but on a limited basis.

Dr. Nies is a provider for most managed care companies that operate in the area. Reimbursement for CPT code 96117 varies among carriers from $44.00 to $77.00. While it is obviously not cost effective to provide services at the $44.00 an hour rate, disenrolling from this particular provider panel would result in disenrollment as a provider from a panel with a favorable fee schedule. Traditional indemnity plans cover 80% to 100% of fees depending on the contract. Reimbursement by Worker's compensation varies by state and fee schedule but, contrary to popular belief, is not always 100%.

Dr. Marcopulos

Dr. Marcopulos works in Staunton, Virginia. Staunton is a small metropolitan area in central Virginia, about 150 miles southwest of Washington, DC, in the Shenandoah Valley, between the Blue Ridge and Allegheny Mountain ranges. Staunton has a population of 24,461 and it is the county seat of Augusta County, which has a population of approximately 55,000. Almost 80% of the residents live in rural areas according to the 1990 U.S. census data. The primary industry is agriculture, with Augusta County ranking second in agricultural sales in Virginia. The state of Virginia has 18.8% African American, 0.2% Native American, 2.6% Asian and 2.6% Hispanic populations. Augusta County and the greater Shenandoah Valley area have far fewer minorities (4.1% non-white) than the state's average and the population consists mostly of white Americans of German, Irish and Scottish descent.

Dr. Marcopulos directs the Neuropsychology Laboratory at Western State Hospital in Staunton, Virginia. Western State Hospital (WSH) is a 350 bed adult psychiatric facility serving clients from central and northern Virginia. The patients served tend to be indigent and from rural areas around central Virginia. The hospital has a wide catchment area and serves Virginia minorities with an average of 20% African American, 2% Hispanic, 0.5% Asian, and 0.2% Native American in-patients in a given month. The hospital catchment area also includes Northern Virginia and urban areas around Washington, DC, but the majority of patients are from rural areas. WSH is affiliated with the University of Virginia School of Medicine, Department of Psychiatric Medicine and it serves as a teaching hospital for medical students, nurses, occupational, physical and speech therapists, psychology graduate students, occupational, physical and speech therapy students, residents and post-doctoral fellows, and psychiatry and neurology residents.

The Neuropsychology Lab is part of the Division of Behavioral Medicine at WSH, which includes Speech Pathology, and Audiology services and is housed in the medical unit building where patients go to other specialty clinics such as neurology, ophthalmology, Podiatry, Dentistry, x-ray, etc. Personnel in the Neuropsychology Lab include one board certified clinical neuropsychologist who holds an appointment of Assistant Professor of Clinical Psychiatric Medicine at the University of Virginia School of Medicine, a post-doctoral fellow in Neuropsychology and predoctoral Clinical Psychology resident or graduate student from the University of Virginia, one full-time Neuropsychology test technician and an executive secretary. The executive secretary does all the scheduling of patients. The test technician and executive secretary do the cost accounting. Patients are not billed directly and cost of the neuropsychological testing is figured into the per diem cost. Most of the patients do not have private insurance.

The typical number of patients seen per week ranges from three to seven. Most referrals come from the five admission wards (three co-ed, one forensic, one geriatric) for diagnostic evaluations, which typically include personality testing. These referrals have the highest priority and are seen within one week of receiving the referral, depending on whether the patient has stabilized enough for testing. Oral or written feedback on preliminary test results are given within 48 hours via phone call, e-mail, or chart note, with the formal written report being completed in seven to ten days. Other referrals come from the extended care wards or specialty programs for deaf, mentally retarded, or substance abusing clients. These evaluations tend to focus more on psychosocial rehabilitative and community re-entry issues, such as eligibility for disability, recommendations for educational or vocational programs or placement in the cognitive remediation program for persistent cognitive deficits in severe mental illness. Severe mental illnesses such as schizophrenia and major depression are commonly accompanied by cognitive deficits, which need to be documented and incorporated into the treatment plans.

Many patients who are referred have a history of head injury, CVA, epilepsy, Huntington's disease, suspected dementia or other neurological illness. The referral question is often phrased: "To what extent do these neurobehavioral syndromes impact on the manifestation of their psychiatric illness? Are there modifications that must be made in the treatment plan to compensate for the cognitive deficits that might accompany these neurological problems? Are there cognitive interventions that may be appropriate?" There are cognitive therapies available in the psychosocial rehabilitation program including cognitive rehabilitation and memory training, which is directed by the neuropsychologist. Dementia work-ups, including a neurology consult and neuropsychological testing, are conducted on all patients entering the geriatric admissions ward. The Neuropsychology Lab has a close working relationship with the Neurology Department at the University of Virginia, which runs a dementia clinic at the hospital once per month. A 'flexible battery' approach is used, but there are established batteries for dementia and patients in the mentally ill/ chemically addicted unit. Tests of malingering are used for patients from the forensic unit who are being evaluated for competency to stand trial or mental status at time of offense. Also, tests of symptom validity are used when testing is for disability secondary to cognitive impairment.

Dr. Marcopulos also works part-time (one or two weekends per month) doing outpatient adult neuropsychological assessment in a group private practice also located in Staunton, VA. This group practice consists of five licensed clinical psychologists, including two board-certified neuropsychologists and one board certified forensic psychologist, a licensed professional counselor, a substance abuse counselor, and four licensed clinical social workers. Dr. Marcopulos sometimes uses a technician and pays her directly at an hourly rate. She pays overhead to the practice for each assessment for space rental, an answering service, transcription service, and a medical billing service. Referrals come primarily from primary care physicians and neurologists for evaluation of suspected dementia, closed head injury and other neurological illnesses. Dr. Marcopulos also receives referrals from attorneys in criminal cases, especially those charged with capital murder. Virginia has the death penalty so neuropsychological testing is often requested as part of the presentencing report for mitigation.

In Dr. Marcopulos's area there are several large managed care organizations (MCOs) providing mental health insurance coverage. MCO's account for 40% of the health insurance for the area and continues to grow at a rapid rate. The largest MCOs in central Virginia for mental health are Sentara (serves all state government employees), Greenspring, Value Behavioral Health, and Merit Behavioral Care. The practice contracts with a medical billing service to collect fees. When a referral is made to the practice, the patient is first directed to talk with the medical billing service to determine whether insurance covers testing, make sure pre-approval has been obtained, set the co-pay, get the proper referral, etc; Clients are expected to pay their insurance co-pay at the time services are rendered. After testing is completed, the billing service submits a bill to their insurance carrier. Reimbursement rates vary from 50% (Medicare) to 100% (some worker's compensation).

Practice Issues for Rural Settings

Epidemiology

There is possibly a greater need for psychological services in rural areas than urban areas as residents in these areas tend to be poorer, older, and have more medical problems than their urban peers (Human & Wasem, 1991). Children in rural communities are particularly affected by lack of special education resources; while women, children, and the elderly are affected by the lack of mental health and social service resources (Hargrove & Breazeale, 1993; Foxhall, 2000). Despite this greater documented need, there are fewer services available. This lack of resources is attributed, in part, to the 'farm crisis'. While the rural population generally has remained steady, the farm population has shown a consistent decline and persistent economic problems. Hargrove (1989) highlighted the cascade of events that followed the farm crisis: loss of jobs, an exodus of young people, a weakened tax base, and loss of financial support for health and human services.

Rural occupations may pose more health risks than urban occupations. There are very few neuroepidemiological studies of rural populations, with the exception of dementia (Brayne & Calloway, 1989). Most epidemiological studies have focused on general psychiatric conditions, rather than conditions of direct concern to a neuropsychologist such as brain injury or stroke. One exception is the Copiah County survey in Mississippi, in which rates of disability for several neurological diseases such as stroke or dementia were found to be greater for rural than urban residents (Haerer, Anderson, & Schoenberg, 1986). Several rural occupations, such as farming and mining, have been associated with greater health risk and disability, including neuropsychologically relevant problems like brain injury and toxic exposure (Leigh & Fries, 1992; Lee, Anderson, & Kraus, 1993; Mulloy, 1996). Farming, mining, and logging are associated with a high frequency of job related injuries, including brain trauma and toxic exposure (Horton & McManus, 1989; Hartman, 1995). Rural residence, drinking well water, and exposure to pesticides have all been implicated as risk factors for Parkinson's Disease (Koller et al., 1990; Hubble, Cao, Hassanein, Neuberger, & Koller, 1993). Exposure to organophosphorous pesticides (whose use is prevalent in rural regions) may result in abnormal neurological changes and behavioral changes (Maroni, Jarvisalo, & LaFerla, 1986). A study completed in Italy found that patients with gliomas were more likely to have been exposed to organic pesticides, fertilizers and herbicides in agriculture activities (Musicco, Filippini, Bordo, Melotto, Morello, & Berino, 1982).

According to several surveys, poverty is more common in rural populations and the unemployment rate is higher compared to urban populations (Cordes, 1989; Horton & McManus, 1989; Porter, 1989). Often, rural/urban differences in base rates of psychiatric or neurological disorders can be explained on the basis of poverty or socioeconomic status (e.g., Schwab, Warheit, & Holzer, 1974; Dohrenwend, 1990). Poverty, in general, has been found to be associated with high rates of severe emotional disturbance in children (Costello, Angold, Burns, Erkanli, Stangl, & Tweed, 1996b). In a survey of children from the southern Appalachian Mountain region of North Carolina, rural/urban rate differences for psychiatric disorder were nonsignificant after controlling for level of poverty (Costello et al., 1996a). Mainous and Kohrs (1995) found that while there were few differences in health status between rural and urban adults, rural elders (age 65 and older) had significantly poorer health than urban elders. Additionally, although persons living in rural areas tend to suffer more medical illnesses, they are less likely than their urban counterparts to have health insurance (Horton & McManus, 1989; Rowlands & Lyons, 1989). There are also far fewer health care professionals, especially for specialized services, and health care facilities in rural areas (US Congress, 1988).

Normative issues

The WAIS-R is one of the few tests that have been analyzed by geographical region. One study failed to find differences between rural and urban residents on IQs or subtests scale scores except for the older age groups (Reynolds, Chastain, Kaufman, & McLean, 1987). Kaufman, McLean and Reynolds (1988), however, found that urban adults ages 55 to 74 years out-performed rural adults on Information, Digit Span, Vocabulary and Arithmetic. These results may be attributed to differences in educational opportunities and the availability of TV and the mass media for this cohort of older rural adults. In general, the rural/urban differences in intelligence have declined, presumably due to a decrease in rural isolation, improved farm technology, and better educational opportunities in rural areas for later cohorts (Neisser et al., 1996).

Education and neuropsychological testing

Individuals who live in rural isolated areas where fishing, mining, or agriculture are the primary occupations may have lower rates of secondary school completion than individuals living in more industrialized, developed areas (Watkins & Watkins, 1984). Therefore, while educational history is important for neuropsychological assessments performed in all settings, educational experiences may be even more salient in a rural setting, especially with older cohorts.

Education has a substantial impact on cognitive test scores (for reviews see Ardila, Rosselli, & Ostrosky-Solis, 1992; Rogoff & Chavajay, 1995; Heaton, Ryan, Grant & Matthews, 1996). For instance, cognitive development studies show that Piaget's stages of formal operation cannot be attained without formal education (Rogoff & Chavajay, 1995). Cole (1990) has suggested that one of the important things students learn in school that has a direct impact on test taking is sorting things into taxonomic categories. Individuals with little formal education tend to sort things according to function rather than semantic category and they do not use clustering strategies to aid memory of word lists (Cole, Gay, Glick, & Sharp, 1971; Scribner, 1974; Cole & Scribner, 1977). Rogoff (1981) reviewed the literature on education and cognitive activities and found that schooling promotes graphic ability, remembering disconnected bits of information, and organizing things into categories. Given that these cognitive functions are some of the ones examined with neuropsychological testing, it is not surprising that education affects neuropsychological test scores.

Literacy and education have an impact on neuropsychological test performance and may even have an impact on brain organization. Lecours et al. (1987, 1988) examined illiterate and schooled aphasics and concluded that illiterates have greater "ambilaterality of language representations" (Lecours et al., 1988, p. 586). The authors underscored the need for educational corrections on aphasia tests. Ardila and colleagues (Ardila, Rosselli, & Rosas, 1989; Rosselli, Ardila, & Rosas, 1990) found that education was a very important predictor of performance on neuropsychological tests measuring language, praxis, memory and visuospatial functions. Ostrosky-Solis, Conseco, Quintara, Navarro, Meneses, and Ardila (1985) found that individuals from lower socioeconomic levels from Mexico City performed poorly on neuropsychological test items measuring complex language, calculation, and organization of motor sequences. The finding of poor fine motor performance was surprising, but explained by the fact that individuals in a higher socioeconomic classes use writing skills more frequently than those individuals in lower socioeconomic classes. Low levels of education have also been found to be associated with increased prevalence of dementia in African Americans age 65 and older (Callahan, Hall, Hui, Musick, Unverzagt, & Hendrie,1996) as well as other samples (e.g., Stern, Gurland, Tatemichi, Tang, Wilder, & Mayeux, 1994; White et al., 1994; Prencipe, Casini, Ferretti, Lattanzio, Fiorelli, & Culasso, 1996).

Cultural Competency

A person's values influence the likelihood that problems will be defined and treatment will be sought. Rural values that are seen as especially problematic, with regard to seeking psychological or other medical services, are those that stress self-reliance, conservatism, a distrust of outsiders, religious beliefs, work-orientation, familism, individualism, and fatalism (Friedl, 1982; Human & Wasem, 1991). Horton (1984) authored an interesting paper on the psychosocial aspects of medical disability based on extensive interviews with individuals with incapacitating headaches and backaches in rural southern West Virginia. The perception of disability for these rural Appalachian residents was quite different from 'mainstream' society. Disability was seen as an inevitable result of age (past 40) and traditional rehabilitation services were not viewed as reasonable options. In addition to an expectation that the individual could never work again and, would therefore, need disability income, the local community and family were expected to support the disabled individual as this is the "goodchristian" thing to do (Horton, 1984, p. 651).

In addition to a thorough knowledge and appreciation of the variety of cultural issues and value systems impacting neuropsychological test performance, a rural practitioner is well advised to obtain guidance regarding the colorful local jargon. Phrases such as 'puny,' which means sick, 'ill' which means hateful or irritable, 'backward' which means shy, 'stoved up' which means any kind of pain, 'pump knot' which is a lump on the head, a 'spell' which may be a seizure, 'breaking bad' which means combative, or 'fit' which is the past tense of fight, may confuse an interviewer. Of the formal assessment tools available to the neuropsychologist, only the WAIS-R allows credit for southern dialectical definitions (e.g., the word 'domestic' on the Vocabulary subtest). While a response such as 'country flower' for a hexagon on a test of confrontation naming may be technically incorrect, for a rural resident with a 4th grade education and an extensive quilting background, it is hardly an indication of language disturbance.

Helms (1992) argues that culture strongly influences cognitive ability testing and proposes a culturalist perspective on test development. Her argument and recommendations focus mainly on black–white differences on intelligence testing, but her argument could be extended to other measures that may not equivalently measure cognitive abilities across groups. For instance, Helms recommends using separate norms for different racial groups. Perhaps specialized local norms should be developed for specific clinical uses. For instance, Marcopulos, McLain, and Giuliano (1997) obtained local norms for some commonly administered neuropsychological tests used for dementia. They found that almost half of their presumably normal elderly subjects with less than ten years of education, from rural central Virginia, scored below established cut-offs for dementia.

Sue and Sue (1990) have defined culture as all those things that people have learned to do, believe, value, and enjoy in their history. It is the totality of ideals, beliefs, skills, tools, customs, and institutions into which each member of a society is born (Sue & Sue, 1990, p. 35). A clinical neuropsychologist needs to learn about the local culture, educational system, religions, common experiences and dialect to ensure that the tests chosen to evaluate cognitive functioning will be valid and have good clinical utility. It is the responsibility of the assessor to determine whether the individuals to whom tests will be administered are from the same or similar groups on which the test was standardized and normed. The neuropsychologist must determine whether the test is culturally equivalent. Questions to ask oneself include: Does the test have the same meaning and measure the same psychological constructs across groups? Is your primary clinical population going to be familiar with the content of the test items? Is the language used in the test familiar to your clinical population? If the test was normed on persons similar in age, ethnic composition, geographical region, gender, and education, it might be appropriate.

Ethical Issues

Several articles have addressed the issue of ethical dilemmas in rural practice. Because relative isolation increases interdependence among rural residents, there appears to be an unavoidable presence of non-sexual dual or multiple relations with clients (Sleek, 1994). Faulkner and Faulkner (1997) suggest that guidelines for avoiding non-sexual multiple relationships may be inadequate or inappropriate in a rural setting. Unless practitioners live in an area distant from their practice, they will see clients in the community. In a rural setting a psychologist's services may be sought out because of a personal relationship. Co-workers, professionals and support staff, may want to support the practice that employs them. While it could be argued that it is clearly inappropriate to see a friend or co-workers in therapy, assessment of co-workers' family members is a gray area. Certainly the diagnosis and referral question must be considered, in addition to the ability of the clinician to be objective and to avoid exploitation. Relationships must be assessed in terms of the current situation, future relationships, and the compatibility of these relationships. Seeking consultation from an objective colleague is recommended, as is discussion with the potential client in terms of the consequences of starting a therapeutic relationship.

Confidentiality

Confidentiality is a complicated issue in a rural area. While privacy is of paramount value, in many instances the patient, in effect, waves their right to confidentiality by greeting the psychologist in the community and talking openly about their treatment. Social or other non-professional contacts with persons who are patients or supervisees are inevitable. Psychologists are advised to address the issue of chance meetings early on in therapy to determine how each individual client would like the situation handled. Also, it is not uncommon for patients within a practice to know one another. Depending on the circumstances, patients may need to be scheduled so that their respective appointments do not coincide with one another. From a practice standpoint, even office location can impact privacy. In this regard it is beneficial to have the office located in a large building with several other businesses, rather than a single office building where a patient's car may be recognized in the parking lot.

Training and Educational Issues

Clinical psychology, and especially neuropsychology, has been criticized for being an urban profession (Murray & Keller, 1991). Although there was a 97% increase in the number of rural psychologists between 1970 and 1981 many of those psychologists were academicians and not trained in neuropsychology (Sladen, Mozdzierz, & Greenblatt, 1986; Sladen & Mozdzierz, 1989).

A perusal of the Neuropsychology programs listed in the 1999–2000 Association of Psychology Postdoctoral and Internship Centers directory revealed that only 7 out of the 43 programs listed 'rural' as a training focus. The comprehensive listing in *The Clinical Neuropsychologist* (Cripe, 2000) shows that most neuropsychology training centers are in large urban centers. Is a specific training program in 'Rural Neuropsychology' necessary to competently practice in rural areas? Perhaps not, as long as the training site provides some formal didactics and supervised clinical experience dealing with the issues outlined in the sections above, (i.e., cultural, language, ethical, and educational considerations in testing). Although these issues are also relevant in non-rural settings and should be a required part of any training program, it seems obvious that if a neuropsychologist seeks to work in a rural setting, training in a large urban setting will not give them exposure to the unique issues facing the rural practitioner. Pursuing an internship or postdoctoral fellowship in the rural geographic area where one may want to practice is recommended. This will enable the nascent practitioner to learn about the particular resources, social structure, customs, and both positive and negative health practices of the local residents.

Practicum and internship experience providing generalized psychological services to a rural population is invaluable experience prior to a post-doctoral fellowship in neuropsychology. Hargrove and Breazeale (1993) propose a strategy for training psychologists working in rural areas. They argue that psychologists working in rural areas should acquire skills working with a wide variety of professionals and institutions (e.g., law enforcement, social services), administrative experience, and be able to collaborate with other professionals and nonprofessionals. Neuropsychologists who choose to work in rural areas need to have broad-based training, in addition to their specialized training in clinical neuropsychology. They may receive referrals from family practitioners and may be asked to respond to a wider variety of psychological issues than cognitive function. Basic competencies in lifespan issues, (i.e., assessment of children and geriatrics) are essential. However, while it is important to have broad-based training, a clinical neuropsychologist cannot be expected to cover all mental health services and needs to effectively communicate to referral sources and clients the parameters of their competency and expertise. The fact that mental health providers have been encouraged to adopt a more ‘generalist’ role does not fit with the highly specialized training required to be a neuropsychologist.

Perhaps an even more important issue than training is how to recruit neuropsychologists to work in rural areas (e.g., Merwin, Goldsmith, & Manderscheid, 1995). Several call to action papers have been published in recent years, imploring psychologists to better address the challenges of rural mental health needs (DeLeon, Wakefield, Schultz, Williams & VandenBos, 1989; Hutner & Windle, 1991; Murray & Keller, 1991; Hargrove & Breazeale, 1993). In 1990, Congress increased funding to the National Health Service Corps, which provides scholarships and loan repayment to health professionals in exchange for service in underserved areas. In 1992, the Health Resources and Services established new criteria for designated areas with shortages of mental health professionals. Despite these actions, however, there has been a trend in rural areas to use Master’s level practitioners. If there is a paucity of qualified psychologists in rural areas, there is most certainly a paucity of qualified neuropsychologists. Master’s level training is insufficient for the practice of neuropsychology.

The practice of rural psychology has received recent attention in The Monitor (Foxhall, 2000; Smith, 2001) and may result in increased interest in this type of work. These articles highlight the benefits as well as the challenges inherent in a rural practice on personal, clinical, and ethical fronts. Students, as well as practicing psychologists who are considering a professional move, are well advised to carefully consider whether they are suited to a career in rural America. Sleek (1994) stated that psychologists who are more likely to be satisfied with rural practice are those who have had extensive experience with dual relationships and multiple personal and professional roles. They appear better able to maintain professional integrity within the changing demands of this unique social environment.

Future Directions

Despite the many challenges, psychologists can play an important role in the future of rural America on several levels (Murray & Keller, 1991). Psychologists are uniquely qualified to continue to research the issues that have been highlighted in this chapter and to debunk myths regarding the rural experience. Neuropsychologists must unite to integrate the use of non-doctoral level practitioners and to combat ignorance and prejudice. Technology (e.g., internet services, teleconferencing) will play an increasingly important role in the lives of patients as well as professionals. Escalating health care costs will require creative solutions in areas where mental health and general medical status have been comprised secondary to poor accessibility and lack of human and fiscal resources. It is recommended that training be offered that takes into account the neuropsychological, cultural, medical, and ethical issues associated with rural populations. The onus will be on the practitioner to provide current and clinically sound service in view of ethically sound cultural and clinical competency.

References

Ardila, A., Rosselli, M., & Ostrosky-Solis, F. (1992). Socioeducational. In A.E. Puente & R.J. McCaffrey (Eds.), *Handbook of neuropsychological assessment: A biopsychosocial perspective* (pp.181–192). New York: Plenum Press.

Ardila, A., Rosselli, M., & Rosas, P. (1989). Neuropsychological assessment in illiterates: Visuospatial and memory abilities. *Brain and Cognition, 11*, 147–166.

Brayne, C., & Calloway, P. (1989). An epidemiological study of dementia in a rural population of elderly women. *British Journal of Psychiatry, 155*, 214–219.

Callahan, C.M., Hall, K.S., Hui, S.L., Musick, B.S., Unverzagt, F.W., & Hendrie, H.C. (1996). Relationship of age, education, and occupation with dementia among a community-based sample of African Americans. *Archives of Neurology, 53*,134–140.

Cole, M. (1990). Cognitive development and formal schooling: The evidence from cross-cultural research. In L. C. Mill (Ed.), *Vygotsky and education* (pp. 89–110). Cambridge: Cambridge University Press.

Cole, M., Gay, J., Glick, J.A., & Sharp, D.W. (1971). *The cultural context of learning and thinking.* New York: Basic Books.

Cole, M., & Scribner, S. (1977). Cross-cultural studies of memory and cognition. In R.V. Kail, Jr. & J.W. Hagen (Eds.), *Perspectives on the development of memory and cognition* (pp. 239–271). Hilldale, NJ: Erlbaum.

Cordes, S. (1989). The changing rural environment and the relationship between health services and rural development. *Health Services Research, 23*, 757–784.
Costello, E.J., Angold, A., Burns, B.J., Erkanli, A., Stangl, D.K., & Tweed, D.L. (1996a). The great smoky mountains study of youth. Functional impairment and serious emotional disturbance. *Archives of General Psychiatry, 53*, 1137–1143.
Costello, E.J., Angold, A., Burns, B.J., Stangl, D.K., Tweed, D.L., Erkanli, A., & Worthman, C.M. (1996b). The great smoky mountain study of youth. Goals, designs, methods, and the prevalence of DSM-III-R disorders. *Archives of General Psychiatry, 53*, 1129–1136.
Cripe, L. (2000). List of training programs in clinical neuropsychology-2000. *The Clinical Neuropsychologist, 14*, 357–448.
DeLeon, P.H., Wakefield, M., Schultz, A.J., Williams, J., VandenBos, G.R. (1989). Rural America. Unique opportunities for health care delivery and health services research. *American Psychologist, 44*, 1298–1306.
Dohrenwend, P. (1990). Socioeconomic status (SES) and psychiatric disorders: Are the issues still compelling? *Social Psychiatry and Psychiatric Epidemiology, 25*, 41–47.
Faulkner, K.K., & Faulkner, T.A. (1997). Managing multiple relationships in rural communities: Neutrality and Boundary Violations. *Clinical Psychology: Science and Practice, 4,* p. 225–234.
Foxhall, K. (2000). Rural life holds particular stressors for women. *Monitor, 31*(11), 30–31 .
Friedl, J. (1982). Explanatory models of black lung: Understanding the health-related behavior of Appalachian coal miners. *Culture, Medicine, and Psychiatry, 6(1)*, 3–10.
Haerer, A.F., Anderson, D.W., & Schoenberg, B.S. (1986). Functional disability associated with major neurologic disorders. Findings from the Copiah county study. *Archives of Neurology, 43*, 1000–1003.
Hargrove, D.S. (1989). Impacts of trade liberalization and restructuring of agriculture on rural communities. *Journal of Agribusiness, 7*, 70–72.
Hargrove, D.S., & Breazeale, R.L. (1993). Psychologists and rural services: Addressing a new agenda. *Professional Psychology: Research and Practice, 24*, 319–324.
Hartman, D.E. (1995). *Neuropsychological toxicology* (2nd ed.). New York: Plenum Press.
Heaton, R.K., Ryan, L., Grant, I., & Matthews, C.G. (1996). Demographic influences on neuropsychological test performance. In I. Grant & K. M. Adams (Eds.), *Neuropsychological assessment of neuropsychiatric disorders* (2nd ed.) (pp. 141–163). New York: Oxford University Press.
Helms, J. (1992). Why is there no study of cultural equivalence in standardized cognitive ability testing? *American Psychologist, 47*, 1083–1101.
Horton, C.F. (1984). Women have headaches, men have backaches: Patterns of illness in an Appalachian community. *Social Science and Medicine, 19*, 647–654.
Horton, C.H., & McManus, M.A. (1989). Background tables on demographic characteristics, health status and health services utilization. *Health Services Research, 23*, 725–756.
Hubble, J.P., Cao, T., Hassanein, R.E., Neurberger, J.S., & Koller, W.C. (1993). Risk factors in Parkinson's disease. *Neurology, 43*, 1693–1697.
Human, J., & Wasem, C. (1991). Rural mental health in America. *American Psychologist, 46*, 232–239.
Hutner, M., & Windle, C. (1991). NIMH support of rural mental health. *American Psychologist, 46*, 240–243.
Jordan, S.A., & Hargrove, D.S. (1987). Implication of an empirical application of categorical definitions of rural. *Journal of Rural Community Psychology, 8(2)*, 14–29.

Kaufman, A.S., McLean, J.E., & Reynolds, C.R. (1988). Sex, race, residence, region, and education differences on the 11 WAIS-R subtests. *Journal of Clinical Psychology, 44(2)*, 231–248.

Kingsport Area Chamber of Commerce. (1998). 2000 Newcomers Guide. Kingsport, TN: Kingsport Area Chamber of Commerce.

Koller, W., Vetere-Overfield, B., Gray, C., Alexander, C., Chin, T., Dolezal, J., Hassanein, R., & Tanner, C. (1990). Environmental risk factors in Parkinson's disease. *Neurology, 40*, 1218–1221.

Lecours, A.R., Mehler, J., Parente, M.A., Beltrami, M.C., Tolipan, L.C., Cary, L., Castro, M.J., Carrono, V., Chagastelles, L., Denhaut, F., Delgado, R., Evangelista, A., Fajgenbaum, S., Fontoura, C., Karmann, D.F., Gurd, J., Torne, C.H. Jakubovicz, R., Kac, R., Lefevre, B., Lima, C., Maciel, J., Mansur, L., Martinez, R., Nobrega, M.C., Osorio, Z., Paciomik, J., Papaterra, F., Penedo, M.A., Saboya, B., Scheuer, C., Silva, A.B., Spinardi, M. & Teixeira, M. (1988). Illiteracy and brain damage — 3: A contribution to the study of speech and language disorders in illiterates with unilateral brain damage (initial testing). *Neuropsychologia, 26*, 575–589.

Lecours, A.R., Mehler, J., Parente, M.A., Caldeira, A., Cary, L., Castro, M.J., Dehaut, F., Delgado, R., Gurd, J., Karmann, D., Jakubovitz, R., Osorio, Z., Cabral, L.S., & Junqueira, A.M.S. (1987). Illiteracy and brain damage — 1. Aphasia testing in culturally contrasted populations (control subjects). *Neuropsychologia, 25*, 231–245.

Lee, T., Anderson, C., & Kraus, J.F. (1993). Acute traumatic injuries in underground bituminous coal miners. *American Journal of Industrial Medicine, 23*, 407–415.

Leigh, J.P., & Fries, J.F. (1992). Disability in occupations in a national sample. *American Journal of Public Health, 82*, 1517–1524.

Mainous, A.G. & Kohrs, F.P. (1995). A comparison of health status between rural and urban adults. *Journal of Community Health, 20*, 423–431.

Marcopulos, B.A., McLain, C.A., & Giuliano, A. J. (1997). Cognitive impairment or inadequate norms? A study of healthy, rural, older adults with limited education. *The Clinical Neuropsychologist, 11*, 111–131.

Maroni, M., Jarvisalo, J., & LaFerla, F. (1986). The WHO-UNDP epidemiological health effects of exposure to organophosphorous pesticides. *Toxicology Letters, 33*, 115–123.

Merwin, E.I., Goldsmith, H.F., & Manderscheid, R.W. (1995). Human resource issues in rural mental health services. *Community Mental Health Journal, 31*, 525–537.

Mulloy, K.B. (1996). Two cases of neurological disease in coal preparation plant workers. *American Journal of Industrial Medicine, 30*, 56–61.

Murray, J.D., & Keller, P.A. (1991). Psychology and rural America. Current status and future directions. *American Psychologist, 46*, 220–231.

Musicco, M., Filippini, G., Bordo, B.M., Melotto, A., Morello, G., & Berino, F. (1982). Gliomas and occupational exposure to carcinogens: a case-control study. *American Journal of Epidemiology, 116*, 782–790.

Neisser, U., Boodoo, G., Bouchard, T.J., Boykin, A.W., Brody, N., Ceci, S. J., Halpern, D.F., Loehlin, J.C., Perloff, R., Sternberg, R.J., & Urbina, S. (1996). Intelligence: Knowns and unknowns. *American Psychologist, 51(2)*, 77–101.

Office of Management and Budget, Statistical Policy Division (1975). Standard metropolitan statistical areas. Revised edition. Washington, DC: U S Government Printing Office.

Ostrosky-Solis, F., Canseco, E., Quintanar, L., Navarro, E., Meneses, S., & Ardila, A. (1985). Sociocultural effects in neuropsychological assessment. *International Journal of Neuroscience, 27*, 53–66.

Peake, T.H., McClain, V.R., Wilson, K., & Orrell, T. (1992). Neuropsychology in the hinterlands. *Medical Psychotherapy, 5*, 29–38.

Porter, K.H. (1989). Poverty in rural America: A national overview. Washington, DC: Center on the Budget and Policy Priorities.

Prencipe, M, Casini, A.R., Ferretti, C., Lattanzio, M.T., Fiorelli, M., and Culasso, F. (1996). Prevalence of dementia in an elderly rural population: effects of age, sex, and education. *Journal of Neurology, Neurosurgery, and Psychiatry, 60*, 628–633.

Reynolds, C.R., Chastain, R.L., Kaufman, A.S., & McLean, J.E. (1987). Demographic characteristics and IQ among adults: Analysis of the WAIS-R standardization sample as a function of the stratification variables. *Journal of School Psychology, 25*, 323–342.

Rogoff, B. (1981). Schooling and the development of cognitive skills. In H.C. Triandis & Heron, G. (Eds.), *Handbook of cross-cultural psychology* (vol. 4, pp. 233–294). Rockleigh, NJ: Allyn & Bacon.

Rogoff, B., & Chavajay, P. (1995). What's become of research on the cultural basis of cognitive development? *American Psychologist, 50*, 859–877.

Rosselli, M., Ardila, A., & Rosas, P. (1990). Neuropsychological assessment in illiterates. II. Language and praxic abilities. *Brain and Cognition, 12*, 281–196.

Rowlands, D., & Lyons, B. (1989). Triple jeopardy: Rural, poor, and uninsured. *Health Services Research, 23*, 975–1004.

Schwab, J.J., Warheit, G.J., & Holzer, C.E. (1974). Mental health: Rural-urban comparisons. *Mental Health and Society, 1*, 265–274.

Scribner, S. (1974). Developmental aspects of categorized recall in a West African society. *Cognitive Psychology, 6*, 475–494.

Sladen, B.J., & Mozdzierz, G.J. (1989). Distribution of psychologists in underserved areas: Changes over time, 1970–1981. *Professional Psychology, 20*, 244–247.

Sladen, B.J., Mozdzierz, G.J., & Greenblatt, R.L. (1986). Geographic distribution of neuropsychological services providers and its correlates. *Professional Psychology: Research and Practice, 17*, 256–259.

Sleek, S. (1994). Ethical dilemmas plague rural practice. *Monitor*, December, 26.

Smith, D. (2001). Collaborating in the country. *Monitor, 32(4)*, 72–73.

Stern, Y., Gurlan, B., Taternichi, T.K., Tang, M.X., Wilder, D., & Mayeux, R. (1994). Influence of education and occupation on the incidence of Alzheimer's disease. *Journal of the American Medical Association, 271*, 1004–1010.

Sue, D.W., & Sue, D. (1990). *Counseling the culturally different.* New York: Wiley.

Troster, A.I., Paolo, A.M., Glatt, S.L., Hubble, J.P., & Koller, W.C. (1995). "Interactive video conferencing" in the provision of neuropsychological services to rural areas. *Journal of Community Psychology, 23*, 85–88.

US Congress. (1988). The rural health care challenge (staff report to the Special Report on Aging. US Senate [100-W]). Washington, DC: US Government Printing Office.

Watkins, J.M., & Watkins, D.A. (1984). *Social policy in the rural setting.* New York: Springer.

White, L., Katzman, R., Losonczy, K., Salive, M., Wallace, R., Berkman, L., Taylor, J., Fillenbaum, G., & Havlik, R. (1994). Association of education with incidence of cognitive impairment in three established studies of the elderly. *Journal of Clinical Epidemiology, 47*, 363–374.

Chapter 18

PRACTICE IN THE SCHOOLS

N. William Walker, Kristie J. Nies, and Rudy Lorber

Introduction

This chapter describes how three practitioners approach the delivery of neuropsychological services to the schools. Provision of these services varies because of differences in their training and experience, and the manner in which their practices are arranged. It is hoped that readers will be able to identify with and profit from these somewhat diverse approaches to a similar setting. After a brief review of the historical perspectives affecting the role of neuropsychologists in the schools, we will describe our individual practices, including referral sources, marketing, billing and collecting, personnel, and other practical aspects of managing each of the three practices. Practical issues common to most neuropsychological practices in the schools will also be discussed. Areas reviewed will include, contractual arrangements, issues in school consultation and collaboration, neuropsychological assessments and reports for the schools and, training issues for neuropsychologists working with the schools. Finally, segments of sample school-appropriate recommendations will be provided as demonstrations of the concepts being covered.

Historical perspective

Psychologists have practiced in the schools for more than 100 years. Responsibilities have typically included assessment and counseling services to students as well as in-service training of school personnel. With the passage of the Education for All Handicapped Children Act of 1975 (P.L. 94-142), psychologists began to more formally address the growing concerns regarding the number of children who were either excluded from receiving public education, or who were receiving inadequate or inappropriate forms of education. In essence PL 94-142 provides for:

> "...a free appropriate education which emphasizes special education and related services designed to meet their unique needs, to assure that the rights of handicapped children and their parents or guardians are protected, to assist States and localities to provide for the education of all handicapped children, and to assess and assure the effectiveness of efforts to educate handicapped children." (P.L. 94-142, Sec. 601[c])

This law is the basis for the classification and provision of services to exceptional children (e.g. learning disabled, educably mentally handicapped, other health impaired, etc.)

In 1990 an additional law, the Individuals with Disabilities Education Act (IDEA) or P.L. 101-476 was passed and holds even more importance for neuropsychologists. IDEA extended the coverage of P.L. 94-142 to children and adolescents with traumatic brain injuries (TBI), making these students eligible for Special Education services in the schools. Because of the provisions of this law, neuropsychologists have an opportunity to become increasingly involved in the assessment and programming of school-age children and adolescents. It is important, however, to note the federal definition of TBI. The current definition is as follows:

> "'Traumatic brain injury' means an acquired injury to the brain caused by an external physical force, resulting in total or partial functional disability or psychosocial impairment, or both, that adversely affects a child's educational performance. The term applies to open or closed injuries resulting in impairments in one or more areas, such as cognition; language; memory; attention; problem solving; sensory, perceptual and motor abilities; psychosocial behavior; physical functions; information processing; and speech. The term does not apply to brain injuries that are congenital or degenerative, or brain injuries induced by birth trauma." (Federal Register, 1992).

Neuropsychologists should make specific note of the last sentence in this definition since it excludes from this classification many school age children we feel should receive special services (e.g. children and adolescents with brain insult caused by seizure disorders, tumors, strokes, disease, etc.). Students with these conditions can, however, receive services under other existing exceptional child classifications such as Specific Learning Disability (SLD), or Other Health Impaired (OHI) depending on the individual circumstances.

In 1992, the Americans with Disabilities Act of 1990 (ADA; PL 101-336) was implemented. As a result, tangible consequences such as wheelchair ramps and handicap parking became apparent. Less visible consequences have also become apparent. The ADA mandates that institutions of higher education also provide accommodations to students with disabilities (see Chapter 13). This includes college students with brain injuries and some disabling psychiatric disorders. This law ensures that reasonable accommodations must be developed for each form of disability. The process of identifying and accommodating disabilities under ADA is described in Gordon and Keiser (1998).

Finally, each state has a Department of Education, Public Instruction, etc. that publishes guidelines for the identification and provision of services to exceptional children and adolescents, usually on an annual basis. These guidelines form the basis of all decisions regarding classification, placement and appropriate programming for these students. In summary, an understanding of the specific laws that affect children with disabilities and the schools is essential for neuropsychologists intending to work in the school setting.

The Authors and their Practices

Dr. Walker received his doctorate in school psychology and secured his neuropsychological training through a two-year fellowship in clinical neuropsychology. One year of this training was in an adult brain-injury rehabilitation hospital with the second year devoted to pediatric neuropsychology within a pediatric neurology division of an acute trauma hospital. Dr. Walker has directed the brain injury rehabilitation programs for a national rehabilitation hospital corporation, and has been in the private practice of neuropsychology, for over 15 years. His private practice experience has usually been as a member of a group practice with pediatric or adult neurologists. Dr. Walker's current role is primarily that of training doctoral students. He is the former training director for an APA accredited doctoral program in Clinical, School and Counseling Psychology, and currently directs the Neuropsychology Clinic at a university-based Human Development Center at James Madison University (JMU), Virginia.

The Human Development Center provides assessment and intervention services to school-age children and adolescents and their families, and college students with suspected learning disabilities. The Human Development Center is located in a primarily rural area. It is the mission of the Center to provide services to the community as part of the training for graduate students in school psychology, counseling psychology and the doctoral program with which Dr. Walker is associated. The Center is located in an on-campus facility featuring several testing and counseling rooms all equipped with video taping devices and observational mirrors. All testing and counseling sessions are taped for supervision by graduate program faculty. Faculty observes and/or co-leads testing and counseling sessions with graduate students. The neuropsychology clinic that Dr. Walker directs is located physically within the Human Development Center. All cases referred to the Human Development Center with suspected neurological complications are triaged through the neuropsychology clinic for possible evaluation and/or intervention.

Dr. Nies has been in private practice (i.e., Psychological Consultants, LLC), serving both children and adults, for 3.5 years. Previous experience includes working in a corporate rehabilitation setting as well as a multispeciality medical practice. For a full description of her training and background see Chapter 17.

Dr. Lorber received his M.S. degree in School Psychology and Ph.D. in Clinical Psychology from the University of Oregon. He has received two Board Certifications from the American Board of Professional Psychology in School Psychology and in Behavioral Psychology. Dr. Lorber is also a Fellow of both the Academy of School Psychology and the Academy of Behavioral Psychology. His neuropsychological training has been an ongoing process including graduate coursework, and a clinical internship at the University of Washington School of Medicine Department of Rehabilitation Medicine and Children's Orthopedic Hospital in the Learning Disabilities Assessment Program. Dr. Lorber's training in behavioral intervention and behavioral assessment/analysis began with his work at the Oregon Social Learning Center in Eugene, Oregon.

Currently, Dr. Lorber is in private practice at Lake Shore Neuropsychological Services located in the northern suburbs of Chicago, Illinois. In addition, he holds staff appointments in the Departments of Psychiatry and Pediatrics at Evanston Northwestern Healthcare. He is an Assistant Professor of Pediatrics at the McGaw Medical Center of Northwestern University, an Adjunct Assistant Professor, Department of Psychology at Northwestern University, and an Instructor at Loyola University of Chicago, Department of Education, where he teaches courses for the school psychology graduate program in neuropsychology and neuropsychological assessment. Previously, Dr. Lorber was the Coordinator of the Behavioral Pediatric Neuropsychology Service in the Department of Pediatrics at Rush-Presbyterian-St. Lukes Medical Center. Other relevant positions include Director of the Evaluation Center for Learning at Evanston Hospital, and Level I Due Process Officer for the state of Illinois.

Dr. Lorber's private practice includes several learning disabilities and educational specialists located in a suite of private offices. The majority of his practice entails conducting comprehensive evaluations of children and adolescents with a variety of neurological, learning, behavioral, and emotional disorders. Dr. Lorber also engages in forensic evaluations involving personal injury and medical malpractice, gives public lectures on assessment, intervention, and parental rights for local organizations (e.g., the Learning Disabilities Association), and when time permits engages in professional writing and research.

Referral sources and marketing

Referral sources and marketing practices reflect the differences in nature of the practices of the three authors. Dr. Walker's is a university-based practice, which limits the necessity for independent marketing, whereas the practices of Drs. Nies and Lorber are more dependent on traditional approaches to marketing. The primary referral sources for Dr. Walker's practice consist of local school systems, parents, local courts and child protective agencies, attorneys, self-referrals (usually college students), and local children's and family service agencies. Dr. Walker triages all clients referred to the university center that are suspected of having a neurological disorder as part of the mission of the neuropsychology clinic. In some cases, children and adolescents who have been seen by the university center for other reasons (e.g. learning or behavior problems) are referred for further screening or evaluation at the neuropsychology clinic due to findings in the initial evaluation that are suggestive of neurological complications. It is a primary mission of the neuropsychology clinic to provide training to graduate students interested in neuropsychology.

The neuropsychology clinic has developed a brochure and an Internet web site as additional marketing tools. The web site (www.cep.jmu.edu/neuroclinic) serves as a vehicle to provide support for schools, parents, survivors, and other interested parties who may be unable to travel to the neuropsychology clinic. Educational information regarding brain injury is provided on this web site along with the opportunity to have specific questions answered by the Clinic staff.

Children and adolescents are referred to Dr. Nies by pediatricians, neurosurgeons, parents, psychiatrists, psychologists, the public school system, and the local university. As is the case with Dr. Lorber, many referrals come by 'word of mouth' particularly since her practice is located in a small community. The group with which she practices has developed a brochure that includes services available for children. Participation in community wellness fairs and injury prevention programs has been an additional means of networking with, and marketing to, other professionals and parents.

Dr. Lorber's primary referral sources include pediatricians, neurologists, psychiatrists, psychologists, other mental health professionals, attorneys, child advocates, and school personnel. Despite many professional referral sources, the majority of referrals come from 'word of mouth.' Dr. Lorber has also developed a brochure describing his practice and the available services. This brochure is available in his waiting room and they are distributed at community talks and school meetings. Brochures are also mailed to potential referral sources and are included with copies of evaluation report that parents request be sent to treating physicians, psychologists, mental health professionals, and child advocates. When requested, a brochure holder filled with brochures is sent to referral sources to keep in their waiting rooms. Currently a web site is under construction for dissemination of information regarding Dr. Lorber's practice.

Personnel, procedures and mechanics of practice

The personnel involved in Dr. Walker's practice are mainly graduate student trainees and interns, and the administrative staff of the Human Development Center, which houses the neuropsychology clinic. After completing course work in neuropsychology and psychophysiology, doctoral students and pre-doctoral interns interested in neuropsychology complete a practicum in the neuropsychology clinic. They gain experience in assessment, school programming and consultation for children and adolescents identified with neurological conditions. Teams of 2–3 students, directly supervised by Dr. Walker, provide all clinical services. In addition to the services rendered, each case seen is used as a training opportunity for students. Student teams are comprised of advanced and beginning doctoral students with more advanced students participating directly in the assessment and report writing and less experienced students playing supportive roles to the team (e.g. school observations). Interpretive sessions with parents are done in a team fashion also to facilitate training. The neuropsychology clinic also consults directly with local schools dealing with traumatic brain injury (TBI) placement issues, including school IEP meetings, school reentry, school personnel training, and academic and behavioral programming for students surviving brain injury. Clients range from preschool-age students to university students. Some adults are seen as well. In addition to directing the Neuropsychology Clinic, Dr. Walker maintains a small therapy caseload of exclusively brain injury survivors. In those cases where clients give permission, students can observe Dr. Walker's therapy sessions to facilitate training.

The theoretical basis for the assessments done through the Neuropsychology Clinic is primarily the Process Approach popularized by Edith Kaplan (1990). This approach appears to be a good match for school evaluations since it uses some assessment techniques already familiar to school personnel and it can provide more context for programming recommendations and training. While a basic core testing protocol is followed in most cases, supplementary evaluation techniques will differ depending on the student's age, initial identification of strengths and weaknesses, and the specific circumstances of the referral, e.g. cognitive vs. social-emotional. Evaluations will typically take 6–8 hours and are completed over 2–3 testing sessions. The interval between evaluations and reports is somewhat slower than desired due to the service-training mission of the Clinic, but most cases are completed in 3–4 weeks. All cases are completed on an outpatient basis.

Dr. Nies uses a technician for all cases seen in the office. The test battery is flexible (i.e., varies depending on the referral question, age of the patient, and insurance status), but is generally completed in six to ten hours inclusive of interview, scoring, record review, and report writing. Often, by the time a child is referred to Dr. Nies they have had multiple evaluations of intellectual and academic functioning. In these cases, the focus is solely on neuropsychological and emotional functioning. Evaluations always include interviews of the child and parent(s) as well as record review. The majority of parent's return for feedback and Dr. Nies attends M-Team meetings on a limited basis.

Several insurance companies require pre-authorization (including a list of planned tests) and many have restrictions regarding the number of hours that will be authorized. Hospital consults are completed in 1-2 hours and generally result in a recommendation for additional evaluation. In general, reports are completed within one week. If a report is going to be delayed, a summary letter is sent within two to three days of the evaluation or by the time the patient is seen by the referral source.

The majority of Dr. Lorber's professional time is spent in the assessment, treatment, consultation, and advocacy of school-age children and adolescents. The professional staff of his clinical practice includes a certified Special Education teacher and a certified Regular Education teacher. A member of his staff is also bilingual in English and Spanish. The professional staff serves two roles. First, they are involved in the administration of parts of the comprehensive test battery (e.g., measures of academic processing). Second, they also provide patients with specialized remedial intervention services. Dr. Lorber personally conducts intake sessions with each new patient's family, begins the evaluation process (i.e., starting with the neuropsychological evaluation), determines the other components and test measures to be administered, and conducts the feedback session(s).

Assessment instruments include measures of intellectual, neuropsychological, academic, and social, emotional, behavioral functioning, and at times adaptive functioning. The philosophy underlying Dr. Lorber's evaluation process is to assess the individual's underlying cognitive strengths and weaknesses across the spectrum of skills underlying academic, social, and daily living skills. The evaluation process includes an intake with parents and a clinical interview with the child/adolescent. Feedback sessions with parents are held to: 1) educate parents about psychometric test data in general, 2) discuss the test findings, and 3) determine specific recommendations for additional assessments, and educational and behavioral interventions at school, e.g. the need for 'Parent Training', as well as private therapies or interventions. At the request of parents, Dr. Lorber attends Multidisciplinary Case Conference (MDC) and Individual Education Program (IEP) meetings at schools to present the assessment data, discuss the clinical impressions and recommendations, and when necessary act as an advocate for the child/adolescent and his or her family. Dr. Lorber may also attend the yearly IEP review meetings or meetings convened during the school year due to specific issues. Periodic educational re-evaluations are conducted (to monitor a student's progress), or for specialized interventions (e.g., double-blind medication trials). Dr. Lorber also provides specific types of student observations (e.g., to determine the appropriateness of an educational settings or interventions strategy) and formal functional behavioral assessments. He also works directly with parents and schools setting up cross-situational behavioral interventions, sometimes employing a social learning parent-training model. Dr. Lorber's board certifications in School Psychology and Behavioral Psychology have proven to be extremely helpful to him, both in his consultation services, as well as in the processes of advocacy and forensic work.

Evaluations are typically conducted over a two and one-half to three-day period. Parental feedback sessions and a separate feedback session for older adolescents occur approximately one to two weeks following the evaluation. For families who have to travel great distances, these feedback sessions can be conducted over the phone. Dr. Lorber's assessment battery includes a core set of test measures, determined by the patient's age and the nature of their disabilities. Additional test measures are added depending upon specific referral questions and the results of initial testing. A core battery also allows for the assessment of a fundamental set of cognitive, academic processing, and social, emotional, and behavioral scores for gaining a holistic understanding of each patient's strengths and weaknesses.

Inherent in Dr. Lorber's evaluation approach is a comprehensive and integrated set of test measures that significantly add to the purpose of solely documenting the presence or absence of neurologically based deficits. Components include intellectual functioning, neuropsychological functioning (with additional emphasis on functions underlying school-related tasks), academic processing skills, and components of one's social, emotional, behavioral, and at times adaptive functioning. Working within schools, the pediatric neuropsychologist must also be able to integrate the findings of the varied professional disciplines that may be involved with children (e.g., occupational therapist, physical therapist, speech and language pathologist, and audiologist), each of whom may speak a different 'language.'

This documentation, often found in existing records, is crucial for demonstrating effectiveness or ineffectiveness of previous interventions and/or environmental adaptations, modifications, or supports/services. The historical record may help to determine if more intensive interventions are needed, or if subtle disabilities have been described for an extended period of time, yet not appropriately addressed. These factors may be crucial when attempting to obtain services for a child under the entitlements of Public Laws.

Dr. Lorber's written reports also contain two additional sections necessary for supporting students within a school setting. First, is a concise summary of the clinical findings, along with specific determination of the Special Education Characteristics identified by the test data, by the findings of other professionals, and the historical record. Second, specific recommendations are provided to address a child's needs by suggesting appropriate interventions that describe the types of educational, cognitive, behavioral, and therapeutic interventions. As neuropsychologists, the better we can educate parents and schools as to what neuropsychologists can do clinically, the better our unique area of expertise can be used. Due to the length and complexity of the evaluation reports, turnaround is approximately six weeks. With rare exception, all evaluations are on an outpatient basis.

Business aspects and physical environment of practice

As mentioned earlier, Dr. Walker's practice takes place in a university-based, neuropsychology clinic. Most assessment and intervention services take place within this setting, although there are many instances where school observations and teacher interviews can provide valuable information regarding a client's performance in the school setting. Doctoral students and other applied graduate program students (e.g. school psychology) carry out these observations and interviews under Dr. Walker's supervision. Much of the intervention and programming work is also done in the client's school setting. Parent training and family therapy, if called for, is usually done at the Neuropsychology Clinic. The staff of the university center provides the Clinic with support services including, secretarial and billing services.

Psychological Consultants, LLC, leases office space that contains five offices, a conference room, a reception area, secretarial, space, and a break room. Dr. Nies shares the cost of a technician (i.e., a Master's level, state licensed Psychological Examiner), including health insurance, with one other psychologist. Each psychologist purchases his or her own test forms and equipment although a very collaborative arrangement exists with regard to test usage. An office manager and one full-time secretary manage the office of Psychological Consultants. They are responsible for the day-to-day operations of answering the telephone, scheduling patients, managing accounts receivable and payable, and verifying insurance, as well as billing and collections. The only outside services employed are those of an accountant (and the lawyer who set up the LLC). Practice members are invoiced bi-monthly for rent, advertising, insurance (medical, malpractice, liability), office supplies, and utilities. This 'overhead' is approximately 30% of collections. Membership dues, journal subscriptions, books, pager, cell phone, supplies, test equipment/forms, disability insurance, and Continuing Education expenses are not included in the office overhead, but, rather are paid by each psychologist independent of the practice. Each member is responsible for paying their own quarterly taxes and funding their own retirements. In total, overhead runs about 45–50%. (It should be noted, however, that using this type of calculation is somewhat deceptive. Some costs are fixed and the overhead percentage, at any one time, varies depending on collections.)

Dr. Lorber's practice takes place primarily in a suite of offices that were designed and constructed uniquely for his clinical practice. The location was specifically chosen to be convenient by either car or commuter railroad. Since some patients come from great distances, families will often need to stay at local hotels while testing is being completed. Thus, the office location was picked to be near restaurants and stores to facilitate a comfortable stay by patients and their families.

When going into private practice, it is important to remember that every paperclip, protocol, phone call, and every minute of electricity use comes out of 'collected' patient fees. Separate malpractice and office liability insurance must be paid, followed by staff and office manager/secretary salaries. Dr. Lorber's practice also employed the services of an attorney to set up his corporation. An attorney and an accountant are also employed to prepare tax forms, deal with legal questions, and conduct fee collections when neces-

Table 1.

Item	Percentage of expenses
Staff salaries	34%
Rent	9%
Taxes	5%
Insurance	1%
Utilities/telephone	2%
Supplies/equipment/printing	3%
Professional development/travel	3%
Practice promotion	1%
Miscellaneous (legal, depreciation, repairs, etc.)	6%
Salary for clinician	36%

sary. The handling of money can be difficult for the new practitioner. Finally, continuing education, continued training, attendance at professional meetings and the purchase of books are undertaken as funds allow. On top of all of these expenses, pro-bono work is also conducted as time permits.

The following breakdown serves as an illustration of a typical apportionment of monies collected in practice. Every collected dollar is apportioned as shown in Table 1. Using the example contained therein, for every dollar collected in an independent private practice, approximately 36-cents gross would be the clinician's salary.

Billing and collection practices

Just as differences in the practices shape the marketing and referral processes in the three practices, billing and collecting procedures also reflect these differences.

The primary mission of Dr. Walker's neuropsychology clinic is the provision of quality services within a training environment. A significant advantage of being part of such a setting is in not having the billing pressures experienced in more traditional settings such as private practice. Billing in the Clinic is done on a sliding scale. Most clients eventually pay little or nothing for these services due to the low SES nature of the rural clientele in the immediate area. Medicare and provider billing for the clients of the neuropsychology clinic is done by the University Center using ICD-DSM codes established specifically for neuropsychological services whenever possible.

There are occasions when faculty members are permitted to use the University Center facilities to carry private cases. In these situations, billing is also done through the University Center with a proportion of the fees going to the Center for operational expenses. In the case of the neuropsychology clinic, one of several sub-clinics at the Center, these funds are diverted to the operational expenses of the Clinic for such things as testing equipment, computer scoring programs, resource books, etc.

Dr. Nies submits billing information, (i.e. CPT and ICD/DSM codes, number of hours involved), to the office staff for preparation of Health Care Finance Administration (HCFA) forms or other billing statements (e.g., in the case of attorneys). Forms are expected to be sent out within 72 hours of provision of service. Pro bono cases are seen, but on a limited basis.

Attorney referred cases are considered forensic and require pre-payment at the typical hourly rate. The patient's health insurance company is not billed for these types of cases. Additional time spent on the case (i.e., preparation, deposition, record review, etc.) is billed at a substantially higher rate. Fees for depositions, trials, or meetings, are due one week in advance and are non-refundable. As previously mentioned, Dr. Nies participates in M-Team meetings on a limited basis. Parents pay out of pocket for this service, at a self-pay rate, as insurance companies do not typically cover M-Team participation.

Dr. Nies is a provider for most managed care companies that operate in the area. Reimbursement for CPT code 96117 varies among carriers from $44.00 to $77.00. While it is obviously not cost effective to provide services at the $44.00 an hour rate, disenrolling from this particular provider panel would result in disenrollment as a provider from a panel with a favorable fee schedule. Traditional indemnity plans cover 80% to 100% of fees depending on the contract.

Given the evaluations typical of Dr. Lorber's private practice, all clinical services provided by his practice are conducted on a fee for service basis. When new patients call, the office secretary conducts a telephone intake regarding referral question, medications, school situation, etc. The services provided are described, fees and payment schedules are explained, and an intake appointment is scheduled with Dr. Lorber. At the intake session, the evaluation process is discussed in detail, parental expectations are determined, and the fees and payment schedule are again discussed. Given that the total professional and staff time for each comprehensive evaluation ranges from 20 to 30 hours, one inclusive fee has been established. This fee covers everything from the intake, testing, scoring and integration of the data, the parental feedback session, and the production and dissemination of the evaluation report. The inclusive evaluation fee is broken into thirds. One third is collected at the intake session; one third is collected at the parental feedback session, and the final third prior to the release of the written report. To facilitate this process, and to assist in collections, patients are asked to sign an agreement regarding their responsibilities with regard to fee collection. If needed, patients can arrange for an extended payment plan (usually to be completed within a 12-month period). Most other fees (e.g., remediation, parent training, and in-office consultations) are requested at the time of service. Payment for school staffings, out-of-office and telephone consultations are expected within 30 days of service. Finally, payment for forensic work usually takes several months from date of billing, as a third-party payer (i.e., insurance company) is usually involved.

It is extremely rare that patients are sent to collections (i.e., approximately 1% of billing). Overdue accounts are turned over to an attorney for collection. After all legal action is completed, usually in several years' time, the practice can expect to recoup approximately 40% percent of the outstanding account.

Although all fees are expected to be paid by the patient, Dr. Lorber's practice assists families in receiving reimbursement from their insurance companies. A computer- generated bill contains all of the necessary information for insurance submission, including dates of service, procedure codes (i.e., CPT codes), hours of service, diagnosis codes, payments made, and the corporation's Federal Tax Identification Number. If needed, a 'pre-determination' letter is produced prior to the provision of clinical services that lists the clinical procedures in detail and describes the referral source and aspects of the referral questions.

Finally, all billing and accounting is conducted within the clinic using a financial computer program. Following each feedback session, Dr. Lorber records the diagnosis codes, and following each consultation the clinical time is recorded and transcribed into the printed bill.

Issues Common to Most School Neuropsychological Practices

This section describes several issues common to almost all neuropsychological practices in the schools regardless of the exact nature of the individual practice.

The contractual agreement

Perhaps the most common arrangement between outside practitioners and the schools is the individual case contractual agreement. In general, schools prefer to handle all of the services they deliver to students using school personnel. The most obvious reason for this is financial. Most school systems simply do not have enough discretionary funds to seek specific expertise for cases that may be beyond the capabilities of their personnel. It is important for outside professionals to recognize this economic fact. It is very possible for neuropsychologists to 'price themselves out of business' thinking schools can pay the same rates as other professional referral sources (e.g., attorneys). Some school systems and states have begun to search for other means to provide neuropsychological services for students with TBI to offset the financial burden inherent in seeking these services by private neuropsychologists. As an example, one state faced with this dilemma has decided to allocate funds to training local school psychologists to provide a major part of the follow-up on these cases as an alternative to paying private neuropsychologists for follow-up evaluations and case consultation (Theye & Walker, 1999).

Schools will, however, subcontract neuropsychological services where specific expertise cannot be provided by school staff and where the neuropsy-

Sample Proposal

To provide neuropsychological services to a select number of students in the Anywhere City School System.

Benefit to the School System

Neuropsychological testing is an objective means by which an individual's ability to function cognitively and succeed in school can be evaluated. This interaction between school/environmental demands and neuropsychological functioning should be considered in most cases of known cerebral trauma (TBI) or other neurological condition. This is particularly true in the case of individuals, who by outward appearance do not show obvious deficits. When these individuals attempt to meet academic demands, subtle deficits become evident that can lead to errors, frustration, depression, anxiety, and possibly behavior problems.

Examples of the Utility of Neuropsychological testing in the Academic Setting

1. Assessment of cognitive functioning in patients with known neurological damage (e.g., traumatic brain injury, stroke, tumor, seizure disorder) to determine the child's ability to participate in a classroom and complete coursework.
2. Assessment of presence and degree of a specific learning disability.
3. Assessment of presence and degree of ADD/ADHD
4. Assessment of autism.

Neuropsychological Assessment

The focus of neuropsychology has evolved from diagnosing the presence of brain injury to assessing the degree of functional deficit associated with everyday living. Most neuropsychologists agree that certain cognitive functions are basic to performing in an academic setting. A comprehensive neuropsychological evaluation will address cognitive strength and weakness, as well as, psychological issues within the context of school demands. A typical assessment battery consists of a clinical interview and a comprehensive set of tests designed to clarify the student's ability to perform the following sample functions. (*Note*. Specific testing goals are determined for each individual student.)

Attention and concentration
Auditory perception and processing
Behavioral monitoring and ability to self-correct
Communication
Decision-making and ability to follow through on plans
Dual processing (e.g., two simultaneous sensory inputs or more than one organizing principle specific to a given task
Judgment (e.g., safety, appropriateness of action choice)
Memory
Orientation
Reasoning
Tactual perception and processing
Visual/spatial perception and processing

Typical Fee Structure

The diagnosis and the referral question as well as the age of the student determine the length and depth of an evaluation. The length of the evaluation is also determined by the speed at which the student can work. Often, the school psychologist or other school personnel have already completed IQ and achievement testing before a student is referred. In these cases, the evaluation can be completed in a shorter amount of time. The fee for a typical neuropsychological evaluation is $ XXX.XX. This cost includes: 1) the preparation of a written report, 2) a meeting with school personnel and/or the student's parents to explain the results, and 3) a follow-up contact with the school.

Figure 1.

Dear Mr./Ms. Disability Services:

Thank you for taking the time to discuss Learning Disabilities and Attention Deficit/Hyperactivity Disorder with me over the phone. Enclosed are my business card and a brochure about our office and the services we provide. In relation to your specific need, I estimate that an evaluation for the type of student you described would last approximately 3.5 hours. Additional time would be needed to score and interpret the tests, and prepare a written report. Using our current rate system this type of evaluation would cost approximately $ XXX.XX. I would like to offer your program a discounted rate of $ XXX.XX, in view of the number of cases that may be involved.

Should your office want to schedule students for an evaluation, please have them contact my office manager who coordinates all new patient referrals.

Sincerely,

Dr. Neuropsychologist

Figure 2.

chologist is sensitive to the cost containment issues of the schools. In offering such services we must also recognize that school personnel often do not know when and how to use neuropsychological expertise. There are many false impressions about neuropsychology that we must dispel or clarify if school personnel are to make appropriate use of neuropsychological services. It is the job of the neuropsychologist to facilitate this educational process. Figure 1 gives an example of a contract for neuropsychological services that provides an educational component describing what neuropsychology is and what can be gained from a neuropsychological evaluation. (*Note to readers*. It has been our experience that establishing flat fees is easier for school systems to deal with as opposed to hourly fee arrangements.)

Another sample 'contract' was developed in response to a request from a local University for neuropsychological and psychoeducational evaluations. Often these evaluations are requested by the university's office of disabilities and can be effective in granting accommodations for students with specific learning disabilities, TBI, and other disorders covered by the Americans with Disabilities Act. A letter such as the one in Figure 2 can serve as the formal contract.

Neuropsychological consultation/collaboration in the schools

Neuropsychologists should be aware that school personnel have become wary of external consultants in general. Perhaps more than any other service agency, school systems are deluged by consultants showing up with offers of services or goods, which often have not proven to be helpful to school personnel. Neuropsychologists should assume that the school systems they are dealing with have had negative interactions with external consultants in the past. At the same time, it is clear that there is a genuine, recognized need for neuropsychological services in the schools. School personnel, as it is implied, may be ill equipped to assess and develop appropriate educational plans for children and adolescents with complex neurological disorders, including severe learning disabilities, ADD/ADHD, seizure disorders and, in particular, students with TBI as defined in the 1990 federal legislation.

By the same token, many neuropsychologists have not been adequately trained to effectively consult with school personnel. They may often lack awareness of the school 'climate,' procedures, guidelines for placement of exceptional children, relevant laws affecting provision of services to children with disabilities, and the range of accommodations, modifications and other support that public schools are required to provide for exceptional children.

Many professionals without specific training in consultation with schools adopt a style similar to the Mental Health Consulting model (Caplan, 1970) wherein consultants present themselves as the 'expert' rendering needed information. While this model can be appropriate in many medical and mental health situations, it is not appropriate for the school setting where exceptional student personnel function as a multidisciplinary team. The essence of the IDEA is that decisions are made by teams, a concept that is mandated in the schools, as opposed to more linear, 'expert' decision models often used in medical settings. Consequently, the Mental Health model of consultation is generally recognized as ineffective in school consultation. Consultation models that emphasize process or collaboration have historically been more successful and better accepted by school personnel. These models appear to be more sensitive to the political/professional climate of the school (Brown, Pryzwansky, & Schulte, 1991).

Perhaps a better alternative is to consider collaborating with 'liaison' school personnel who are better able to navigate the school climate and relevant procedures. In most cases, the most effective point of contact would be the school psychologist. There are some states where school psychologists have received extensive training in brain injury in order to meet the need for the identification of students with TBI. Two such states are North Carolina and Wisconsin (Theye & Walker, 1999). Although somewhat different in their respective approaches to the problem of identifying students with TBI, both states have adopted training systems that focus on the role of the school psychologist in providing some of the testing and intervention services required in TBI cases.

There are many possible scenarios available to the neuropsychologist in collaborating with the school psychologist. Collaboration can be particularly effective if the school system is too great a distance for on-site consultation. One method of collaboration involves sharing the testing responsibilities for a specific case. This alternative has the advantage of 'leaving something behind' in that the neuropsychologist will be in a position to teach the school psychologist about neuropsychology and how best it can be used. In this arrangement, the school psychologist can conduct some of the basic testing procedures, e.g., intellectual or achievement, and the neuropsychologist can provide the additional assessment data that is necessary for a comprehensive understanding of the child's deficits and unique needs. Another approach to collaboration involves suggesting specific supplementary tests the school psychologist can add to the school battery. Adding supplementary tests to the typical school psychological test battery can result in identifying many potential effects of TBI that might otherwise go unnoticed. A typical example is memory functioning. Memory is often not assessed or under-assessed in the typical school psychologist's battery. Memory testing is crucial in helping to identify aspects of a brain-injured student's most effective mode of learning, a valuable asset for academic programming recommendations to teachers.

It is also possible for the consulting neuropsychologist to help the school psychologist interpret test data that they have collected in a different way, using a 'neuropsychological perspective.' Using such a perspective, it is possible to sensitize the school psychologist to additional ways of analyzing information obtained from typically administered tests such as the WISC III. Analyzing individual subtest responses with a neuropsychological perspective can be used to support hypotheses about the effects of specific brain injury (Walker, 1997). Kaplan's methods of interpreting subtle error differences on the Block Design subtest to support suspected left or right hemisphere damage is an example of this approach (Kaplan, 1990).

Other contractual approaches for involving neuropsychologists in the schools include the use of agreements wherein the neuropsychologist provides services for a school system in an arrangement similar to a retainer fee. This contractual arrangement differs from the individual case contract in that it can form the basis for an ongoing relationship with the school system. In this arrangement, the neuropsychologist can be used in many ways by the school system including evaluations, case consultation, training, etc. for any situation the school system identifies. These contracts can be developed in a per hour, per case, or per diem arrangement, or on an annual retainer fee format.

As another possible variation on this theme, some school systems have begun to hire neuropsychologists with school backgrounds as the 'system neuropsychologist.' Positions such as these would be very appealing to neuropsychologists who received their initial training and/or degree in school psychology, although any neuropsychologist with sufficient school training and/or experience might find such a position appealing.

Neuropsychological assessments for the schools

As with other specific sites, school-based neuropsychological evaluations require subtle modifications. As a part of their preparation for school-based assessments, neuropsychologists will need to become familiar with the strengths and constraints of the typical school psychological placement battery.

As presently conceptualized, the testing procedures used by school psychologists to identify exceptional students for appropriate classification are not designed to address the intricacies inherent in evaluating students with complex neurological disorders. Telzrow (1987) suggests that school psychologists evaluating students who have experienced brain trauma such as a TBI should follow an assessment approach similar to that found in neuropsychological evaluations, i.e. a domain approach. Although the evaluations conducted by school psychologists may currently follow this approach, the domains assessed tend to be very specific to the definitions of special education categories, e.g. Specific Learning Disability or Other Health Impaired. Typical assessment domains found in school psychological assessment batteries include general cognitive/intellectual functioning, some additional, specific cognitive areas, e.g. psychomotor functioning, academic achievement levels, and, depending on the referral question, some aspects of social, emotional or behavioral functioning. In comparison, the domains typically covered in a neuropsychological assessment battery include some variation of the following: A complete medical history, sensory/perceptual functioning, attention and concentration, fine motor abilities, visuoperceptual, visuoconstruction, and graphomotor functioning, memory and learning, language, executive functions, and social, emotional, and behavioral functioning.

Depth and/or comprehensiveness are also differences found in the two batteries. While a typical school psychological battery may include some information or clues to areas generally covered in neuropsychological batteries, neuropsychological test instruments typically describe cognitive functioning in greater depth and at more complex levels for the purpose of determining the specific effects of the brain insult on functioning. Neuropsychological assessment is highly dependent on the functional interpretation of measures of brain integrity and the expertise of the neuropsychologist in translating test results into meaningful and appropriate recommendations.

It should be noted that these comments are not intended to criticize school psychologists. The testing batteries they use are typically designed to provide the information necessary for placement decisions. Heavy caseloads, budget, and time restrictions can often prohibit all but the most basic evaluations. It seems clear also that most school psychologists have only a rudimentary knowledge of neuropsychology, brain function, and the effects of brain injury. This information is not usually taught in school psychology training programs (Walker, Boling, & Cobb, 1999).

Neuropsychological reports for the schools

It is probably an understatement to say that school personnel have been known to complain that the information some neuropsychologists render in their reports is difficult to understand and generally of little practical use for the school setting. Specifically, they complain that these reports can be full of irrelevant jargon and unmindful of the school setting and the legal responsibilities of schools to provide an 'appropriate' education to disabled students. Since we have experienced the range of services available in hospitals and rehab facilities, it is likely that we may expect schools to provide services that are well beyond their capabilities. Simply stated, our reports are seen as not 'user friendly.' Some neuropsychological consultants continue to generate reports that, although useful in one setting, may be of little utility to consultees in another setting. As an example, a report that may be appropriate for a medical setting is probably of little use in the school setting. It is also important to remember that under special education law, school districts do not have to *accept* independent evaluations; they must only demonstrate that they have *considered* them. Therefore, for our services to be most effective for our clients, neuropsychological reports must reflect an understanding of the criteria for qualifying children for special education services. They must also reflect recognition of the rights and constraints public school systems deal with in providing these services. While a detailed description of this information is beyond the scope of this chapter, issues in the application of neuropsychological test data to school consultation and school advocacy can be found in Lorber and Yurk (1999), who state that, in general, school-based neuropsychological reports and consultations should include:

1. A clear, concise picture of the child's strengths and deficits designed to facilitate educating parents and school personnel about the disabled child's immediate and future needs.
2. Clear and simplified terminology to facilitate and reinforce an understanding of the complexity of the child's functioning by parents and school personnel.
3. An approach to school consultation that is both professional and respectful of the school's areas of expertise.
4. Recommendations specific to a child's needs that directly stem from the neuropsychological test results. These recommendations should be specific enough to easily translate into measurable goals and objectives within the framework of the child's Individual Education Program (IEP), which allows the schools as well as parents to be active and creative participants in this process.
5. Given that the revision of special education law stipulates that individuals with expertise in the interpretation of specific types of test data need to be present at the IEP meeting, the neuropsychologist's presence at such meetings is often crucial.
6. Reports should relate neurological findings to specific issues with which teachers are familiar. For example, describing how a child with a central auditory processing deficit and memory retrieval deficit cannot retrieve, process, or manipulate phonic sounds, and (most importantly) how these deficits might impact the acquisition of reading skills.

Training neuropsychologists to work in the school setting

It should be a given that the individual interested in practicing neuropsychology in the schools must have training and or experience with pediatric populations and with schools. One should not assume that training and experience exclusively with adults would be sufficient. The ability to assess children and adolescents, to determine appropriate forms of intervention, and to assist schools with establishing proper educational environments, requires training that is often not part of most clinical psychology or neuropsychology graduate training programs. We should not assume that children are just little adults. Working with pediatric populations in a neuropsychological context requires a thorough knowledge of child development, in general, and the impact brain insult can have on the developing cognitive functions (Dennis, 1988).

As a start, the pediatric neuropsychologist who chooses to consult with schools, as well as advocate for children in public school systems, needs to understand the rights and entitlements of children with 'disabilities.' Knowledge of these laws is invaluable. One way a neuropsychologist can gain insight into how state and federal guidelines affect the lives of school-age children and adolescents with disabilities is by observing school due process hearings. Individual clinicians can check with their states for scheduled hearings, and, with parental permission, they can learn more about how schools operate through these hearings. As an example, Dr. Lorber has served as a Level I Due Process Officer for the state of Illinois. This opportunity has provided him with additional training and experience in working with the laws that address children with disabilities in public school settings.

Summary

School-based neuropsychology is a relatively new concept, and it is one that requires specific approaches and preparation. Neuropsychologists, who have come into the field with previous training and/or experience in a school-related field, e.g., school psychology, special education, will find such a practice relatively comfortable. Others will have to learn those aspects of schools that will help ensure their success. It is clear, however, that practitioners should not underestimate the demands of such a practice. As a start, neuropsychologists aspiring to develop a school-based practice must learn those federal and state laws that govern the placement and programming of exceptional children. Federal laws basic to school practice are PL 94-142, the Individuals with Disabilities Education Act (IDEA) or P.L. 101-476, and the Americans with Disabilities Act of 1990 (PL 101-336). In addition, neuropsychologists should become familiar with their state's published guidelines for placement and programming of exceptional children, including local interpretations of these laws. It is impossible to practice effectively in the schools without this information. Neuropsychologists will lose credibility with school personnel if they are not familiar with these laws and guidelines.

Neuropsychological reports should be designed with schools in mind. School personnel often complain that neuropsychological reports are not 'user friendly.' Eliminating jargon and recognizing the constraints schools are under in providing services to exceptional children will enhance the credibility of the neuropsychologist. Special emphasis should be placed on making recommendations that are easy to translate into school programming interventions.

The importance of pediatric experience in general, knowledge of child and adolescent development, and the specific effects traumatic brain injury can have on the developing child's functioning are crucial foundations. Understanding schools and how they operate is equally important. Observing Due Process Hearings and taking part in school meetings and presentations can be very valuable in this regard.

Future Directions

It would appear that the opportunities for neuropsychologists to become involved in school-based practices are developing rapidly. It is fertile ground for neuropsychologists trained in pediatric issues. There is perhaps, no better access to children and adolescents than the schools. It seems clear that neuropsychological principles are currently being applied to disorders that were not being considered only a short while ago, e.g. learning disabilities and autism. These new directions along with the advent of federal laws providing Special Education services for students with traumatic brain injury suggest that schools have a growing need for neuropsychological services. Schools are searching for ways to effectively address these needs. One example of this is the relatively recent addition of neuropsychologists to school professional staffs.

It is also clear that schools have not used the TBI legislation effectively. If we can believe the epidemiological evidence available on the incidence of TBI, 1 in every 200 school-age child has suffered a traumatic brain injury (Lehr, 1990). A cursory check of our schools, however, does not reflect an incidence anywhere near that suggested by the epidemiological data. Why is this so? The fact that students with TBI are not being identified or served appropriately may reflect the schools' lack of knowledge and expertise with regard to brain injury. Therefore, neuropsychologists can be an important educational resource to schools and parents in helping them understand the impact of brain injury and in helping identify needy students.

Finally, it is probably true that many professionals with less than desirable training and experience in schools and children will vie for the 'brass ring' that a school-based practice may hold. It is incumbent upon our field us to determine how best to monitor these situations and how best to inform schools with regard to what expectations they should have for such services.

References

Brown, D., Pryzwansky, W.B., & Schulte, A.C. (1991). *Psychological consultation: Introduction theory and practice.* Needham Heights, Mass.: Allyn and Bacon.

Caplan, G. (1970). *The theory and practice of mental health consultation.* New York: Basic Books.

Dennis, M. (1988). Language and the young damaged brain. In T. Boll & B.K. Bryant (Eds.*), Clinical neuropsychology and brain function: Research, measurement, and practice* (pp. 85–123). Washington, DC: American Psychological Association.

Federal Register. (1992). 57, 44802.

Gordon, M. & Keiser, S. (1998). *Accommodations in higher education under the Americans with Disabilities Act (ADA): A no-nonsense guide for clinicians.* GSI Publications, Dewitt: NY.

Kaplan, E. (1990). The process approach to neuropsychological assessment of psychiatric patients. *Journal of Neuropsychiatry and Clinical Neurosciences, 2,* 72–87.

Lehr, E. (1990). *Psychological management of traumatic brain injuries in children and adolescents.* Rockville, Maryland: Aspen Publishers, Inc.

Lorber, R. & Yurk, H., (1999). Special pediatric issues: neuropsychological applications and consultations in schools. In J.J. Sweet (Ed.), *Forensic neuropsychology: Fundamentals and practice.* Lisse, Netherlands: Swets and Zeitlinger.

Telzrow, C.F. (1987). Management of academic and educational problems in head injury. *Journal of Learning Disabilities, 20,* 536–545.

Theye, F. W. and Walker, N. W. (1999). Pediatric neuropsychology and departments of public instruction. *Pediatric Neuropsychology Interest Group Newsletter,* 6, 6–9.

Walker, N.W. (1997). *Best practices in assessment and programming for TBI students.* Raleigh, NC: North Carolina Department of Public Instruction.

Walker, N.W., Boling, M. S., & Cobb, H. (1999). The training of school psychologists in Neuropsychology and Traumatic Brain Injury (TBI): Results of a national survey of training programs. *Child Neuropsychology, 5,* 137–142.

CONTRIBUTORS ADDRESS LIST

John T. Beetar, Ph.D.
The Ohio State University and Children's Hospital
Columbus, OH

Linas A. Bieliauskas, Ph.D.
V.A. Medical Center, University of Michigan Health System
Ann Arbor, MI

David S. Bush, Ph.D.
Independent Practice
Palm Beach Gardens, FL

Andrew N. Colvin, Ph.D.
The Ohio State University and Children's Hospital
Columbus, OH

John C. Courtney, Psy.D.
Clinical Neuropsychology, P.C.
South Bend, IN

Richard C. Delaney, Ph.D.
Gaylord Hospital
Wallingford, CT
Yale University School of Medicine
New Haven, CT

M. Frank Greiffenstein, Ph.D.
Psychological Systems, Inc.
Royal Oak, MI

Robert L. Heilbronner, Ph.D.
Independent Practice
Chicago, IL

Greg J. Lamberty, Ph.D.
Noran Neurological Clinic
Minneapolis, MN

Rudy Lorber, Ph.D.
Chicago, IL

Bernice A. Marcopulos
Western State Hospital
Staunton, VA

Michael McCrea, Ph.D.
Waukesha Memorial Hospital
Waukesha, WI

Paul J. Moberg, Ph.D.
University of Pennsylvania Medical Center
Philadelphia, PA

Kristie J. Nies, Ph.D.
Independent Practice
Kingsport, TN

David C. Osmon, Ph.D.
University of Wisconsin-Milwaukee
Milwaukee, WI

Edward A Peck, Ph.D.
Neuropsychological Services of Virginia, Inc.
Richmond, VA

Neil H. Pliskin, Ph.D.
University of Illinois, Chicago
Chicago, IL

Joseph H. Ricker, Ph.D.
University of Pittsburgh,
Pittsburgh, PA

Anthony H. Risser, Ph.D.
University of Houston
Houston, TX
University of Pennsylvania School of Medicine
Philadelphia, PA

Michael Schmidt, Ph.D.
Independent Practice
Colorado Springs, CO

Brett A. Steinberg, Ph.D.
University of Connecticut
Storrs, CT

Yana Suchy, Ph.D.
Evanston Northwestern Healthcare Medical Group
Evanston, IL

Jerry J. Sweet, Ph.D.
Evanston Northwestern Healthcare Medical Group
Evanston, IL

Ivan Torres, Ph.D.
Simon Fraser University
Burnaby, BC, Canada

N. William Walker, Ed.D.
James Madison University
Harrisonburg, VA

Keith O. Yeates, Ph.D.
The Ohio State University and Children's Hospital
Columbus, OH

SUBJECT INDEX

AUTHOR INDEX

STUDIES ON NEUROPSYCHOLOGY, DEVELOPMENT, AND COGNITION

1. *Fundamentals of Functional Brain Imaging: A Guide to the Methods and their Applications to Psychology and Behavioral Neuroscience.* Andrew C. Papanicolaou
   1998. ISBN 90 265 1528 6

2. *Forensic Neuropsychology: Fundamentals and Practice.* Edited by Jerry J. Sweet
   1999. ISBN 90 265 1544 8

3. *Neuropsychological Differential Diagnosis.* Konstantine K. Zakzanis, Larry Leach and Edith Kaplan
   1999. ISBN 90 265 1552 9

4. *Minority and Cross-Cultural Aspects of Neuropsychological Assessment.* Edited by F. Richard Ferraro
   2002. ISBN 90 265 1830 7

5. *Ethical Issues in Clinical Neuropsychology.* Edited by Shane S. Bush and Michael L. Drexler
   2002. ISBN 90 265 1924 9

6. *Practice of Child-Clinical Neuropsychology: An Introduction.* Byron P. Rourke, Harry van der Vlugt and Sean B. Rourke
   2002. ISBN 90 265 1929 X

7. *The Practice of Clinical Neuropsychology: A Survey of Practices and Settings.* Greg J. Lamberty, John C. Courtney and Robert L. Heilbronner
   2003. ISBN 90 265 1940 0